ADOLESCENT MEDICINE: STATE OF THE ART REVIEWS

Hot Topics in Adolescent Health

GUEST EDITORS

Cynthia Holland-Hall, MD, MPH

Paula K. Braverman, MD

August 2014 • Volume 25 • Number 2

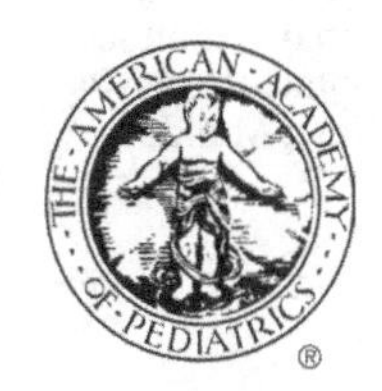

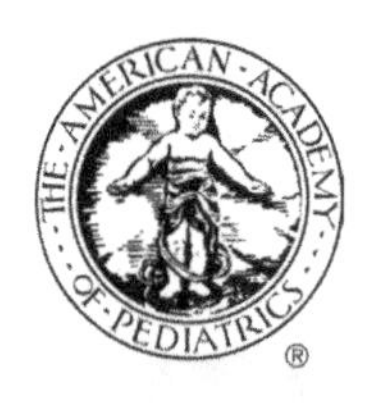

ADOLESCENT MEDICINE:
STATE OF THE ART REVIEWS
August 2014
Editor: Carrie Peters
Marketing Manager: Marirose Russo
Production Manager: Shannan Martin
eBook Developer: Houston Adams

Volume 25, Number 2
ISBN 978-1-58110-785-2
ISSN 1934-4287
MA0666
SUB1006

The recommendations in this publication do not indicate an exclusive course of treatment or serve as a standard of medical care. Variations, taking into account individual circumstances, may be appropriate.

Statements and opinions expressed are those of the author and not necessarily those of the American Academy of Pediatrics.

Products and Web sites are mentioned for informational purposes only. Inclusion in this publication does not imply endorsement by the American Academy of Pediatrics. The American Academy of Pediatrics is not responsible for the content of the resources mentioned in this publication. Web site addresses are as current as possible but may change at any time.

Every effort has been made to ensure that the drug selection and dosage set forth in this text are in accordance with the current recommendations and practice at the time of publication. It is the responsibility of the health care provider to check the package insert of each drug for any change in indications and dosage and for added warnings and precautions.

Adolescent Medicine: State of the Art Reviews is published three times per year by the American Academy of Pediatrics, 141 Northwest Point Blvd, Elk Grove Village, IL 60007-1019. Periodicals postage paid at Arlington Heights, IL.

POSTMASTER: Send address changes to American Academy of Pediatrics, Department of Marketing and Publications, Attn: AM:STARs, 141 Northwest Point Blvd, Elk Grove Village, IL 60007-1019.

Subscriptions: Subscriptions to *Adolescent Medicine: State of the Art Reviews* (AM:STARs) are provided to members of the American Academy of Pediatrics' Section on Adolescent Health as part of annual section membership dues. All others, please contact the AAP Customer Service Center at 866/843-2271 (7:00 am–5:30 pm Central Time, Monday–Friday) for pricing and information.

Adolescent Medicine: State of the Art Reviews

Official Journal of the American Academy of Pediatrics
Section on Adolescent Health

EDITORS-IN-CHIEF

VICTOR C. STRASBURGER, MD, Distinguished Professor of Pediatrics, Founding Chief, Division of Adolescent Medicine, University of New Mexico, School of Medicine, Albuquerque, New Mexico

DONALD E. GREYDANUS, MD, Dr HC (ATHENS), Professor & Founding Chair, Department of Pediatric & Adolescent Medicine, Western Michigan University School of Medicine, Kalamazoo, Michigan

GUEST EDITORS

CYNTHIA HOLLAND-HALL, MD, MPH, Associate Professor of Clinical Pediatrics, The Ohio State University, College of Medicine, Nationwide Children's Hospital, Columbus, Ohio

PAULA K. BRAVERMAN, MD, Professor of Pediatrics, Cincinnati Children's Hospital Medical Center, University of Cincinnati College of Medicine, Cincinnati, Ohio

CONTRIBUTORS

JESSICA BAUMAN, MD, Fellow in Hematology-Oncology, Massachusetts General Hospital, Harvard Medical School, Boston, Massachusetts

SARAH J. BEAL, PhD, Division of Adolescent and Transition Medicine, Cincinnati Children's Hospital Medical Center, Cincinnati, Ohio

ELISE D. BERLAN, MD, MPH, Division of Adolescent Medicine, Nationwide Children's Hospital, Columbus, Ohio; Department of Pediatrics, The Ohio State University College of Medicine, Columbus, Ohio; Center for Clinical and Translational Research, The Research Institute at Nationwide Children's Hospital, Columbus, Ohio

PAULA K. BRAVERMAN, MD, Professor of Pediatrics, Cincinnati Children's Hospital Medical Center, University of Cincinnati College of Medicine, Cincinnati, Ohio

GALE R. BURSTEIN, MD, MPH, Erie County Department of Health, Buffalo, New York, and Department of Pediatrics, SUNY at Buffalo School of Medicine and Biomedical Sciences, Buffalo, New York

DEBORAH CHRISTIE, DipClinPsych, PhD, Consultant Clinical Psychologist & Reader in Paediatric and Adolescent Health, Department of Child and Adolescent Psychological Services, University College Hospital London NHS Foundation Trust, London, United Kingdom

CASEY B. COTTRILL, MD, Division of Adolescent Medicine, Nationwide Children's Hospital, Columbus, Ohio

JACQUELINE DOYLE, DClinPsych, PhD, Clinical Psychologist, Department of Child and Adolescent Psychological Services, University College Hospital London NHS Foundation Trust, London, United Kingdom

MICHELLE FORCIER, MD, MPH, Associate Professor of Clinical Pediatrics, Alpert School of Medicine, Brown University, Providence, Rhode Island

CATHERINE M. GORDON, MD, MSc, Hasbro Children's Hospital, Alpert Medical School of Brown University, Providence, Rhode Island

STEFANO GUANDALINI, MD, Professor and Chief Section of Gastroenterology, Hepatology and Nutrition, Department of Pediatrics, University of Chicago Medicine, Chicago, Illinois; Founder and Medical Director, University of Chicago Celiac Disease Center

ANDREA J. HOOPES, MD, Division of Adolescent Medicine, University of Washington Department of Pediatrics, Seattle, Washington

THOMAS H. INGE, MD, PhD, Division of Pediatric Surgery, Cincinnati Children's Hospital Medical Center, Cincinnati, Ohio

HILARY JERICHO, MD, Assistant Professor, Section of Gastroenterology, Hepatology and Nutrition, Department of Pediatrics, University of Chicago Medicine, Chicago, Illinois

MANMOHAN K. KAMBOJ, MD, Associate Professor, Wexner Medical Center at The Ohio State University, Section of Endocrinology, Metabolism and Diabetes, Department of Pediatrics, Nationwide Children's Hospital, Columbus, Ohio

DEBRA K. KATZMAN, MD, FRCPC, Professor of Pediatrics, Senior Associate Scientist, Research Institute, The Hospital for Sick Children and University of Toronto, Toronto, Ontario, Canada

SARAH KIDD, MD, MPH, Division of STD Prevention, National Center for HIV/AIDS, Viral Hepatitis, STD and TB Prevention, Centers for Disease Control and Prevention, Atlanta, Georgia

ROBERT D. KIRKCALDY, MD, MPH, Division of STD Prevention, National Center for HIV/AIDS, Viral Hepatitis, STD and TB Prevention, Centers for Disease Control and Prevention, Atlanta, Georgia

LINDA M. KOLLAR, RN, CNP, CBN, Division of Pediatric Surgery, Cincinnati Children's Hospital Medical Center, Cincinnati, Ohio

CORINNE E. LEHMANN, MD, MEd, Division of Adolescent and Transition Medicine, Department of Pediatrics, Cincinnati Children's Hospital Medical Center, Cincinnati, Ohio; University of Cincinnati College of Medicine, Cincinnati, Ohio

INGA MANSKOPF, BS, Coordinator, Prevention WINS Coalition, Division of Adolescent Medicine, Seattle Children's, Seattle, Washington

STEVEN C. MATSON, MD, Division of Adolescent Medicine, Nationwide Children's Hospital, Columbus, Ohio; Department of Pediatrics, The Ohio State University College of Medicine, Columbus, Ohio

ERIN R. MCKNIGHT, MD, Division of Adolescent Medicine, Nationwide Children's Hospital, Columbus, Ohio

TANYA L. KOWALCZYK MULLINS, MD, MS, Division of Adolescent and Transition Medicine, Department of Pediatrics, Cincinnati Children's Hospital Medical Center, Cincinnati, Ohio; University of Cincinnati College of Medicine, Cincinnati, Ohio

ABIGAIL NYE, MD, Division of Adolescent and Transition Medicine, Cincinnati Children's Hospital Medical Center, Cincinnati, Ohio; College of Medicine, University of Cincinnati, Cincinnati, Ohio

JOHANNA OLSON, MD, Assistant Professor of Clinical Pediatrics, USC Keck School of Medicine, Los Angeles, California

ROLLYN M. ORNSTEIN, MD, Associate Professor of Pediatrics, Division of Adolescent Medicine and Eating Disorders, Penn State Hershey Children's Hospital/College of Medicine, Hershey, Pennsylvania

SHERINE PATTERSON-ROSE, MD, MPH, Assistant Professor of Pediatrics, Cincinnati Children's Hospital Medical Center, Cincinnati, Ohio

DAVID R. REPASKE, MD, PhD, Professor, Wexner Medical Center at The Ohio State University, Section of Endocrinology, Metabolism and Diabetes, Department of Pediatrics, Nationwide Children's Hospital, Columbus, Ohio

BENJAMIN N. SHAIN, MD, PhD, Vice Chair, Department of Psychiatry, Head, Division of Child and Adolescent Psychiatry, NorthShore University HealthSystem, Deerfield, Illinois

JENNIFER M. SHOREMAN, MD, Division of Adolescent and Transition Medicine, Cincinnati Children's Hospital Medical Center, Cincinnati, Ohio; College of Medicine, University of Cincinnati, Cincinnati, Ohio

TREGONY SIMONEAU, MD, Connecticut Children's Medical Center, University of Connecticut School of Medicine, Hartford, Connecticut

EARL J. SOILEAU JR, MD, Assistant Professor of Family Medicine, Louisiana State University Health Sciences Center, New Orleans at Lake Charles, Louisiana

VICTOR C. STRASBURGER, MD, Distinguished Professor of Pediatrics, Founding Chief, Division of Adolescent Medicine, Department of Pediatrics, University of New Mexico School of Medicine, Albuquerque, New Mexico

DARCEY L. THORNTON, MD, Division of Adolescent and Transition Medicine, Cincinnati Children's Hospital Medical Center, Cincinnati, Ohio; College of Medicine, University of Cincinnati, Cincinnati, Ohio

DZUNG X. VO, MD, FAAP, Assistant Clinical Professor, Division of Adolescent Health and Medicine, Department of Pediatrics, University of British Columbia and British Columbia Children's Hospital, Vancouver, British Columbia, Canada

LESLIE WALKER, MD, Chief, Division of Adolescent Medicine, Seattle Children's, Director, University of Washington LEAH (Leadership Education in Adolescent Health), Professor, Vice Chair of Faculty Affairs, University of Washington Department of Pediatrics, Seattle, Washington

LORI WIRTH, MD, Medical Director of the Center for Head and Neck Cancers, Massachusetts General Hospital, Boston, Massachusetts; Assistant Professor, Department of Medicine, Division of Medical Oncology, Massachusetts General Hospital, Boston, Massachusetts

JASON F. WOODWARD, MD, MS, Division of Adolescent and Transition Medicine, Cincinnati Children's Hospital Medical Center, Cincinnati, Ohio; College of Medicine, University of Cincinnati, Cincinnati, Ohio

CONTENTS

Over the last 10 years, there has been an explosion of data about vitamin D—including findings related to both supplementation and bone health as well as the extraskeletal effects of this vitamin. Adolescence is a critical time for the accrual of peak bone mass, necessitating adequate intake of vitamin D and maintenance of an adequate vitamin D status. However, many disease processes affect adolescents, and each may be influenced by vitamin D status. Specific diseases and certain medications also may alter vitamin D metabolism and thus change the requirements needed to maintain adequate circulating vitamin D concentrations. In this review, we discuss the current recommendations and guidelines for supplementation as well as some of the extraskeletal effects of vitamin D that are particularly pertinent to adolescents.

American adolescents are trying opioids, being admitted for opioid dependence treatment, and dying from opioid overdose at ever increasing rates. Given the chronic and life-threatening nature of opioid dependence, interventions that will prevent the development and progression of the disease of addiction must be utilized. Before medication-assisted treatment (MAT), the success of treating opioid dependence was abysmal. Now, there is a powerful tool to help young drug-addicted patients experience sobriety and realize their full potential in life. MAT is a way for physicians to make a difference in patients experiencing the serious chronic disease of addiction.

Adolesc Med 025 (2014) xvii

Preface

Hot Topics in Adolescent Health

The 21st century has brought with it a renewed focus on the health of adolescents and young adults. This issue of *Adolescent Medicine: State of the Art Reviews, Hot Topics in Adolescent Health*, brings the reader up to date on a variety of rapidly evolving aspects in the field.

The *Diagnostic and Statistical Manual of Mental Disorders*, Fifth Edition (DSM-5), published in 2013, includes updated diagnostic criteria for several disorders affecting adolescents. Bipolar disorder and the new DSM-5 diagnosis of disruptive mood dysregulation disorder are discussed, including the controversies surrounding these diagnoses in children and adolescents. Criteria for diagnosing eating disorders such as anorexia nervosa and bulimia nervosa have been modified to be more applicable to males and younger adolescents, and a new diagnosis of Avoidant/Restrictive Food Intake Disorder has been added. Attention-deficit/hyperactivity disorder criteria have similarly been adapted to facilitate diagnosis in later adolescence and young adulthood; other diagnostic modalities and new stimulant medications have been brought to market as well and are described herein.

Evolving nutritional issues in adolescents include the role of vitamin D in skeletal and extraskeletal health, and the current guidelines for screening for and treating vitamin D deficiency. Exciting advances are being made in the diagnosis and treatment of celiac disease; furthermore, gluten-free diets are being widely adopted by those without serologic or histologic evidence of this disease. Contributions on these topics will help physicians address patient questions about these nutrients in an informed and up-to-date manner. Obesity among adolescents continues to increase and along with it the prevalence of metabolic syndrome. The significance of this syndrome versus its individual components in adolescents is explored, as well as the use of bariatric surgical procedures to address adolescent obesity and its medical consequences.

Providing reproductive health for adolescents poses a challenge for some pediatric physicians. Articles on sexually transmitted infections (STIs) and human immunodeficiency virus (HIV) present the reader with current guidelines on screening for and treatment of these infections, as well as tips on incorporating STI and HIV testing into a busy office setting. Long-acting reversible contraceptives (LARCs) are widely recommended for use in adolescents because of their superior efficacy; a contribution on this topic helps physicians counsel patients on these methods and addresses barriers to their widespread use. Human papillomavirus (HPV) is now known to cause a high proportion of oropharyngeal cancers, and acquisition through oral sexual contact has been demonstrated. It is postulated, but remains to be proven, that widespread vaccination against HPV could dramatically lessen the incidence of these cancers.

High-risk behaviors including substance abuse and violence contribute significantly to morbidity and mortality among adolescents and young adults. There has been increasing use of opiates in terms of both illegal drugs such as heroin and prescription medications.

 ISSN 1934-4287

One article in this issue addresses the medical treatment of opiate addiction while another examines the influence of violence in the media on adolescent behavior and health.

New and evolving issues often bring with them more questions than answers. The legalization of medical and recreational marijuana in some states is likely to impact adolescent health; experts from Washington state provide us with their perspective on the possible ramifications of these policy changes. Mindfulness, a "hot topic" that has been practiced by some for more than 2000 years, encompasses techniques that are now widely encouraged in the treatment of chronic physical and mental health conditions. Adaptations of these techniques for incorporation into the care of adolescents are described, along with the current state of the evidence supporting their use. Transitioning between pediatric and adult care presents numerous challenges for healthy adolescents and is particularly difficult for those with chronic illnesses. This issue includes an article outlining a framework for transitioning youth into the health care system. With the evolving changes in our society, transgender and gender nonconforming youth are increasingly presenting to their health care physicians. The development of gender identity along with the medical and mental health care needs of these youth are addressed.

Among the hot topics presented in this issue, some will have an immediate impact on patient care, some may stimulate physicians to consider future changes in their approach to adolescent patients, and some may simply inform readers of new developments in the field. All will hopefully, eventually, help us to improve the health and well-being of adolescents.

Paula K. Braverman, MD
Professor of Pediatrics
Cincinnati Children's Hospital Medical Center
University of Cincinnati College of Medicine

Cynthia Holland-Hall, MD, MPH
Associate Professor of Clinical Pediatrics
The Ohio State University, College of Medicine
Nationwide Children's Hospital

Adolesc Med 025 (2014) 239–250

Vitamin D: Recent Recommendations and Discoveries

Tregony Simoneau, MD[a];
Catherine M. Gordon, MD, MSc[b*]

[a]Connecticut Children's Medical Center, University of Connecticut School of Medicine, Hartford, Connecticut; [b]Hasbro Children's Hospital, Alpert Medical School of Brown University, Providence, Rhode Island

INTRODUCTION

Hundreds of articles have been published in the last 10 years about vitamin D and its effect on health. Initially, the literature focused on bone health, trying to identify the rates of vitamin D deficiency and the effect of that deficiency in terms of bone loss, osteoporosis, or fractures. From there, supplementation requirements have been studied in infants, children, adolescents, and adults. Along the way, vitamin D has been implicated in various disease processes, ranging from autoimmune diseases, such as multiple sclerosis, to asthma, diabetes mellitus, coronary heart disease, and cancer. In this review, we discuss the literature in this area that has been published over the past decade, with a focus on topics pertinent to the health and care of adolescents. We will begin with an overview of articles investigating contemporary rates of vitamin D insufficiency and deficiency. We will then review the current recommendations for vitamin D screening and supplementation. Finally, we will review the outcomes and associations with vitamin D deficiency in terms of bone health but also will discuss other disease processes pertinent to adolescents.

Vitamin D has long been recognized as a hormone necessary for the regulation of calcium and phosphate metabolism.[1] Different from any other hormone, vitamin D is made in the skin from exposure to sunlight. The vitamin D made in the skin is cholecalciferol (or vitamin D_3). Vitamin D also can be absorbed from the diet, either as ergocalciferol (vitamin D_2) or cholecalciferol, but few foods

*Corresponding author:
E-mail address: catherine_gordon@brown.edu

 ISSN 1934-4287

naturally contain vitamin D. In the United States, milk and some other foods are fortified with vitamin D, but enteral vitamin D primarily comes in the form of supplements. The primary role of vitamin D is to maintain calcium homeostasis by facilitating intestinal absorption of calcium. The active form of vitamin D is 1,25-dihydroxyvitamin D [1,25$(OH)_2$ D]. Vitamin D that comes from the skin or diet is biologically inert and requires hydroxylation in the liver to 25-hydroxyvitamin D [25(OH)D] and then further hydroxylation to the active form in the kidney. The active form interacts with the vitamin D nuclear receptor most avidly and has been shown to be present in the small intestine, kidneys, respiratory epithelium, and other tissues.[2] The 25(OH)D metabolite is the circulating form of vitamin D and has a half-life of 2 to 3 weeks. The circulating 25(OH)D concentration is the most accurate marker of vitamin D status, reflecting both dietary and cutaneous sources.[3]

Lack of vitamin D can result in elevated parathyroid hormone (PTH) levels, causing calcium to be resorbed from bone in order to maintain normal calcium homeostasis. This ultimately results in rickets, abnormal mineralization of the skeletal growth plates in children, and, in longstanding cases, bone deformities.[4] Achievement of optimal vitamin D levels is critical during adolescence, because this is the time when more than 50% of the adult skeleton is formed and peak mineral bone density is reached.[5] Therefore, it is important to determine what the optimal serum 25(OH)D concentration is and how best to achieve it. Based on the underlying pathophysiology, it would be reasonable to define the optimal serum 25(OH)D concentration based on where PTH levels normalize. Several studies have demonstrated an inverse relationship between PTH and 25(OH)D levels.[6-9] However, studies have shown that this relationship varies among individuals, making it difficult to define the optimal 25(OH)D concentration.[10] In a large study of children and adolescents, the 25(OH)D concentration associated with a plateau for PTH secretion was not easily identified.[11] Additionally, a large study by Valcour et al[12] found an age effect on the PTH–25(OH)D relationship with no identifiable PTH plateau. However, few studies have examined the optimal 25(OH)D level needed to confer benefit from the extraskeletal effects of vitamin D. Given the sparse and sometimes conflicting data that are available, there is, understandably, controversy surrounding target 25(OH)D concentrations. A study in 2006 by Bischoff-Ferrari et al[13] suggested that the optimal level of 25(OH)D in terms of bone mineral density (BMD), fall risk, fractures, and colorectal cancer is between 36 and 40 ng/mL (90-100 nmol/L), with the benefits beginning at a 25(OH)D concentration of 30 ng/mL (75 nmol/L). The Institute of Medicine (IOM)[5] report identified vitamin D sufficiency at a lower threshold of 20 to 50 ng/mL (50-125 nmol/L), with risk of insufficiency occurring within the range from 12 to 19 ng/mL (30-49 nmol/L) and risk of deficiency occurring at levels less than 12 ng/mL (<30 nmol/L). However, the Endocrine Society Guidelines define vitamin D deficiency as a 25(OH)D concentration less than 20 ng/mL (50 mmol/mL) and insufficiency as a 25(OH)D concentration between 20 and 29 ng/mL, with a therapeutic goal to maintain a concentration more than

30 ng/mL.[14] It is important to consider the intent of each of these guidelines. The IOM recommendations were aimed at a general pediatric and adult population, whereas the Endocrine Society guidelines were developed for children or adults known to be at risk for lack of bone accretion or bone loss, or who are at risk for vitamin D deficiency itself. The Endocrine Society panel recommends aiming for a slightly higher 25(OH)D threshold for individuals with a known low bone mass or medical condition associated with bone loss.

Observations Among Healthy Children and Adolescents

Despite the variability in the definition of deficiency, several studies have demonstrated that the rates of vitamin D deficiency and insufficiency are quite high within the pediatric population. A study of Hispanic and black adolescents in Boston revealed 52% had 25(OH)D concentrations less than 15 ng/mL.[15] NHANES data analyzed by Kumar et al[16] demonstrated that 9% of the US pediatric population between 2001 and 2004 was vitamin D deficient (25(OH)D <15 ng/mL) with 61% being insufficient (25(OH)D <30 ng/mL), representing 50.8 million US children and adolescents. Among adolescents alone, the highest rates of insufficiency were found in Mexican American girls and boys, 69% and 79% respectively.[16] Grinde et al[17] went on to show that vitamin D levels declined over the last decade since NHANES III in 1988 to 1994. Similarly, rates of deficiency have climbed, with a 3-fold increase in the prevalence of 25(OH)D in a range less than 10 ng/mL.[17] The problem is not unique to the United States; many other countries have noted similar prevalence rates. Vierucci et al[18] found 45.9% of Italian children and adolescents were vitamin D deficient, with 25(OH) D concentrations less than 20 ng/mL. Risk factors for low vitamin D levels include obesity, regular use of sunscreen, blood samples drawn during winter, low vitamin D intake (through either diet or supplementation), and decreased outdoor activity.[15-20]

The ongoing reports of the high prevalence of vitamin D deficiency and insufficiency have led to the recommendation for daily supplementation starting prenatally and continuing through childhood into adulthood. However, the actual amount of supplementation required remains a source of controversy both for healthy adolescents as well as for those who are considered at risk for vitamin D deficiency. The IOM recommendations from 2009 included 600 international units (IU) daily from age 1 year through 70 years (and 400 IU daily for infants 0-12 months).[5] A few studies have suggested that 400 IU/day may be enough to prevent rickets and maintain 25(OH)D levels more than 20 ng/mL.[21,22] However, other studies have suggested that higher doses are required to maintain levels above the recommended goal of 30 ng/mL.[23,24] Importantly, the study by Maalouf et al[23] in 2008 showed no safety concerns with supplementation dosed at 14,000 IU/week for 1 year in boys and girls aged 10 to 17 years. Additionally, the clinical trial by Putman et al[25] demonstrated no safety concerns with a supplementation dose of 1000 IU given daily to healthy adolescents. Therefore, the

Endocrine Society Practice Guidelines published in 2011 recommend 600 to 1000 IU/day for adolescents, but they recognize that more than 1000 IU/day may be needed to maintain 25(OH)D concentrations more than 30 ng/mL.[14] Furthermore, these guidelines recommend that certain groups of patients require even higher supplementation doses (Table 1). Obese adolescents and those receiving anticonvulsant medications, glucocorticoids, antifungals, and medications for AIDS may require 2 to 3 times more vitamin D. Currently, there is no recommendation for routine screening of 25(OH)D concentrations in healthy adolescents, but those considered at risk for vitamin D deficiency should be screened and may require significant supplementation above that recommended for healthy individuals (Table 1). The Endocrine Society Practice Guidelines recommend a replacement regimen for individuals 1 to 18 years old found to be vitamin D deficient of 2000 IU of D2 or D3 daily or 50,000 IU

Table 1
Conditions that place adolescents at risk for vitamin D deficiency

Bone disease
Rickets Osteomalacia Osteoporosis Hyperparathyroidism
Kidney/liver disease
Chronic kidney disease Kidney transplant Hepatic failure and/or cholestasis
Malabsorption syndromes
Cystic fibrosis Inflammatory bowel disease Celiac disease
Medication-induced
Chronic glucocorticoid requirement Antiseizure medications Antifungal therapy Antiretroviral therapy
Granulomatous disorders
Tuberculosis Sarcoidosis
Dietary restriction
Lactose intolerance Parenteral nutrition Obese children (body mass index >30 kg/m^2) Black and Hispanic children

weekly for 6 weeks.[14] A repeat 25(OH)D level should be checked within 2 to 3 weeks after completion of the vitamin D treatment course.

Following these supplementation and screening guidelines, and attempting to maintain an adequate vitamin D status are important for many reasons, including bone health. Fractures are a common complication of osteoporosis among the elderly, but it has been postulated that a 10% increase in peak bone mass could result in a 50% decrease in the relative risk of hip fracture.[26,27] Given that 80% to 90% of peak bone mass is reached during the teenage years, optimizing bone health during these critical years could have a significant effect on bone health later in life.[28,29] However, the relationship between 25(OH)D concentration during adolescence and BMD does not seem to be a simple one. In a study of 14- to 16-year-old Finnish adolescents, 25(OH)D level did not correlate with BMD at baseline but was shown to correlate with change in lumbar spine BMD 3 years later.[30,31] Furthermore, calcium intake, in addition to vitamin D status, is likely to be an important factor in the development of peak bone mass.[9] A meta-analysis of the 6 randomized controlled trials that examined the relationship between vitamin D supplementation and BMD found that only for those children with low 25(OH)D levels (<35 nmol/L) did supplementation significantly increase bone mineral content and BMD.[32,33] Bone density has been shown to be a risk factor for fracture, specifically forearm fracture in children,[34-36] but a direct link between vitamin D and fracture has not yet been demonstrated.

EXTRASKELETAL EFFECTS OF VITAMIN D

Many of the extraskeletal effects of vitamin D stem from the effects of vitamin D on the immune system, both innate and adaptive. Many of the cells comprising the innate immune system express the vitamin D receptor (VDR).[37] Macrophages and dendritic cells are also capable of enzymatic activation of the circulating vitamin D precursor.[38,39] Activation of toll-like receptors, which are important for pattern recognition of certain pathogens, results in the production of cathelicidin and ß-defensin-2, both of which are important for bacterial killing.[40,41] In the adaptive immune system, the intracrine activation of vitamin D by dendritic cells results in overall T-cell suppression,[42] promotion of T-regulatory cells (Tregs), and suppression of the proinflammatory cytokine interleukin (IL)-17.[43] It is through this anti-inflammatory pathway that vitamin D is thought to be protective against autoimmune disease (reviewed by Szodoray et al[44]).

Vitamin D and Type 1 Diabetes Mellitus

Several studies have demonstrated high rates of vitamin D deficiency in children at the time of diagnosis of type 1 diabetes mellitus (T1DM).[45-48] Furthermore, a decreased risk of T1DM with vitamin D supplementation during infancy also has been suggested.[49] A meta-analysis of the available case control and cohort studies regarding vitamin D supplementation and risk of developing T1DM revealed 8 studies assessing the effect of vitamin D supplementation during infancy or childhood.[50-56] Five of the 8 studies reported a reduction in risk of T1DM with vitamin D intake, whereas the other 3 found no association. The pooled odds ratio was 0.71 (95% confidence interval, 0.51-0.98), suggesting that vitamin D intake during early life is associated with a reduced risk of type 1 diabetes.[57]

Vitamin D and Infectious Diseases

Cathelicidin is a potent antimicrobial peptide capable of killing *Mycobacterium tuberculosis,* which causes tuberculosis (TB). For this reason, vitamin D has long been used as a treatment of TB. Several studies have demonstrated lower serum 25(OH)D concentrations in individuals with TB compared with controls.[58,59] A study by Williams et al[60] in 2008 looked specifically at 25(OH)D concentrations in children with TB and found that 86% had inadequate vitamin D concentrations. A recent randomized controlled trial found a treatment benefit of vitamin D supplementation in terms of clinical and radiographic improvement in subjects who initially were vitamin D deficient.[61] In addition to its association with TB, low vitamin D concentrations have been associated with influenza A infection. A randomized controlled study of children receiving 1200 IU of vitamin D daily through the winter had significantly lower rates of influenza A infection.[62] In addition, a prospective study in adults found vitamin D levels greater than 38 ng/mL resulted in a 2-fold reduction in the risk of respiratory tract infection.[63]

Vitamin D and Chronic Disease

Several chronic diseases have been found to have associations with vitamin D deficiency. Cystic fibrosis (CF) and inflammatory bowel disease (IBD) are 2 of the illnesses that have undergone more recent investigation into the effects of vitamin D. CF is a disease characterized by recurrent lung infections with progressive bronchiectasis and decline in pulmonary function. Most people with CF are pancreatic insufficient and require pancreatic enzyme replacement in order to absorb fat. Vitamins A, D, E, and K are fat-soluble vitamins. Therefore, the CF Foundation recommends routine daily supplementation with CF-specific vitamins containing ADEK.[64] Despite these recommendations, several studies have found high rates of vitamin D insufficiency and deficiency despite routine supplementation.[65,66] Given the previously described effects of vitamin D on the immune system and inflammation, it would make sense that adequate vitamin D levels would improve respiratory outcomes in patients with CF. However, few studies have thoroughly explored this association. A pilot study by Grossman et al[67] showed increased survival and hospital-free days in the year after receipt of a 1-time dose of 250,000 IU of D3. Another study demonstrated an association between low 25(OH)D concentrations and increased rates of rejection and infection in lung transplant patients.[68]

IBD includes both Crohn disease and ulcerative colitis, both diseases of immune dysregulation within the intestinal tract.[69] Several studies have demonstrated a high prevalence of vitamin D insufficiency and deficiency among patients with IBD, including pediatric populations.[70,71] These data have been derived primarily from clinical samples from gastroenterology practices. However, the link between vitamin D status and disease severity has not been consistent among studies. Two cross-sectional studies showed no relationship between vitamin D levels and disease severity,[72,73] whereas a large prospective study recently demonstrated that vitamin D deficiency was associated with increased rates of surgery and hospitalization.[74] In addition, a few trials have demonstrated improved outcomes with daily vitamin D supplementation.[75-77] A recent trial has also demonstrated the difficulty experienced in trying to prevent vitamin D deficiency and achieve an optimal vitamin D level in this patient group.[78] Given these studies, the Endocrine Society clinical practice guidelines recommend screening individuals with IBD for vitamin D insufficiency.[14] A recent guideline has also been developed that includes recommendations for optimal vitamin D supplementation for pediatric patients with IBD, in addition to routine screening for vitamin D status and bone health.[79]

Vitamin D and Critical Illness

There is a rapidly growing body of literature demonstrating a connection between vitamin D status and critical illness, among both children and adults. Beginning with a study published in 2009 on vitamin D levels in young children admitted to the hospital with acute lower respiratory tract infections, the patients who required intensive care had significantly lower 25(OH)D concentrations at the time of admission.[80] These findings were further supported by 2 large subsequent studies that showed high rates of vitamin D deficiency among patients admitted to pediatric intensive care units, along with some association between lower vitamin D levels and increased illness severity.[81,82] However, no association has been found between low vitamin D levels and increased mortality risk.[83] These results are promising but need to be expanded to prospective, interventional trials.

Vitamin D and Asthma and Allergy

Asthma is a disease that shares several risk factors with vitamin D deficiency, such as obesity, black ethnicity, and inner-city residence.[84] Because of this association and the previously described effects of vitamin D on the immune system, several observational studies have examined the relationship between vitamin D levels and asthma. Several adult studies have not found an association between vitamin D deficiency and asthma,[85,86] whereas a study looking specifically at black children and adolescents found significantly lower 25(OH)D concentrations in the subjects with asthma compared to healthy control subjects.[87] Similarly, a birth-cohort study showed that maternal dietary intake of vitamin D was associated with a decreased risk of asthma in 5-year-old children.[88] A few studies have shown a correlation between low serum vitamin D levels

(25(OH)D <30 ng/mL) and asthma exacerbations.[89,90] One small interventional study showed a decrease in severe asthma exacerbations in children treated with vitamin D supplementation.[91]

Given the evidence for vitamin D deficiency playing a pathophysiologic role in asthma, a logical next step would be to examine the association of vitamin D status and other atopic diseases, such as food allergies. However, the data exploring the association between vitamin D status and food allergies are both limited and contradictory. In part, the challenge lies in the timing of vitamin D measurement. To date, most studies have included birth cohorts that examine maternal vitamin D intake or levels. The NHANES data revealed that vitamin D deficiency is associated with elevated specific immunoglobulin E (IgE) to food and environmental allergens in children and adolescents.[92] However, at least 1 birth-cohort study found no association between vitamin D deficiency and food allergen sensitization,[93] whereas others showed more of a U-shaped association, with both low and high maternal vitamin D levels associated with higher rates of food allergies.[94] These contradictory results emphasize that a prospective study is needed, and several studies currently are ongoing. The results of these studies will represent important contributions to the field.

SUMMARY

The evidence continues to mount for the important role of vitamin D as a hormone that provides protective benefits to the immune system. Guidelines have been developed recommending routine vitamin D supplementation in order to optimize bone health, including aiming for a goal 25(OH)D concentration greater than 30 ng/mL among select patient groups who are at risk for skeletal deficits or vitamin D deficiency itself. Whether this level is the optimal one that confers the extraskeletal benefits of vitamin D remains unknown. Whether healthy children and adolescents may benefit from maintenance of 25(OH)D levels at higher thresholds also is unknown and under study. Adolescence is a critical time for the accrual of peak bone mass, and optimizing vitamin D during this important developmental period and throughout the life cycle may be beneficial for and beyond the skeleton. Although routine screening of 25(OH)D levels is not currently recommended, those individuals at higher risk for insufficiency/deficiency should be screened and appropriately supplemented.

References

1. Reichel H, Koeffler HP, Norman AW. The role of the vitamin D endocrine system in health and disease. *N Engl J Med.* 1989;32(15):980-991
2. Christakos S, DeLuca HF. Minireview: vitamin D: is there a role in extraskeletal health? *Endocrinology.* 2011;152(8):2930-2936
3. Brannon PM, Yetley EA, Bailey RL, Picciano MF. Vitamin D and health in the 21st century: an update. Proceedings of a conference held September 2007 in Bethesda, Maryland. *Am J Clin Nutr.* 2008;88(2):483S-592S

4. Shore RM, Chesney RW. Rickets: part I. *Pediatr Radiol.* 2013;43(2):140-151
5. Institute of Medicine (IOM). *Dietary Reference Intakes for Calcium and Vitamin D.* Washington, DC: The National Academies Press; 2011
6. Grinde AA, Wolfe P, Camargo CA, Schwartz RS. Defining vitamin D status by secondary hyperparathyroidism in the U.S. population. *J Endocrinol Invest.* 2012;35(1):42-48
7. Okazaki R, Sugimoto T, Haji H, et al. Vitamin D insufficiency defined by serum 25-hydroxyvitamin D and parathyroid hormone before and after oral vitamin D3 load in Japanese subjects. *J Bone Miner Metab.* 2011;29(1):103-110
8. Carpenter TO, Herreros F, Zhang JH, et al. Demographic, dietary and biochemical determinants of vitamin D status in inner-city children. *Am J Clin Nutr.* 2012;95(1):137-146
9. Esterle L, Nguyen M, Walrant-Debray O, Sabatier JP, Garabedian M. Diverse interaction of low-calcium diet and low 25(OH)D levels on lumbar spine mineralization in late-pubertal girls. *J Bone Miner Res.* 2010;25:2392-2398
10. Dawson-Hughes B, Harris SS, Dallal GE. Plasma calcidiol, season, and serum parathyroid hormone concentrations in healthy elderly men and women. *Am J Clin Nutr.* 1997;65:67-71
11. Hill KM, McCabe GP, McCabe LD, Gordon CM, Abrams SA, Weaver CM. An inflection point of serum 25-hydroxyvitamin D for maximal suppression of parathyroid hormone is not evident from multi-site pooled data in children and adolescents. *J Nutr.* 2010;140(11):1983-1988
12. Valcour A, Blocki F, Hawkins DM, Rao SD. Effects of age and serum 25-OH-vitamin D on serum parathyroid hormone levels. *J Clin Endocrinol Metab.* 2012;97(11):3989-3995
13. Bischoff-Ferrari HA, Giovannucci E, Willett C, Dietrich T, Dawson-Hughes B. Estimation of optimal serum concentrations of 25-hydroxyvitamin D for multiple health outcomes. *Am J Clin Nutr.* 2006;84(1):18-28
14. Holick MF, Binkley NC, Bischoff-Ferrari HA, et al. Evaluation, treatment, and prevention of vitamin D deficiency: an Endocrine Society Clinical Practice Guideline. *J Clin Endocrinol Metab.* 2011;96:1911-1930
15. Gordon CM, DePeter KC, Feldman HA, Grace E, Emans SJ. Prevalence of vitamin D deficiency among healthy adolescents. *Arch Pediatr Adolesc Med.* 2004;158(6):531-537
16. Kumar J, Muntner P, Kaskel FJ, Hailpern SM, Melamed ML. Prevalence and associations of 25-hydroxyvitamin D deficiency in US children: NHANES 2001-2004. *Pediatrics.* 2009;124(3): e362-e370
17. Grinde AA, Liu MC, Camargo CA. Demographic differences and trends of vitamin D insufficiency in the US population, 1998-2004. *Arch Intern Med.* 2009;169(6):626-632
18. Vierucci F, Del Pistoia M, Fanos M, et al. Vitamin D status and predictors of hypovitaminosis D in Italian children and adolescents: a cross-sectional study. *Eur J Pediatr.* 2013;172:1607-1617
19. Kemp FW, Neti PV, Howell RW, Wenger P, Louria DB, Bogden JD. Elevated blood lead concentrations and vitamin D deficiency in winter and summer in young urban children. *Environ Health Perspect.* 2007;115(4):630-635
20. Wortsman J, Matsuoka LY, Chen TC, Lu Z, Holick MF. Decreased bioavailability of vitamin D in obesity. *Am J Clin Nutr.* 2000;72(3):690-693
21. Aksnes L, Aarskog D. Plasma concentrations of vitamin D metabolites in puberty: effect of sexual maturation and implications for growth. *J Clin Endocrinol Metab.* 1982;55:94-101
22. Gultekin A, Ozalp I, Hasanodlu A, Unal A. Serum 25-hydroxycholecalciferol levels in children and adolescents. *Turk J Pediatr.* 1987;29:155-162
23. Maalouf J, Nabulski M, Vieth R, Kimball S, El-Rassi R, et al. Short- and long-term safety of weekly high-dose vitamin D3 supplementation in school children. *J Clin Endocrinol Metab.* 2008;93:2693-2701
24. El-Hajj Fuleihan G, Nabulsi M, Tamim H, et al. Effect of vitamin D supplementation on musculoskeletal parameters in school children: a randomized controlled trial. *J Clin Endocrinol Metab.* 2006;91:405-412
25. Putman MS, Pitts SA, Milliren CE, Feldman HA, Reinold K, Gordon CM. A randomized clinical trial of vitamin D supplementation in healthy adolescents. *J Adolesc Health.* 2013;52(5):592-598
26. Hernandez CJ, Beaupre GS, Carter DR. A theoretical analysis of the relative influences of peak BMD, age-related bone loss and menopause on the development of osteoporosis. *Osteoporos Int.* 2003;14:843-847

27. Cummings SR, Black DM, Nevitt MC, et al. Bone density at various sites for prediction of hip fractures. The Study of Osteoporotic Fractures Research Group. *Lancet.* 1993;341:72-75
28. Bailey DA, McKay HA, Mirwald RL, Crocker PR, Faulkner RA. A six-year longitudinal study of the relationship of physical activity to bone mineral accrual in growing children: the University of Saskatchewan bone mineral accrual study. *J Bone Miner Res.* 1999;14:1672-1679
29. Henry YM, Fatayerji D, Eastell R. Attainment of peak bone mass at the lumbar spine, femoral neck and radius in men and women: relative contributions of bone size and volumetric bone mineral density. *Osteoporos Int.* 2004;15:263-273
30. Cheng S, Tylavsky F, Kroger H, et al. Association of low 25-hydroxyvitamin D concentrations with elevated parathyroid hormone concentrations and low cortical bone density in early pubertal and prepubertal Finnish girls. *Am J Clin Nutr.* 2003;78:485-492
31. Lehtonen-Veromaa MK, Mottonen TT, Nuotio IO, Irjala KM, Leino AE, Viikari JS. Vitamin D and attainment of peak bone mass among peripubertal Finnish girls: a 3-year prospective study. *Am J Clin Nutr.* 2002;76:1446-1453
32. Winzenberg T, Powell S, Shaw KA, Jones G. Effects of vitamin D supplementation on bone density in healthy children: systematic review and meta-analysis. *Br Med J.* 2011;342:c7254
33. Winzenberg TM, Powell S, Shaw KA, Jones G. Vitamin D supplementation for improving bone mineral density in children. *Cochrane Database Syst Rev.* 2010;10:CD006944
34. Ma D, Jones G. The association between bone mineral density, metacarpal morphometry, and upper limb fractures in children: a population-based case-control study. *J Clin Endocrinol Metab.* 2003;88:1486-1491
35. Goulding A, Cannan R, Williams SM, Gold EJ, Taylor RW, Lewis-Barned NJ. Bone mineral density in girls with forearm fractures. *J Bone Miner Res.* 1998;13:143-148
36. Goulding A, Jones IE, Taylor RW, Williams SM, Manning PJ. Bone mineral density and body composition in boys with distal forearm fractures: a dual-energy X-ray absorptiometry study. *J Pediatr.* 2001;139:509-515
37. Provvedini DM, Tsoukas CD, Deftos LJ, Manolagas SC. 1,25-Dihydroxyvitamin D3 receptors in human leukocytes. *Science.* 1983;221:1181-1183
38. Fritsche J, Mandal K, Ehrnsperger A, Andreesen R, Kreutz M. Regulation of 25-hydroxyvitamin D3–1 alpha-hydroxylase and production of 1 alpha, 25-hydroxyvitamin D3 by human dendritic cells. *Blood.* 2003;102:3314-3316
39. Monkawa T, Yoshida T, Hayashi M, Saruta T. Identification of 25-hydroxyvitamin D3 1 alpha-hydroxylase gene expression in macrophages. *Kidney Int.* 2000;58:559-568
40. Schauber J, Dorschner RA, Coda AB, et al. Injury enhances TLR2 function and antimicrobial peptide expression through a vitamin D-dependent mechanism. *J Clin Invest.* 2007;117:803-811
41. Liu PT, Stenger S, Li H, et al. Toll-like receptor triggering of a vitamin D-mediated human antimicrobial response. *Science.* 2006;311:1770-1773
42. Hewison M, Freeman L, Hughes SV, et al. Differential regulation of vitamin D receptor and its ligand in human monocyte-derived dendritic cells. *J Immunol.* 2003;170:5382-5390
43. Jeffery LE, Wood AM, Qureshi OS, et al. Availability of 25-hydroxyvitamin D3 to APCs controls the balance between regulatory and inflammatory T cell responses. *J. Immunol.* 2012;189:5155-5164
44. Szodoray P, Nakken B, Gaal J, et al. The complex role of vitamin D in autoimmune diseases. *Scand J Immunol.* 2008;68:261-269
45. Mutlu A, Mutlu GY, Ozsu E, Cizmecioglu FM, Hatun S. Vitamin D deficiency in children and adolescents with type 1 diabetes. *J Clin Res Pediatr Endocrinol.* 2011;3:179-183
46. Janner M, Ballinari P, Mullis PE, Fluck CE. High prevalence of vitamin D deficiency in children and adolescents with type 1 diabetes. *Swiss Med Wkly.* 2010;140:w13091
47. Bin-Abbas BS, Jabari MA, Issa SD, Al-Fares AH, Al-Muhsen S. Vitamin D levels in Saudi children with type 1 diabetes. *Saudi Med J.* 2011;32:589-592
48. Franch B, Piazza M, Sandri M, Mazzei F, Maffeis C, Boner AL. Vitamin D at the onset of type 1 diabetes in Italian children. *Eur J Pediatr.* 2014;173(4):477-482
49. The EURODIAB Substudy 2 Study Group. Vitamin D supplement in early childhood and risk for type I (insulin-dependent) diabetes mellitus. *Diabetologia.* 1999;42:51-54
50. Stene LC, Ulriksen J, Magnus P, Joner G. Use of cod liver oil during pregnancy associated with lower risk of type I diabetes in the offspring. *Diabetologia.* 2000;43:1093-1098

51. Hypponen E, Laara E, Reunanen A, Jarvelin MR, Virtanen SM. Intake of vitamin D and risk of type 1 diabetes: a birth-cohort study. *Lancet.* 2001;358:1500-1503
52. Stene LC, Joner G. Use of cod liver oil during the first year of life is associated with lower risk of childhood-onset type 1 diabetes: a large, population-based, case-control study. *Am J Clin Nutr.* 2003;78:1128-1134
53. Visalli N, Sebastiani L, Adorisio E, et al; IMDIAB Group. Environmental risk factors for type 1 diabetes in Rome and province. *Arch Dis Child.* 2003;88:695-698
54. Tenconi MT, Devoti G, Comelli M, et al. Major childhood infectious diseases and other determinants associated with type 1 diabetes: a case-control study. *Acta Diabetol.* 2007;44:14-19
55. Ahadi M, Tabatabaeiyan M, Moazzami K. Association between environmental factors and risk of type 1 diabetes: a case-control study. *Endokrynol Pol.* 2011;62:134-137
56. Simpson M, Brady H, Yin X, et al. No association of vitamin D intake or 25-hydroxyvitamin D levels in childhood with risk of islet autoimmunity and type 1 diabetes: the Diabetes Autoimmunity Study in the Young (DAISY) *Diabetologia.* 2011;54:2779-2788
57. Dong J, Zhang W, Chen JJ, Zhang Z, Han S, Qin L. Vitamin D intake and risk of type 1 diabetes: a meta-analysis of observational studies. *Nutrients.* 2013;5(9):3551-3562
58. Gibney KB, MacGregor L, Leder K, et al. Vitamin D deficiency is associated with tuberculosis and latent tuberculosis infection in immigrants from sub-Saharan Africa. *Clin Infect Dis.* 2008;46(3): 443-446
59. Nnoaham KE, Clarke A. Low serum vitamin D levels and tuberculosis: a systematic review and meta-analysis. *Int J Epidemiol.* 2008;37(1):113-119
60. Williams B, Williams AJ, Anderson ST. Vitamin D deficiency and insufficiency in children with tuberculosis. *Pediatr Infect Dis J.* 2008;27:941-942
61. Salahuddin N, Ali F, Hasan Z, Rao N, Aqeel M, Mahmood F. Vitamin D accelerates clinical recovery from tuberculosis: results of the SUCCINCT Study [Supplementary Cholecalciferol in recovery from tuberculosis]. A randomize, placebo-controlled, clinical trial of vitamin D supplementation in patients with pulmonary tuberculosis. *BMC Infect Dis.* 2013;13:22
62. Urashima M, Segawa T, Okazaki M, Kurihara M, Wada Y, Ida H. Randomized trial of vitamin D supplementation to prevent seasonal influenza A in schoolchildren. *Am J Clin Nutr.* 2010;91:1255-1260
63. Sabetta JR, DePetrillo P, Cipriani RJ, Smardin J, Burns LA, Landry ML. Serum 25-hydroxyvitamin D and the incidence of acute viral respiratory tract infections in healthy adults. *PLoS One.* 2010;5(6):e11088
64. Tangpricha V, Kelly A, Stephenson A, et al. An update on the screening, diagnosis, management, and treatment of vitamin D deficiency in individuals with cystic fibrosis: evidence-based recommendations from the Cystic Fibrosis Foundation. *J Clin Endocrinol Metab.* 2012;97:1082-1093
65. Grey V, Atkinson S, Drury D, et al. Prevalence of low bone mass and deficiencies of vitamins D and K in pediatric patients with cystic fibrosis from 3 Canadian centers. *Pediatrics.* 2008;122:1014-1020
66. Rovner AJ, Stallings VA, Schall JI, Leonard MB, Zemel BS. Vitamin D insufficiency in children, adolescents, and young adults with cystic fibrosis despite routine oral supplementation. *Am J Clin Nutr.* 2007;86:1694-1699
67. Grossmann RE, Zughaier SM, Kumari M, et al. Pilot study of vitamin D supplementation in adults with cystic fibrosis pulmonary exacerbation: a randomized, controlled trial. *Dermatoendocrinol.* 2012;4:191-197
68. Lowery EM, Bemiss B, Cascino T, et al. Low vitamin D levels are associated with increased rejection and infections after lung transplantation. *J Heart Lung Transplant.* 2012;31:700-707
69. Abraham C, Cho JH. Inflammatory bowel disease. *N Engl J Med.* 2009;361:2066-2078
70. Pappa HM, Gordon CM, Saslowsky TM, et al. Vitamin D status in children and young adults with inflammatory bowel disease. *Pediatrics.* 2006;118:1950-1961
71. Pappa HM, Langereis EJ, Grand RJ, Gordon CM. Prevalence and risk factors for hypovitaminosis D in young patients with inflammatory bowel disease. *J Pediatr Gastroenterol Nutr.* 2011;53: 361-364
72. El-Matary W, Sikora S, Spady D. Bone mineral density, vitamin D, and disease activity in children newly diagnosed with inflammatory bowel disease. *Dig Dis Sci.* 2011;56:825-829

73. Joseph AJ, George B, Pulimood AB, Seshadri MS, Chacko A. 25(OH) Vitamin D level in Crohn's disease: association with sun exposure & disease activity. *Indian J Med Res.* 2009;130:133-137
74. Ananthakrishnan AN, Cagan A, Gainer VS, et al. Normalization of plasma 25-hydroxy vitamin D is associated with reduced risk of surgery in Crohn's disease. *Inflamm Bowel Dis.* 2013;19:1921-1927
75. Jorgensen SP, Agnholt J, Glerup H, et al. Clinical trial: vitamin D3 treatment in Crohn's disease: a randomized double-blind placebo-controlled study. *Aliment Pharmacol Ther.* 2010;32:377-383
76. Miheller P, Muzes G, Hritz I, et al. Comparison of the effects of 1,25 dihydroxyvitamin D and 25 hydroxyvitamin D on bone pathology and disease activity in Crohn's disease patients. *Inflamm Bowel Dis.* 2009;15:1656-1662
77. Yang L, Weaver V, Smith JP, Bingaman S, Hartman TJ, Cantorna MT. Therapeutic effect of vitamin D supplementation in a pilot study of Crohn's patients. *Clin Transl Gastroenterol.* 2013;4:e33
78. Pappa HM, Mitchell PD, Jiang H, et al. Treatment of vitamin D insufficiency in children and adolescents with inflammatory bowel disease: a randomized clinical trial comparing three regimens. *J Clin Endocrinol Metab.* 2012;97(6):2134-2142
79. Pappa H, Thayu M, Sylvester F, Leonard M, Zemel B, Gordon CM. Skeletal health of children and adolescents with inflammatory bowel disease. *J Pediatr Gastroenterol Nutr.* 2011;53(1):11-25
80. McNally JD, Leis K, Matheson LA, Karuananyake C, Sankaran K, Rosenberg AM. Vitamin D deficiency in young children with severe acute lower respiratory infection. *Pediatr Pulmonol.* 2009;44(10):981-988
81. Madden K, Feldman HA, Smith EM, et al. Vitamin D deficiency in critically ill children. *Pediatrics.* 2012;130(3):421-428
82. McNally JD, Kusum M, Chakraborty P, et al; Canadian Critical Care Trials Group. The association of vitamin D status with pediatric critical illness. *Pediatrics.* 2012;130(3):429-436
83. Rey C, Sánchez-Arango D, López-Herce J, et al. Vitamin D deficiency at pediatric intensive care admission. *J Pediatr (Rio J).* 2014;90(2):135-142
84. Paul G, Brehn JM, Alcorn JF, Holguín F, Augla SJ, Celedon JC. Vitamin D and asthma. *Am J Respir Crit Care Med.* 2012;185(2):124-132
85. Hypponen E, Sovio U, Wjst M, et al. Infant vitamin D supplementation and allergic conditions in adulthood: northern Finland birth cohort 1966. *Ann N Y Acad Sci.* 2004;1037:84-95
86. Devereux G, Wilson A, Avenell A, McNeill G, Fraser WD. A case-control study of vitamin D status and asthma in adults. *Allergy.* 2010;65:666-667
87. Freishtat RJ, Iqbal SF, Pillai DK, Klein CJ, Ryan LM, Benton AS, Teach SJ. High prevalence of vitamin D deficiency among inner-city African American youth with asthma in Washington, DC. *J Pediatr.* 2010;156:948-952
88. Erkkola M, Kaila M, Nwaru BI, et al. Maternal vitamin D intake during pregnancy is inversely associated with asthma and allergic rhinitis in 5-year-old children. *Clin Exp Allergy.* 2009;39:875-882
89. Brehm JM, Celedon JC, Soto-Quiros ME, et al. Serum vitamin D levels and markers of severity of childhood asthma in Costa Rica. *Am J Respir Crit Care Med.* 2009;179:765-771
90. Brehm JM, Schuemann B, Fuhlbrigge AL, et al. Serum vitamin D levels and severe asthma exacerbations in the Childhood Asthma Management Program study. *J Allergy Clin Immunol.* 2010;126:52-58 e5
91. Majak P, Olszowiec-Chlebna M, Smejda K, Stelmach I. Vitamin D supplementation in children may prevent asthma exacerbation triggered by acute respiratory infection. *J Allergy Clin Immunol.* 2011;127:1294-1296
92. Sharief S, JariwalaS, Kumar J, et al. Vitamin D levels and food and environmental allergies in the United States: results from the National Health and Nutrition Examination Survey. *J Allergy Clin Immunol.* 2011;127:1195-1202
93. Liu X, Wang G, Hong X, et al. Gene–vitamin D interactions on food sensitization: a prospective birth cohort study. *Allergy.* 2011;66:1442-1448
94. Rothers J, Wright AL, Stern DA, et al. Cord blood 25 hydroxyvitamin D levels are associated with aeroallergen sensitization in children from Tucson, Arizona. *J Allergy Clin Immunol.* 2011;128:1093-1099

Adolesc Med 025 (2014) 251–265

Medication-Assisted Treatment of Opioid Use Disorder in Adolescents and Young Adults

Casey B. Cottrill, MD[a1*]; Steven C. Matson, MD[a,b2]

[a]*Division of Adolescent Medicine, Nationwide Children's Hospital, Columbus, Ohio;*
[b]*Department of Pediatrics, The Ohio State University College of Medicine, Columbus, Ohio*

THE OPIOID EPIDEMIC

Each day, American teenagers expose themselves to illicit substances at alarming rates. According to a Substance Abuse and Mental Health Services Administration (SAMHSA) report, on an average day, 4,348 American teenagers will use an illicit drug, 2,517 will use pain relievers nonmedically, and 86 will use heroin for the first time in their lives.[1] According to the 2013 Monitoring the Future Study, high school seniors are reporting lifetime use of heroin at 1%, any prescription drug used nonmedically at 21.5%, and any narcotic other than heroin at 11.1%. This survey also documents the use of Vicodin and OxyContin within the past year by high school seniors to be 5.3% and 3.6%, respectively.[2] These striking numbers highlight the need for appropriate recognition and treatment of this growing problem within the United States.

Not only are American teenagers using opioids at increasing rates, but admissions to facilities receiving federal state drug or alcohol funds for substance abuse treatment and overdose deaths involving opioid medications are increasing. In 2007, the Treatment Episode Data Set (TEDS), which tracks national admission rates for substance abuse for the US Department of Health and Human Services, reported that of the 1.82 million admissions for substance

---

[1] No financial disclosures to make.
[2] Teaching advocate for Reckitt Benckiser, the maker of Suboxone. Dr. Matson has given 1 CME presentation on the use of Suboxone to treat opioid dependence.

*Corresponding author:
E-mail address: Casey.Cottrill@NationwideChildrens.org

 ISSN 1934-4287

abuse, 11.4% (206,911) were for patients younger than 19 years. In this age group, 8.1% (11,542) of these admissions were because of heroin and other opiates.[3] The Centers for Disease Control and Prevention (CDC) reports that deaths related to opioid drugs rose from 4,030 in 1999 to 16,651 in 2010. This trend of increasing opioid overdose death rates occurred for the 11th consecutive year as of 2010.[4] As shown in Figure 1, in adolescents, deaths from opioid medications exceed those from all other illegal drugs.[5] These statistics help to clarify the gravity of this situation for American youth; not only are they trying opioids and being admitted for opioid use disorder treatment, but they also are dying from opioid overdose at ever increasing rates.

Although there are many deaths because of opioid abuse, there are also many adolescents who go on to develop a chronic relapsing relationship with opioids. For these adolescents with long-term addiction careers, the outcomes are very stark. One study that followed a sample of 697 daily opioid users 12 years after they entered treatment found 25% of the subjects were still engaging in daily opioid use. The overall length of addiction for this sample, defined as the time between first and last daily opioid use, ranged from 1 to 35 years. Specifically, 28% were addicted for 1 to 5 years, 33% for 6 to 11 years, 36% for 12 to 20 years, and 4% for more than 20 years, with the average length of time addicted being 9.9 years. The results of this study demonstrate that some individuals will never resolve their dependence on opioid drugs.[6] Given the potentially chronic and life-threatening nature of opi-

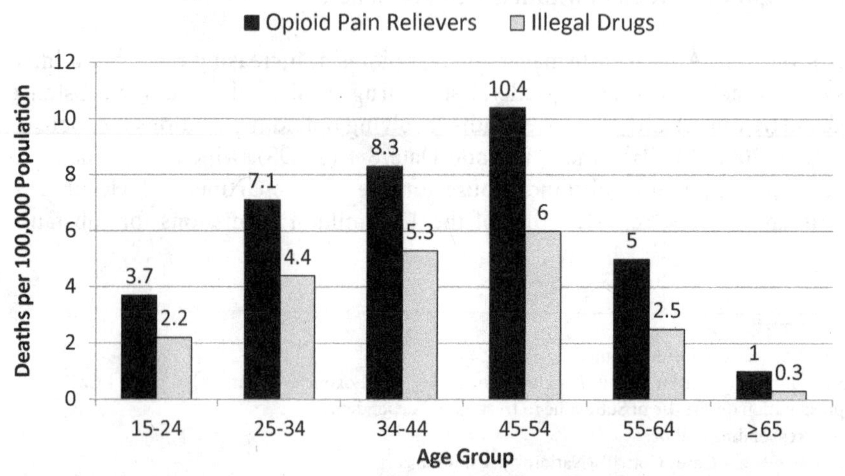

Fig 1. Drug overdose death rates. (From Centers for Disease Control and Prevention. Vital signs: overdoses of prescription opioid relievers—United States, 1999-2008. *MMWR*. 2011;60[43]:1487-1492.)

oid dependence, interventions and treatments that will prevent the development and progression of the disease of addiction must be found.

THE HISTORY AND SCIENCE OF ADDICTION MEDICINE

The modern scientific definition of addiction states that addiction is a chronic, relapsing brain disease that is characterized by compulsive drug-seeking behaviors and use, despite harmful consequences. This modern definition differs greatly from the early teachings of addiction, which held that addiction was a reflection of moral depravity or otherwise the etiology or symptom of a mental illness. One of the first to write about addiction as a disease was Dr Benjamin Rush (1746-1813), a member of the Continental Congress, a signer of the Declaration of Independence, and Physician General of the Continental Army. Rush broke with the traditional view of alcoholism and wrote that alcoholism should be viewed as a self-contained disease and that continued abstinence from alcohol was the only hope for treatment.[7,8] Despite Dr Rush's progressive disease characterization and treatment suggestions, as early as the 1800s and even into the 20th century, scientists studying addiction behaviors still worked with the basic assumption that people addicted to drugs were morally flawed and lacking in sufficient willpower. Those views shaped society's responses to drug abuse, treating it as a moral failing rather than a health problem. The linkage of addiction and moral corruption led to an emphasis on punitive rather than preventive and therapeutic actions.[9]

The contemporary view of addiction focuses on the physiologic changes occurring during addiction, especially with regard to the neurotransmitter dopamine. Early studies established that dopamine was the neurotransmitter of pleasure and that dopamine modulated the pleasure of eating and sexual behavior.[10-15] Di Chiara and Imperato demonstrated that drugs abused by humans increased extracellular dopamine concentrations, especially in the nucleus accumbens. The nucleus accumbens, also known as "the pleasure center of the brain," is 1 part of the mesolimbic pathway that controls dopaminergic systems in the brain. It traverses from the ventral tegmental area (VTA) to the nucleus accumbens and finally to the prefrontal cortex (Figure 2). Because the mesolimbic pathway has been shown to be associated with feelings of reward and desire, this pathway is heavily implicated in neurobiologic theories of addiction.[16,17]

To connect the mesolimbic, dopaminergic reward pathway with opioid use, it is important to remember that opioids act as a powerful agonist at the mu-opioid receptor subtype. Binding and activation at the mu receptor site inhibits the release of gamma-aminobutyric acid (GABA) from the nerve terminal, reducing the inhibitory effect of GABA on dopaminergic neurons. The decreased inhibition, leading to increased activation of dopaminergic neurons, causes a release of dopamine into the synaptic cleft and results in sustained activation of the postsynaptic membrane. Continued activation of the dopaminergic reward

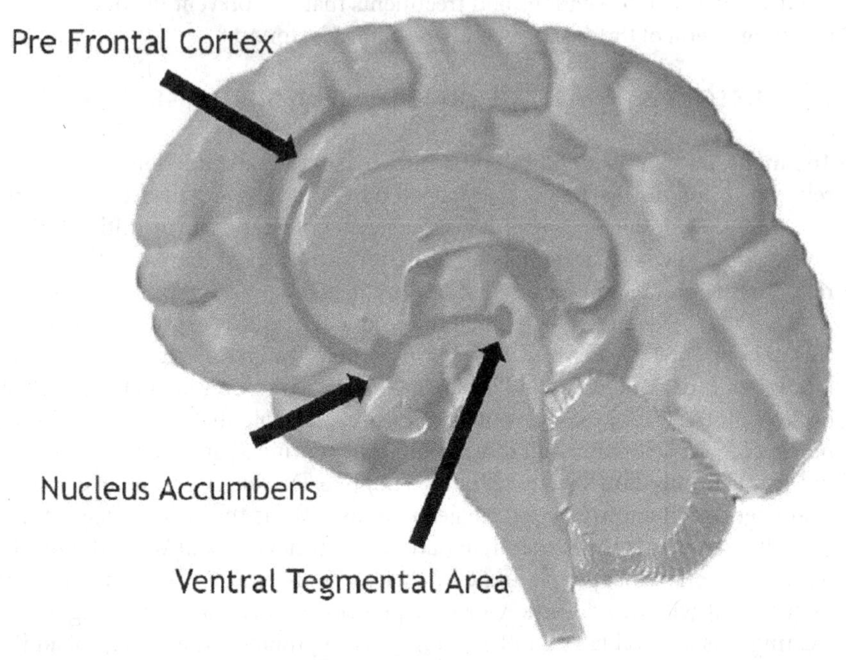

Fig 2. The major structures are highlighted: the ventral tegmental area (VTA), the nucleus accumbens, and the prefrontal cortex.

pathway leads to the feelings of euphoria and the "high" associated with opioid use (Figure 3).[18] It is now understood that addiction is a hijacking of the pleasure systems of the brain and involves significant alterations to the brain's anatomy and chemistry, making it very difficult to resist using more drugs. Even once abstinence is achieved, many of the neurochemical changes can take months to years to return to normal.[19,20]

DIAGNOSIS OF OPIOID USE DISORDER

In past editions of the *Diagnostic and Statistical Manual of Mental Disorders,* patients with serious opioid addiction were diagnosed as opioid dependent; however, in the newly-published fifth edition (*DSM-5*) patients will be placed within a continuum of use under the term opioid use disorder. Opioid use disorder is defined as a problematic pattern of opioid use leading to clinically significant impairment or distress, as manifested by at least 2 out of a possible 11 diagnostic criteria occurring within a 12-month period. Criteria include craving, tolerance, withdrawal, risky behavior, and psychosocial consequences of use. Opioid use disorder is mild if there are 2 to 3 symptoms, moderate with 4 to 5, and severe if there are 6 or more symptoms. Also newly added to the DSM-5 are specifiers created to aid in describing the patient's addiction in more detail and classifying remission status.[21]

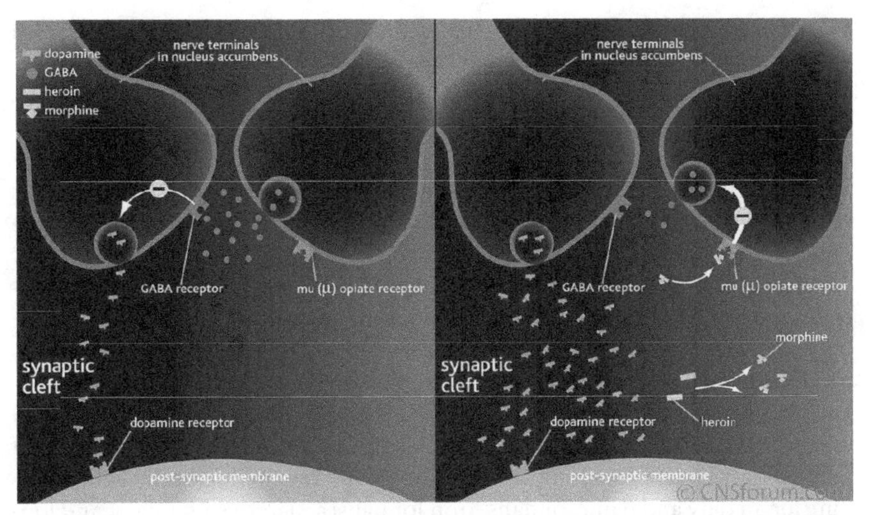

Fig 3. Heroin modifies the action of dopamine in the nucleus accumbens and the ventral tegmental area of the brain—these areas form part of the brain's 'reward pathway'. http://www.cnsforum.com/educationalresources/imagebank/substance_abuse/moa_heroin_mu

TREATMENT OF OPIOID USE DISORDER

In 2000, Congress passed the Drug Abuse Treatment Act of 2000 (DATA 2000), which allowed physicians to prescribe specially approved opioid-based medications for the treatment of opioid dependence. Buprenorphine/naloxone (BUP/NAL) combination therapy (Suboxone) and buprenorphine (BUP) monotherapy (Subutex) became the first medications approved by DATA 2000. They were approved by the US Food and Drug Administration (FDA) in October 2002 and are still the only Schedule III, IV, or V medications with FDA approval for outpatient opioid use disorder treatment. Buprenorphine is a semisynthetic opioid that is a partial mu-opioid agonist displaying high affinity for and slow dissociation from the mu-opioid receptor. The BUP/NAL combination product is designed to decrease the potential for abuse. With proper sublingual administration, little to no naloxone is absorbed, but if BUP/NAL is solubilized and injected, the naloxone released is sufficient enough to induce immediate withdrawal.

In order to prescribe buprenorphine, physicians must become certified for outpatient opioid dependence treatment in accordance with the regulations set forth by DATA 2000. Certification is accomplished by completing 1 of several courses available from the American Academy of Addiction Psychiatry (www.aaap.org/education-and-training/buprenorphine-web-based-training) or from the American Society of Addiction Medicine (www.asam.org/). Following training conclusion, an X number is provided by the DEA to recognize the physician as a buprenorphine provider. For the first year the physician is a certified provider, there is limit of 30 buprenorphine patients, but this limit may be increased to 100 patients after 1 year of clinical experience.

MEDICATION ASSISTED TREATMENT

Empirically derived guidelines describing the optimal treatment for adolescents struggling with opioid dependence are lacking because of the dearth of longitudinal research in this area. In the absence of such guidelines, we present our clinical experience treating this patient population. Over the past 5 years, physicians at our adolescent Medication Assisted Treatment (MAT) Clinic have observed that admission to an inpatient unit for opioid withdrawal typically is needed only when the patient is obtunded because of overdose. In our experience, many patients present to an emergency department (ED) solely looking to relieve withdrawal symptoms rather than presenting truly for treatment of addiction. Patients presenting to the ED are treated symptomatically with clonidine for anxiety and panic, ondansetron for nausea, naproxen for pain, and loperamide for diarrhea. Typically, this will suffice until the patient can present to the outpatient program for a more thorough and controlled evaluation.

A team approach works best for the treatment of adolescents with opioid dependence. At a minimum, a dedicated nurse, a social worker, and a buprenorphine certified physician are needed to properly care for this patient population. Social workers are often the first contact for new patients, and they can explain that MAT is just one component of the treatment plan. Patients seeking treatment are advised of the need for participation in behavioral rehabilitative programming, the requirement of providing a witnessed urine specimen for a drug screen at each visit, and the recommendation to attend 1 to 2 12-step meetings (Alcoholics Anonymous or Narcotics Anonymous) before the intake appointment. Appointments are made as soon as possible, usually within 1 week, to take advantage of the patient's desire to begin addiction treatment.

THE INITIAL VISIT

Patients are referred to the program from other medical professionals, substance abuse treatment programs, drug courts, or self-referral. At the initial MAT visit, all patients undergo a full substance abuse assessment, and a diagnosis of opioid use disorder is confirmed using DSM–5 criteria. The patient's preferred opioid and method of delivery are specified as oral ingestion, nasal snorting, smoking, or injecting either subcutaneously, intramuscularly, or intravenously of solubilized tablets or heroin. Additionally, the substance abuse assessment determines all drugs ever used and details their use by assessing the age of initiation, frequency, maximal use, and routes of delivery. The Teen Addiction Severity Index (T-ASI), a validated and reliable tool to guide obtaining a substance abuse history, is available online for public use. It is a semistructured interview serving as a standardized instrument for periodic evaluation of adolescent substance abuse and can assist in identifying a past and present history of mental health disorders.[22,23]

In addition to self-report of substance abuse history obtained in the comprehensive drug assessment, our clinic references each patient's state prescription drug monitoring program (PDMP) report at the initial visit and before each subsequent visit. The information in the PDMP is derived from electronic databases, which collect information on statewide prescription of controlled substances. PDMPs were developed to promote the public health and welfare by detecting diversion, abuse, and misuse of prescription medications and are available in most states. This is an invaluable tool that allows the MAT physician to ensure that no other controlled medications are being prescribed to the patient. The review of the PDMP report should be noted in the patient's chart at each visit.

After the drug assessment is completed and the PDMP is reviewed, a complete medical history is obtained, including, but not limited to, past medical and surgical history, allergies, medications, family history, review of systems, pregnancy history, and sexual history. A complete physical examination is conducted, with special attention to conditions such as injection track marks, abscesses, skin excoriations because of "picking," and hepatomegaly.

A witnessed point-of-care urine drug test is collected during this visit and at all subsequent visits. This test should have the ability to detect amphetamine, benzodiazepine, cocaine, methadone, opiates, methamphetamine, oxycodone, and tetrahydrocannabinol (THC). Importantly, the test utilized should detect buprenorphine and will serve to monitor MAT adherence at future visits. Any positives noted on point-of-care testing will be a trigger for the urine to be sent for mass spectrometry/gas chromatography confirmatory testing and THC quantification. The quantified THC level is utilized to judge the chronicity of use of marijuana and to follow for decreasing levels while the patient participates in treatment. Any test identifying possible adulteration of urine specimens is beneficial and usually measures urine temperature, pH, and presence of bleach, nitrite, and creatinine. Failure of any adulteration test component results in the declaration of an unacceptable urine specimen or a "dirty urine" and appropriate modification of treatment recommendations. Although our program focuses on sobriety from opioids, we also recommend and monitor for all substance sobriety for patients involved in MAT. We believe that any continued use of other drugs of abuse is detrimental to the future sobriety of the patient.

Initial laboratory testing on all patients should include gonorrhea, chlamydia, trichomonas, human immunodeficiency virus (HIV), and rapid plasma reagin (RPR). Patients also should have confirmation of both immunity to and infection by hepatitis A, B, and C, including Hep A IgG, Hep A IgM, Hep B core antibody, Hep B surface antibody, Hep B surface antigen, Hep C antibody, and, for any Hep C antibody-positive patients, Hep C qualitative polymerase chain reaction (PCR). Patients found to be lacking immunity to hepatitis A and/or B should be reimmunized in order to protect the liver from these infections. Patients with a positive hepatitis C antibody and a negative qualitative PCR either may have cleared the infection or may be early in the infection. Repeat testing in 6 to 8 weeks is suggested to further define the infection. Patients with a positive hepatitis C antibody and positive qualitative PCR are considered to have active hepatitis C infection and should receive further testing, including a quantitative Hep C PCR, liver function testing, and hepatitis C virus typing and subtyping. If the patient has an active hepatitis C infection, a referral to a gastroenterologist within 2 to 3 months of demonstrated sobriety will be made. The reason for this slight delay in referral is because, in our experience, most gastroenterologists require their patients to demonstrate an active commitment to sobriety before initiation of treatment for hepatitis C.

After the comprehensive psychosocial and medical intake evaluation, a recommendation for the level of substance abuse treatment is made. This recommendation is driven by the American Society of Addiction Medicine's Patient Placement Criteria for the Treatment of Substance-Related Disorders.[24] Patients may be recommended for outpatient treatment, intensive outpatient treatment (IOP), or residential treatment, in increasing order of treatment intensity. If a patient is recommended for outpatient treatment and MAT is considered to be potentially beneficial, the patient or the minor's family member signs a contract of expectations that are to be followed in order for the patient to remain enrolled in the MAT program. If a patient is younger than 18 years, we require a parent or other responsible, sober caregiver to sign the treatment contract and agree to active participation as a supervisor of the adolescent in MAT. The expectations set forth in the contract involve regular attendance at medical and behavioral treatment appointments, clean urine drug screening results, and other elements to aid the patient in achieving sobriety. A sample contract is available from the authors on request. If outpatient treatment is not sufficient, then IOP is recommended, which involves 3-4 hour treatment sessions occurring approximately 3 times a week for 6 to 8 weeks to provide extensive addiction education and treatment. For those patients struggling greatly with addiction, the recommendation will often be for a residential placement, which typically involves a 1- to 3-month stay at a facility specializing in addiction treatment.

MEDICATION ASSISTED TREATMENT INDUCTION

Strict protocols exist for in-office buprenorphine induction.[25] Starting patients on a low dose of BUP/NAL under direct observation and gradually increasing the dose over many hours with a goal of resolution of withdrawal is recommended. However, this requires that buprenorphine be stored on site and delivered by the prescribing physician over many hours, which is not amenable to most outpatient practices. Instead, our adolescent MAT program has found that almost all patients can be counseled on how to start the medicine and be sent home to transition onto

BUP/NAL. Most patients are heavily using opiates and will require 8 mg/2 mg films of BUP/NAL twice per day; however, patients taking opiates orally a few times a week may be started on 8 mg/2 mg film of BUP/NAL once per day. Although the BUP/NAL could be taken once a day, twice-a-day dosing has been found to be better tolerated at the beginning of treatment. The initiation of BUP/NAL is best started 12 to 24 hours after the last use of opioids to avoid inducing opioid withdrawal. Most opioids will clear a patient's system within 36 to 48 hours and will be metabolized to low enough levels to start BUP/NAL within 12 to 24 hours. However, if methadone is present, because of its long half-life, initiation of BUP/NAL must be delayed until it clears the system to prevent the patient from experiencing strong withdrawal symptoms.

To further ease the process of transitioning to BUP/NAL, the following prescriptions may be provided: ondansetron 4 to 8 mg by mouth (PO) 3 times per day as needed for nausea, trazodone 50 to 200 mg PO at bedtime as needed for sleep, and polyethylene glycol 17 g mixed with 8 ounces of liquid once or twice daily as needed for constipation. To properly take BUP/NAL, the following instructions are recommended[26]:

1. Take a drink of water to moisten your mouth.
2. Open the foil package and place the film under one side of the tongue (Figure 4).[27]
3. Put your tongue down on the film and do not move your tongue for 10 minutes.

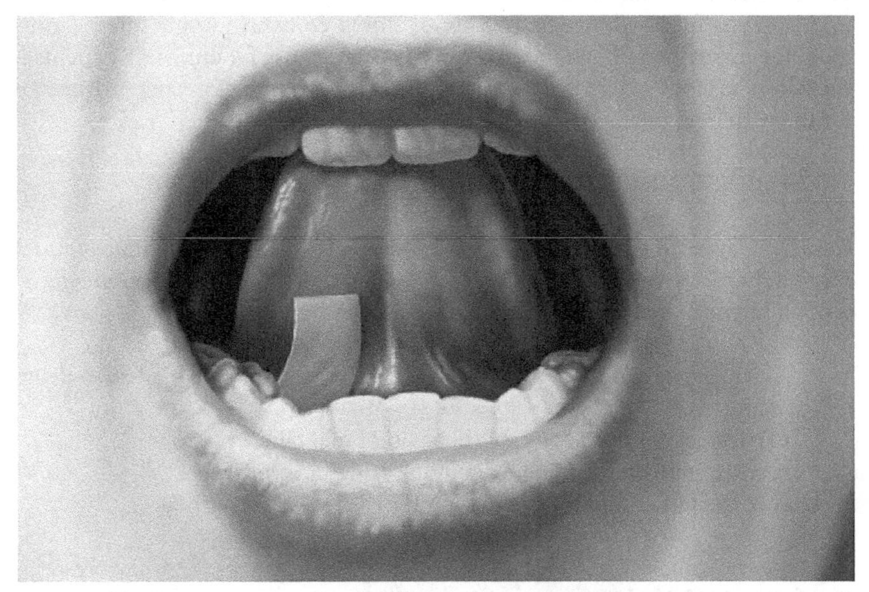

Fig 4. Correct BUP/NAL film placement. Available at www.suboxone.com/content/pdfs/Medication_Guide.pdf. Accessed June 23, 2014. Reprinted by permission of Reckitt Benckiser.

4. Do not talk, eat, smoke, or drink during the time period.
5. Less medicine will be absorbed if you try to speed absorption with extra saliva.
6. After 10 minutes, rinse out the mouth since any leftover film contains no active medication.

Families are told to observe all doses and not to give the patient any future doses to hold and be taken later. Patients are instructed to ***NEVER*** take the medicine any other way than prescribed. If the patient or family feels that they need a change of the buprenorphine, the clinic must be contacted. It is suggested that patients and families store the buprenorphine in a locked storage area to reduce the risk of lost or stolen medication. Part of the patient contract states that "lost" medication will not be replaced and that, if the medication is stolen, a police report is required for replacement medication. Patients are told that they are never to contact the "on call" doctor for changes in dose or refill. Buprenorphine has very high street value, so care needs to be taken to reduce diversion for unintended use. As a secondary tactic to decrease diversion, patients are required to return all of the used film wrappers at follow-up visits so that the films can be counted and the number of wrappers returned verified as the number prescribed.

During the initiation and transition to buprenorphine, a home lockdown of the patient is advised, only allowing the patient to attend school, work, or a rehabilitative program. Confiscation of the patient's cell phone and removal of all current contacts followed by a restriction of stored contacts to only direct family members is advised. The most common cause of relapse for our MAT patients is the failure to stop associating with drug-using friends; therefore, the early goal is for the patient to be under watchful eyes as much as possible.

SUBSEQUENT VISITS

Initially, follow-up visits occur every 7 to 14 days to insure proper clinic requirement adherence and participation in behavioral treatment. Requirements to remain in good standing in the program include:

1. A urine drug screen positive for BUP/NAL and negative for all other drugs of abuse.
2. Participation in an acceptable behavioral rehabilitative program.
3. A clean state prescription drug monitoring program report.
4. A correct used film wrapper count for each dose prescribed.

Patients who adhere with all of the above are given a new 7- to 14-day prescription for the BUP/NAL. Typically, visits occur every 2 weeks for the first 2 months. Once the patient is consistently attending behavioral treatment and maintaining abstinence, the visits are spread out to every 3 weeks for another 2 months. Finally, visits transition to once a month for patients exhibiting excellent program participation. All patients are seen at least monthly while receiving MAT. If the patient begins to falter, visit frequency is increased and behavioral treatment is intensified.

The best way to deliver MAT for this younger, still-developing population has yet to be definitively established. Abstinence and rehabilitative program attendance are primary goals for patients of our MAT program. Anecdotally, even when they are not engaging in behavioral treatment, we find that our MAT patients use illicit substances less frequently and function better in day-to-day life. The benefits of overall decreased illicit substance abuse and improved quality of life for patients engaged in MAT, regardless of behavioral rehabilitative engagement, have been confirmed by several research studies.[28-30] This harm reduction paradigm for MAT may be 1 future focus of youth addiction treatment; however, at this time, we believe that abstinence is the best goal for MAT, and a harm reduction treatment MAT model is best delivered separately.

Although some patients struggle with the program requirements and require higher-level addiction treatment, those who are successful seem to do so with the help of the relationships they build with program providers. For many of the patients, it has been a long time since anyone has given praise and encouragement for their accomplishments. This positive reinforcement carries an incredible power to heal. Patient incentives such as anniversary wrist bands, devotional books, and bus vouchers acknowledge successes and promote continued dedication to sobriety.

CONTINUING TREATMENT

After 4 to 6 weeks of successful treatment and abstinence from opioids, the team re-evaluates the mental health of our patients. This cleansing period allows the team to separate out depression and anxiety associated with chronic drug use from a true mental health disorder. Even after time away from the effects of opioid abuse, many patients will have significant depression, anxiety, attention-deficit/hyperactivity disorder (ADHD), and other mental health concerns. Treating depression, anxiety, and insomnia seems to help patients maintain abstinence.[31] Many of the patients have extreme social phobia and panic that requires high doses of a selective serotonin reuptake inhibitor (SSRI) for maximal benefit. It is important to be careful about using stimulants with these patients, but our MAT clinic has seen improvement when treating the patients most seriously affected by ADHD with a less abuseable stimulant such as a delayed- or sustained-release product that cannot be crushed or solubilized. It is very helpful having a relationship with a psychiatrist who has a special interest in drug abuse seeing the patients with more complex mental health concerns.

LONG-TERM CARE

During treatment, especially given the prolonged nature of addiction treatment, each patient will experience various unique challenges that may become treatment complications. Although each patient's treatment experience is unique, several common clinical scenarios and pitfalls are experienced by many of our MAT patients. These common scenarios and suggested clinical responses are listed in Table 1. Even though we recognize that each patient has his or her own personal set of barriers to sobriety, we have found that the retention and active participation of patients in the MAT program are the most important predictors of long-term success. In a study conducted within our MAT clinic, we found that after 1 visit to initiate MAT, 75% of patients returned for a second visit. Subsequently, when examining retention rates at 60 days into MAT, we found that 45% of patients were still actively participating, and by 1 year 9% were still active in

Table 1
Clinical scenarios and complications commonly addressed with MAT patients

Common problems and responses	
Lack of access to effective and affordable substance abuse treatment programs	Many patients cannot access quality services because of the scarcity and/or the exorbitantly high costs of programs. Often behavioral rehabilitative programs are not covered even by the best insurance plans. For these patients and families, a patchwork program of individual counseling and 12-step meetings may be tried in lieu of a more organized, and often cost-prohibitive, treatment program.
Short-term relapses	Most effectively treated with increased frequency of visits and more intensive drug counseling. If patients have already completed treatment, they may need to repeat an intensive outpatient treatment (IOP) or, at a minimum, receive regular counseling and increase 12-step meeting attendance.
Absence of BUP/NAL in urine drug screen	An ominous finding that is not to be ignored. Buprenorphine has such a long half-life that it is virtually impossible for it not to be found even with "missed doses." Medication technique should be reviewed to ensure that the medication is being absorbed, followed by a frank discussion of possible diversion concerns. Virtually all of the patients who are negative for BUP/NAL on drug screens are not doing well with rehabilitative efforts and need more intensive treatment.
Patients struggling repeatedly to meet program requirements	Patients who are continuously nonadherent with program expectations are given several chances to change their behavior, but a large number are not able to succeed, such that after 3 months only about 25%-30% of patients are still active within the NCH MAT program. If a patient is asked to leave the program, the patient is encouraged to try it his or her way for a while but is made to feel free to return if he or she is willing to re-engage in treatment and meet clinic expectations. Each time a patient experiences a period of drug-free living, he or she moves closer to successful sobriety, and many of NCH MAT's most successful patients failed treatment several times before they achieved long-lasting sobriety.

the program.[32] Developing interventions to improve retention rates will be exceedingly important for the success of future MAT programs.

The long-term treatment goal for MAT patients is for them to be taking the lowest dose of BUP/NAL required to maintain sobriety. Almost all patients are started on 16 mg/4 mg of BUP/NAL daily. For many patients, by 6 to 8 months they have completed the initial phases of their behavioral rehabilitative program and are encouraged to consider tapering their dose. No patients are forced to taper their dose until they feel ready to do so. If they feel ready to taper, we decrease the daily dose only by 2 mg/0.5 mg of BUP/NAL per month; patients often need more than 1 month between tapers. BUP/NAL is available in 12 mg/3 mg, 8 mg/2 mg, 4 mg/1mg, and 2 mg/0.5 mg films, making every possible dose easy to prescribe. In many patients, the BUP/NAL daily dose is slowly weaned to 8 mg/2 mg or less by 1 year. Considering the chronic nature of this disease and the brain chemistry involved, some patients may need a consistent lower dose of BUP/NAL for years in order to maintain sobriety.[19,20] Patients wishing to come off the BUP/NAL continue to wean to an eventual dose of 2 mg/0.5 mg daily or even every 2 to 3 days. At this point, the patient is allowed to make the decision to continue on a low dose or to stop the BUP/NAL entirely. Several of our MAT patients have transitioned off the BUP/NAL after 2 to 3 years of treatment and continue to do well. Perhaps the most difficult long-term problem is helping these young patients to accept that they have a lifelong chronic disease with a tendency to revert back to old habits when faced with life's struggles. For extended success, each patient needs to find a way to acknowledge his or her disease and get the help needed to maintain sobriety.

CONCLUSION

The science of drug addiction has come a long way in the last 300 years. It is now known that addiction is a physiologic brain disease involving genetics and environmental influences rather than merely having a lack of moral fortitude. The biochemical and anatomic changes that occur require serious intervention and lifelong learning with a strong dedication to sobriety. The developing adolescent brain is most certainly more susceptible to the deleterious effects of drugs of abuse.[33,34] Relapses are to be expected in the course of addiction and do not necessarily lead to negative overall outcomes.[35] Although we have made advancements in addiction knowledge, understanding, and treatment, much research is still needed. Well-designed and meticulously conducted studies providing longitudinal data will be needed as MAT continues to be utilized and explored. These data will help structure MAT for adolescents and young adults with a foundation of high-quality, evidence-based guidelines. Although further exploration is needed, we do know that before MAT, the success of treating opioid dependence was abysmal.[36] Now, a powerful tool to help these young addicted patients to get sober and realize their full potential in life is available. MAT is a way that physicians can truly make a difference for patients with the serious chronic disease of addiction.

References

1. Substance Abuse and Mental Health Services Administration, Office of Applied Studies. *The OAS Report: A Day in the Life of American Adolescents: Substance Use Facts.* Rockville, MD: Substance Abuse and Mental Health Services Administration, Office of Applied Studies; 2007
2. Johnston L, O'Malley P, Bachman J, Schulenberg J. American teens more cautious about using synthetic drugs. 2013. Available at: www.monitoringthefuture.org. Accessed January 24, 2014
3. Sustance Abuse and Mental Health Services Administration, Office of Applied Studies. *Treatment Episode Data Set (TEDS): 1996-2006. National Admissions to Substance Abuse Treatment Services.* Rockville, MD: Substance Abuse and Mental Health Services Administration, Office of Applied Studies; 2008
4. Centers for Disease Control and Prevention. Press release: opioids drive continued increase in drug overdose deaths. 2013. Available at: www.cdc.gov/media/releases/2013/p0220_drug_overdose_deaths.html. Accessed January 26, 2014
5. Centers for Disease Control and Prevention. *Vital Signs: Overdoses of Prescription Opioid Pain Relievers – United States, 1999-2008. MMWR Morb Mortal Wkly Rep.* 2011;60(43):1487-1492
6. Simpson D, Sells S. *Opioid Addiction and Treatment: A 12-Year Follow-Up.* Malabar, FL: Robert E. Krieger Publishing Co., Inc.; 1990
7. Bynum W. Chronic alcoholism in the first half of the 19 th century. *Bull Hist Med.* 1968;42(2):160-185
8. White WL. *Slaying the Dragon: The History of Addiction Treatment and Recovery in America.* Bloomington, IL: Chestnut Health Systems/Lighthouse Institute; 1998
9. National Institute on Drug Abuse. *Drug, Brain, and Behavior: The Science of Addiction.* Rockville, MD: US Department of Health and Human Services, National Institutes of Health; 2010
10. Di Chiara G, Tanda G, Cadoni C, Acquas E, Bassareo V, Carboni E. Homologies and differences in the action of drugs of abuse and a conventional reinforcer (food) on dopamine transmission: an interpretative framework of the mechanism of drug dependence. *Adv Pharmacol.* 1998;42:983-987
11. Wenkstern D, Pfaus J, Fibiger H. Dopamine transmission increases in the nucleus accumbens of male rats during their first exposure to sexually receptive female rats. *Brain Res.* 1993;618(1):41-46
12. Fiorino D, Coury A, Phillips A. Dynamic changes in nucleus accumbens dopamine efflux during the Coolidge effect in male rats. *J Neurosci.* 1997;17(12):4849-4855
13. Fiorino D, Phillips A. Facilitation of sexual behavior and enhanced dopamine efflux in the nucleus accumbens of male rats after D-amphetamine-induced behavioral sensitization. *J Neurosci.* 1999;19(1):456-463
14. Robbins T, Cador M, Taylor J, Everitt B. Limbic-striatal interactions in reward-related processes. *Neurosci Biobehav Rev.* 1989;13(2-3):155-162
15. Salamone J. Complex motor and sensorimotor functions of striatal and accumbens dopamine: involvement in instrumental behavior processes. *Psychopharmacology (Berl).* 1992;107(2-3):160-174
16. Diaz J. *How Drugs Influence Behavior: A Neurobehavioral Approach.* Upper Saddle River, New Jersey: Prentice Hall College Div; 1996
17. Di Chiara G, Imperato A. Drugs abused by humans preferentially increase synaptic dopamine concentrations in the mesolimbic system of freely moving rats. *Proc Natl Acad Sci U S A.* 1988; 85(14):5274-5278
18. CNSforum of the Lundbeck Institute. CNSforum: image bank: other: substance abuse. 2011. Available at: www.cnsforum.com/. Accessed November 8, 2013
19. Krasnova I, Justinova Z, Ladenheim B, et al. Methamphetamine self-administration is associated with persistent biochemical alterations in striatal and cortical dopaminergic terminals in the rat. *PLoS One.* 2010;5(1):e8790
20. Volkow N, Chang L, Wang G, et al. Loss of dopamine transporters in methamphetamine abusers recovers with protracted abstinence. *J Neurosci.* 2001;21(23):9414-9418
21. American Psychiatric Association. *Diagnostic and Statistical Manual of Mental Disorders.* 5th ed. Arlington, VA: American Psychiatric Association; 2013

22. European Monitoring Centre for Drugs and Drug Addiction. Teen Addiction Severity Index (T-ASI). 2009. Available at: www.emcdda.europa.eu/html.cfm/index4004EN.html. Accessed December 10, 2013
23. Kaminer Y, Bukstein O, Tarter R. The Teen-Addiction Severity Index: rationale and reliability. *Int J Addict.* 1991;26(2):219-226
24. American Society of Addiction Medicine. *ASAM Patient Placement Criteria for the Treatment of Substance-Related Disorders.* Chevy Chase, MD: American Society of Addiction Medicine; 2001
25. Center for Substance Abuse Treatment. *Clinical Guidelines for the Use of Buprenorphine in the Treatment of Opioid Addiction.* Rockville, MD: Substance Abuse and Mental Health Services Administration, US Department of Health and Human Services; 2004
26. Reckitt Benckiser Pharmaceuticals Inc. Film pack insert: package insert. Richmond, VA: Reckitt Benckiser Pharmaceuticals Inc; 2013
27. Zuckerman C. Suboxone film administration. Richmond, VA: Reckitt Benckiser Pharmaceuticals Inc; 2013
28. Tkacz J, Severt J, Cacciola J, Ruetsch C. Compliance with buprenorphine medication-assisted treatment and relapse to opioid use. *Am J Addict.* 2012;21(1):55-62
29. Schackman B, Leff J, Polsky D, Moore B, Fiellin D. Cost-effectiveness of long-term outpatient buprenorphine-naloxone treatment for opioid dependence in primary care. *J Gen Intern Med.* 2012;27(6):669-676
30. Soeffing J, Martin L, Fingerhood M, Jasinski D, Rastegar D. Buprenorphine maintenance treatment in a primary care setting: outcomes at 1 year. *J Subst Abuse Treat.* 2009;37(4):426-430
31. Nunes E, Sullivan M, Levin F. Treatment of depression in patients with opiate dependence. *Biol Psychiatry.* 2004;56(10):793-802
32. Matson S, Hobson G, Abdel-Rasoul M, Bonny A. A retrospective study of retention of opioid-dependent adolescents and young adults in an outpatient buprenorphine/naloxone clinic. *J Addict Med.* In press.
33. Rezvani A, Levin E. Adolescent and adult rats respond differently to nicotine and alcohol: motor activity and body temperature. *Int J Dev Neurosci.* 2004;22(5-6):349-354
34. Spear LP. The adolescent brain and age-related behavioral manifestations. *Neurosci Biobehav Rev.* 2000;24(4):417-463
35. Brown R, Lawrence A. Neurochemistry underlying relapse to opiate seeking behaviour. *Neurochem Res.* 2009;34(10):1876-1887
36. Hunt G, Odoroff M. Followup study of narcotic drug addicts after hospitalization. *Public Health Rep.* 1962;77:41-54

Adolesc Med 025 (2014) 266–278

Update on HIV Testing, Management, and Prevention in Adolescents and Young Adults

Tanya L. Kowalczyk Mullins, MD, MS[a,b*]; Corinne E. Lehmann, MD, MEd[a,b]

[a]*Division of Adolescent and Transition Medicine, Department of Pediatrics, Cincinnati Children's Hospital Medical Center, Cincinnati, Ohio;*
[b]*University of Cincinnati College of Medicine, Cincinnati, Ohio*

EPIDEMIOLOGY OF HUMAN IMMUNODEFICIENCY VIRUS INFECTION IN THE UNITED STATES

Of the 1.1 million people estimated to be living with human immunodeficiency virus (HIV) in the United States, nearly 1 in 6 (15.8%) is unaware of the infection.[1] The incidence of HIV in the United States has stayed stable—around 50,000 estimated new infections per year—for decades despite advances in testing and treatment. Although rates of new diagnoses have decreased or remained steady in most age groups, rates have *increased* in the age ranges from 20 to 24 years and from 25 to 29 years.[2] Certain populations bear a greater burden of HIV infection, especially young men of all ethnicities who are bisexual and men who have sex with men (MSM). In 2010, the estimated number of new HIV infections among MSM was 29,800, a significant 12% increase from the previous 2 years.[3] Although white MSM of all ages continued to account for the largest number of new HIV infections (11,200), they were almost equaled by the number of new infections in black MSM (10,600).[3] The estimated number of new HIV infections in MSM was greatest in the youngest group aged 13 to 24 years (8018). Black MSM in this age group accounted for 45% of new HIV infections among all black MSM and 55% of new HIV infections among young MSM overall.[3] Hispanics/Latinos are also disproportionately affected by HIV, accounting

*Corresponding author:
E-mail address: tanya.mullins@cchmc.org

 ISSN 1934-4287

for 21% of new HIV infections but representing only 16% of the population in 2010.[3] The rate of new HIV infections for Latino males was 2.9 times that for white males, and the rate of new infections for Latinas was 4.2 times that for white females.[3] Among the geographic regions in the United States, the highest rates of new diagnoses are found in the South. In contrast to the rising rates of new HIV infections among men, rates among women fell 21% from 2008 to 2010. Intravenous drug use also diminished as a mode of transmission for new infections by 54% during this time period.[3]

CURRENT HIV TESTING RECOMMENDATIONS

In 2006, the Centers for Disease Control and Prevention (CDC) published its most recent HIV testing recommendations for health care settings. These guidelines recommend routine opt-out testing for all patients 13 to 64 years of age unless the prevalence of undiagnosed HIV is less than 0.1%. Patients should be informed that HIV testing is being performed. Although delivery of HIV prevention counseling is no longer required in conjunction with testing, it remains an important part of anticipatory guidance. Repeat testing is recommended annually for those at high risk of acquiring HIV, including MSM or heterosexual patients who themselves, or whose partners, have had more than 1 partner since their most recent HIV test.[4] The American Academy of Pediatrics (AAP) recommends routine screening of all adolescents at least once by the age of 16 to 18 years in regions where HIV prevalence is greater than 0.1% as per the CDC; otherwise, routine testing for HIV should be performed for all sexually active adolescents and those with other risk factors for HIV, including injection drug use. The AAP recommends annual screening for youth who are at high risk for acquiring HIV, including those with multiple sexual partners, MSM, injection drug users, and those who participate in transactional sex.[5] The AAP does not recommend an interval for HIV testing for adolescents who are not at high risk.[5] Despite these recommendations, only 27.5% of pediatricians reported recommending HIV testing to all of their sexually active patients.[6]

HIV TESTING UPDATES

Rapid HIV Testing

Clinical Laboratory Improvement Amendments (CLIA)-waived, second-generation rapid HIV tests, such as the OraQuick ADVANCE or Uni-Gold Recombigen, can be used as point-of-care tests, delivering results in 20 minutes or less.[7] Because many adolescents fail to return for HIV test results, rapid tests improve the receipt of results in this population.[8] Rapid testing is preferred by youth. In 1 study, 70% of adolescents opted to receive a rapid test when offered their choice of HIV testing method.[8] In addition, rapid testing in conjunction with routine HIV testing may increase adolescent acceptance of testing.[9] Rapid testing in pediatric emergency departments is acceptable to adolescents as well[10,11] and is recommended by the AAP in high-prevalence areas.[5] The performance of rapid tests may be improved by using fingerstick blood samples,[12] although both the sensitivity and specificity of oral fluid testing are greater than 99%.[13] Positive results on rapid testing must be followed by confirmatory testing (eg, Western blot or immunofluorescent assay) in order to make a diagnosis of HIV infection. No further testing is required in the case of negative rapid test results.[14]

Home Testing

Two in-home HIV tests have been approved by the US Food and Drug Administration (FDA). The Ora-Quick oral fluid test (approved for home testing in 2012 for ages 17 and older) is the same test used in clinical settings. The result is interpreted by the user.[15] The Home Access HIV-1 Test System (approved in 1996 for ages 18 and older) allows a user to collect a fingerstick blood sample at home, which is then mailed to the laboratory for testing. The user receives his or her result by phone.[15] A recent literature review found that, overall, adolescent and adult users can correctly perform and interpret home tests of various types.[16] Adult MSM who used home HIV testing kits described them as easy to use, and subjects found that using the tests with potential sexual partners raised awareness of their risk behaviors and consequently led to less risky behavior.[17,18]

Fourth-Generation Combined Antigen/Antibody Testing

Two FDA-approved fourth-generation HIV tests detect both the HIV p24 antigen and antibodies to HIV-1/HIV-2. These tests can identify HIV infection sooner than the prior generation of tests (median: 6.2-7.4 days after HIV-1 RNA is detectable, which is estimated to be about 10 days after infection).[7] Because these newer tests detect p24 antigen, identification of acute HIV infection is now faster,[7] thereby allowing for counseling of newly infected patients to help prevent transmission from these individuals, who have high viral loads, to uninfected partners.

HIV Testing Algorithms

In light of recent advances in HIV testing methodology, the CDC is revising its HIV testing algorithm. Currently, the diagnostic algorithm consists of testing for HIV antibodies (or antibodies and antigen), followed by supplemental testing with either Western blot or indirect immunofluorescence assay.[19] However, in an effort to improve detection of acute HIV infection, the new algorithm being proposed by the CDC (which has not been finalized as of May 2014) recommends that the initial test be a fourth-generation combined HIV antigen/antibody test. Because the fourth-generation test does not distinguish between HIV-1 and HIV-2, reactive samples would undergo further scrutiny using a second-generation HIV-1/HIV-2 antibody differentiation test to determine which HIV is present. If both tests are reactive, the patient would be considered

HIV infected. If the second-generation test is nonreactive, the sample would undergo HIV RNA testing. If the results of RNA testing are positive, the patient would be considered HIV infected.[20] Western blot testing would no longer be a part of the testing algorithm. This proposed algorithm seems to detect more HIV infections compared to the existing testing algorithm.[21,22]

MANAGEMENT UPDATES

Treatment Updates for Newly Diagnosed HIV Infection

Because treatment guidelines for both adults and children with HIV change almost yearly in the United States, the reader is advised to consult www.aidsinfo.nih.gov for the latest guidelines. For adolescents who have not completed puberty, the treatment guidelines for children should be consulted. Also, some treatments mentioned in the adolescent and adult guidelines may not be approved by the FDA for patients younger than 18 years. HIV treatment has evolved over time, resulting in recommendations to start treatment sooner in the course of the illness. The December 2009 Adolescent and Adult HIV Treatment Guidelines changed from previous versions to recommend starting antiretroviral (drug) therapy (ART) when CD4 counts reach 350 to 500 cells/mm^3 rather than waiting for the CD4 count to fall below 350 cells/mm^3. In addition, the advisory panel consensus in 2009 was nearly split in terms of advocating treatment for all HIV-infected patients regardless of CD4 count.[23] As further evidence emerged regarding the positive outcomes of treatment in persons with CD4 counts greater than 500 cells/mm^3, the 2012 guidelines stated that ART could be initiated for all persons with HIV. The strength of the evidence for treatment is noted for each CD4 range (Table 1).[24] For many years, it has been recommended that patients who are pregnant, have an AIDS-defining illness, have hepatitis B coinfection, or have nephropathy begin ART at any CD4 count.[24]

New Formulations and Medications

Because treatment regimens have been simplified as a result of better pharmacokinetics, new formulations, and fewer side effects, starting a naïve patient on a drug regimen is less daunting than it was 5 or 10 years ago. Three 1-pill-once-a-day combination ART pills are available to treat patients with HIV. A genotype test usually is requested in all patients newly diagnosed with HIV to determine whether patients have acquired a resistant virus. Up to 18% of adolescents and young adults were resistant to 1 class of HIV medications at the time of diagnosis in a 2006 study.[25] Atripla (tenofovir [TDF], emtricitabine [FTC], efavirenz) once daily was approved for use in 2006. In 2011, Complera (TDF, FTC, rilpivirine) was the second 1-pill-daily option approved in the United States; it is rated category B in pregnancy. In 2012, Stribild (TDF, FTC, cobicistat, elvitegravir) was approved. Elvitegravir belongs to the newest class of HIV medications, the integrase inhibitors. Raltegravir, another drug in the integrase inhibitor class, is approved for use

Table 1
Initiating antiretroviral therapy in treatment-naïve individuals, updated May 1, 2014

Antiretroviral therapy (ART) is recommended for all HIV-infected individuals to reduce the risk of disease progression.
The strength and evidence for this recommendation vary by pretreatment CD4 cell count:
- CD4 count <350 cells/mm³ **(AI)**
- CD4 count 350–500 cells/mm³ **(AII)**
- CD4 count >500 cells/mm³ **(BIII)**

ART also is recommended for HIV-infected individuals for the prevention of transmission of HIV.
The strength and evidence for this recommendation vary by transmission risks:
- Perinatal transmission **(AI)**
- Heterosexual transmission **(AI)**
- Other transmission risk groups **(AIII)**

Patients starting ART should be willing and able to commit to treatment and understand the benefits and risks of therapy and the importance of adherence **(AIII)**.
Patients may choose to postpone therapy, and providers, on a case-by-case basis, may elect to defer therapy on the basis of clinical and/or psychosocial factors.
Rating of Recommendations: *A = strong; B = moderate; C = optional*
Rating of Evidence: *I = data from randomized controlled trials; II = data from well-designed nonrandomized trials or observational cohort studies with long-term clinical outcomes; III = expert opinion.*

Adapted from Panel on Antiretroviral Guidelines for Adults and Adolescents. *Guidelines for the use of antiretroviral agents in HIV-1-infected adults and adolescents.* Department of Health and Human Services. March 28, 2012; updated. Available at: aidsinfo.nih.gov/contentfiles/lvguidelines/adultandadolescentgl.pdf. Page E-1. Accessed June 23, 2014

in adults and patients younger than 18 years but currently has twice-a-day dosing. This new medication class is helpful for patients with multiclass drug resistance.

When selecting and starting any HIV treatment regimen, the medical background of the patient, resistance patterns, and potential adherence factors must be considered. Factors that place an adolescent at risk for acquiring HIV, such as homelessness and drug use, also put them at risk for nonadherence; therefore, the current guidelines acknowledge that it may be better to defer ART while aggressively addressing the social factors that can lead to poor adherence in an effort to prevent development of medication resistance.[24] Physicians also may avoid ART that has a lower genetic resistance barrier, such as the nonnucleoside reverse transcriptase inhibitors (NNRTIs) class.[24] A 10-year study of ART use in children and adolescents showed a 76% reduction in mortality with a protease inhibitor (PI)–based regimen compared with other regimens.[26] Although a 1-pill-once-a-day regimen can be tempting to use, some US physicians select PI-based regimens of several pills dosed once a day in an attempt to prevent resistance in adolescents and young adults at risk for adherence issues.

Common Drug Interactions

Although many physicians would not initiate HIV treatment without the involvement of a specialist, primary care physicians should be aware of drug interactions between ART and common medications used in adolescent medicine practice. The interactions between ART classes and other types of medications are not always straightforward and can be difficult for a physician to memorize. If a physician is unsure about a potential ART and drug interaction, he or she should consult an online medication interaction reference or the patient's pharmacist. However, there are a few common interactions of which the physician should be aware when prescribing to patients on ART. Antacids, H2 receptor antagonists, and proton pump inhibitors can interact with the ART class of PIs. Antifungals, antimycobacterials, and anticonvulsants can interact with PIs and NNRTIs, and they should be chosen with care and with pharmacist input (Table 2). Another common drug interaction involves the use of ART and hormonal contraception in women. PIs can decrease the estrogen levels of combined hormonal oral contraceptives.[27] NNRTIs can either increase or decrease estrogen levels in those taking combined hormonal oral contraceptives, but the clinical significance of these effects are unknown.[24,28] Studies have not shown a significant interaction between the progesterone-only injectable contraceptive depot medroxyprogesterone acetate (DMPA) or the levonorgestrel implant system and most ART.[28] However, failure of etonogestrel implants in 2 patients taking efavirenz has been reported.[29] Because of the overall lack of data in this area, the World Health Organization and the CDC have not recommended restrictions on any form of birth control in HIV-infected women.[30,31] Physicians who are concerned that a patient's ART may affect contraception can more strongly recommend the use of condoms or other barrier methods to prevent pregnancy and HIV transmission.

SPECIAL ISSUES FOR PERINATALLY INFECTED ADOLESCENTS

Many perinatally infected youth have survived as a result of the advent of combination ART over the last 2 decades, and these patients are now aging and transitioning into the adult care system. By the end of 2010 in the United States, 10,798 persons were living with perinatally acquired HIV.[2] As with other chronic care populations, these patients will need special attention and assistance when they transition from pediatric to adult systems, and several guidelines and tools exist to help physicians and patients prepare for this transition.[32,33] These adolescents and young adults can face medical challenges similar to those of older adults with acquired HIV infection. These patients may not have received ART for several years, or they may have been placed on 1- or 2-drug ART regimens or on more complicated dosing regimens in the 1990s, perhaps leading to HIV drug resistance. Accurate pharmacokinetic and dosing information in pediatric and adolescent medicine has not been readily available for most ART.[34]

Because of the longer duration of HIV infection and medication side effects, perinatally HIV-infected youth may experience medical complications, such as cognitive dysfunction.[35] Perinatally infected patients also seem to be at higher risk for mental health disorders, but researchers suspect there are multifactorial

Table 2
Common drug interactions for adolescent HIV-infected patients on antiretrovirals

Drug or class	Comments
Protease inhibitors (PIs)	
Antacids	May need to space antacid dosing away from PI dose; can block absorption of PIs
H2 receptor antagonists	Different maximum doses of the H2 receptor antagonist
Proton pump inhibitors (PPIs)	*Use not recommended*; if necessary, different maximum doses of PPIs
Antifungals	High doses may not be recommended or may need antifungal drug levels to guide dosing
Anticonvulsants	May increase or decrease anticonvulsant levels depending on specific interaction; monitor anticonvulsant levels and effects carefully
Antimycobacterials	Prolonged QTc; may decrease antimycobacterial levels
St. John's wort	Do not coadminister with PIs
Hormonal contraceptives	Decreased hormone levels; consider using 35 mcg or higher estrogen dosing, as well as barrier method
Nonnucleoside reverse transcriptase inhibitors (NNRTIs)	
Antifungals	May need to increase antifungal dose Hepatotoxicity
Anticonvulsants	Monitor clinical and drug levels of anticonvulsants Some prohibited combinations of NNRTIs and anticonvulsants
Antimycobacterials	Decreased NNRTI and antibiotic levels Some prohibited combinations of NNRTIs and antibiotics
St. John's wort	Do not coadminister with NNRTIs
Hormonal contraceptive	Generally increased estrogen levels; clinical significance not known

Adapted from Panel on Antiretroviral Guidelines for Adults and Adolescents. *Guidelines for the use of antiretroviral agents in HIV-1-infected adults and adolescents.* Department of Health and Human Services. March 28, 2012; updated. Available at: aidsinfo.nih.gov/contentfiles/lvguidelines/adultandadolescentgl.pdf. Pages L7 to 23. Accessed June 23, 2014

causes that may not be attributable to HIV infection alone.[36] These complications can be more pronounced among "sicker" patients, especially among those diagnosed with AIDS. HIV infection in adults has been associated with pulmonary hypertension and accelerated atherosclerosis. ART in adults has been associated with body fat redistribution (lipodystrophy) and the development of metabolic syndrome consequences, including insulin resistance and hyperlipidemia. Body fat redistribution and hyperlipidemia have also been seen in some studies of children and adolescents on ART. It is important to consider atherosclerosis if a perinatally infected patient has a cardiovascular event.[37] Bone loss is another concern in perinatally infected youth. Again, multifactorial reasons probably are at play in bone loss because HIV-infected patients with lower income status exhibit decreased bone mineral density (BMD) in studies.[38] In the United States, perinatally infected patients have lower BMD compared with uninfected peers. Also, the various ART medications have different effects on bone. Although there is no guideline to check bone density in perinatally infected patients, physicians should maximize their patient's bone health with healthy lifestyle guidance. Because vitamin D deficiency is common, attention should be focused on vitamin D and calcium intake by these patients.[38]

NEW BIOMEDICAL HIV PREVENTION STRATEGIES

Medical Male Circumcision

In recent randomized trials conducted in Africa, medical male circumcision (MMC) decreased the risk of HIV acquisition among heterosexual circumcised men by 51% to 60% at up to 2 years of follow-up.[39-41] Despite hypothetical concerns that men may practice riskier sexual behavior after circumcision because they may feel protected from acquiring HIV infection, no increase in risky behavior was noted among the circumcised men.[40,41] Long-term follow-up from these studies (up to 6 years) demonstrated post-trial effectiveness of 58% to 73% in decreasing HIV acquisition among circumcised men.[42,43] However, the effectiveness of MMC in preventing transmission from HIV-infected male partners to HIV-uninfected female partners is less clear. One trial found a nonstatistically significant decrease in transmission between circumcised HIV-infected men and their HIV-uninfected female partners (compared with noncircumcised HIV-infected men and their female partners).[44] Another study noted no significant difference in HIV acquisition among the female partners of circumcised HIV-infected men compared with noncircumcised men, although there was a higher rate of transmission among those couples who resumed sexual activity before full wound healing.[45] No data currently exist about the effect of MMC on HIV transmission via oral sex or anal sex or for MSM populations.[46]

Nonoccupational Postexposure Prophylaxis

Nonoccupational postexposure prophylaxis (nPEP) is the use of a short course of oral antiretrovirals following potential exposure to HIV, such as through consensual sexual activity or injection drug use. This option remains a fairly underutilized prevention strategy in the context of possible HIV exposure during consensual activities, although it is often used following possible nonconsensual exposure to HIV (eg, in cases of sexual assault or abuse). In a recent study of HIV health care providers, only 49% had ever prescribed nPEP, and 78% reported having rarely or never had patients request nPEP.[47] Prescribing of nPEP among other US physicians is likely even lower given that HIV medical providers typically would be more familiar with HIV prevention methods and would be more comfortable with the medications used for nPEP.[47] Awareness of nPEP is also fairly low. Among MSM surveyed in 6 US cities, only 48% had ever heard of nPEP,[48] and use of nPEP also is low (2%-3%).[48,49] Despite HIV care providers concerns about patient adherence to nPEP and potential promotion of riskier sexual behaviors,[47] a recent meta-analysis found an overall adherence rate of

78%,[50] and nPEP use was not associated with an increase in risky behaviors.[48,51] To date, no studies have examined the use of nPEP specifically among adolescents. According to the 2005 CDC nPEP recommendations, nPEP is recommended for people with substantial risk of HIV exposure (defined as "exposure of the vagina, rectum, eye, mouth, or mucous membranes, non-intact skin, or percutaneous contact" with "blood, semen, vaginal/rectal secretions, breast milk," or bloody body fluid) who present for care within 72 hours of exposure *and* for whom the source is known to be HIV infected.[52] Information about the source's history of ART and current viral load is helpful for tailoring the choice of nPEP regimen and for counseling about the risk of HIV transmission. nPEP is not recommended in cases of negligible risk of HIV exposure or when individuals present for care more than 72 hours after exposure. In all other cases, including cases in which the HIV status of the source is unknown, the determination to start nPEP should be approached on a case-by-case basis. Recommendations for baseline testing, selection of a regimen, and follow-up are provided in the CDC nPEP guidelines.[52] The national PEP Hotline (1-888-448-4911) provides assistance to clinicians who are considering prescribing nPEP.

Preexposure Prophylaxis

Preexposure prophylaxis (PrEP)—the use of antiretroviral medications in patients who are at high risk for acquiring HIV in order to prevent infection—is a relatively new prevention strategy. PrEP was effective in reducing new HIV infections by 44% to 75% among adult MSM,[53] heterosexuals,[54,55] and injection drug users[56] taking daily oral antiretroviral drugs. Because people taking PrEP may become infected with HIV, there is concern about potential development of viral resistance to the PrEP drugs in this situation.[57] The US Public Health Service and CDC released clinical practice guidelines in May 2014 for physicians considering PrEP for patients who are at high risk for acquiring HIV through sexual transmission (both MSM and heterosexually active adults) or injection drug use that establish the eligibility of a patient for PrEP as well as the initiation, monitoring, and discontinuation of PrEP.[58] On July 16, 2012, the FDA approved the combination pill TDF/FTC for PrEP in adults at high risk for sexually acquired HIV infection. Although PrEP is an acceptable intervention for young adults,[59] awareness among potential users seems to be fairly low.[60,61] A substantial proportion of potential users would be willing to take PrEP, although such willingness varies by cost, the potential for side effects, and the level of protection afforded by the medication.[60,62] PrEP was an acceptable intervention for a cohort of adolescent MSM, and, similar to the findings in studies of adults,[63] there was no evidence that PrEP use was associated with an increase in riskier sexual behaviors in this group.[64] Limited data are available about physician attitudes toward PrEP, which is likely to be a key determinant in the success of this strategy. Among US HIV care providers in 2011, only 19% had ever prescribed PrEP.[65] HIV health care provider concerns about the use of PrEP include possible development of HIV viral resistance, potential increase in risky behaviors, lack of adherence, and high cost.[57]

"Test and Treat"

Recent treatment guideline changes have allowed the concept of *test and treat*, in which all patients are tested regularly for HIV, and all HIV-infected persons are immediately started on ART to emerge as a strategy to decrease transmission of HIV. Because patients with lower viral loads are less likely to transmit the virus to their partners, rates of new HIV infections may decrease if all HIV-infected patients are taking ART.[66] However, patients still must maintain adherence to ART to prevent transmission. Only about 25% of HIV-infected patients in the United States are at the goal for therapy: an undetectable viral load.[67] It is imperative to test patients for HIV and then link them to appropriate care, if they are infected, in order for *test and treat* to work as a strategy for both HIV care and prevention.[68]

References

1. Centers for Disease Control and Prevention. Monitoring selected national HIV prevention and care objectives by using HIV surveillance data—United States and 6 dependent areas—2011. HIV Surveillance Supplemental Report 2013;18(No. 5). October 2013. Available at: www.cdc.gov/hiv/library/reports/surveillance/. Accessed January 27, 2014
2. Centers for Disease Control and Prevention. HIV Surveillance Report, 2011; vol. 23. Available at: www.cdc.gov/hiv/topics/surveillance/resources/reports/. Accessed January 11, 2014
3. Centers for Disease Control and Prevention. Estimated HIV incidence in the United States, 2007–2010. HIV Surveillance Supplemental Report 2012;17(No. 4). December 2012. Available at: www.cdc.gov/hiv/topics/surveillance/resources/reports/#supplemental. Accessed January 27, 2014
4. Branson BM, Handsfield HH, Lampe MA, et al. Revised recommendations for HIV testing of adults, adolescents, and pregnant women in health-care settings. *MMWR Morb Mortal Wkly Rep.* 2006;55(RR-14):1-17
5. American Academy of Pediatrics Committee on Pediatric AIDS. Adolescents and HIV infection: the pediatrician's role in promoting routine testing. *Pediatrics.* 2011;128(5):1023-1029
6. Henry-Reid LM, O'Connor KG, Klein JD, Cooper E, Flynn P, Futterman DC. Current pediatrician practices in identifying high-risk behaviors of adolescents. *Pediatrics.* 2010;125(4):e741-e747
7. Centers for Disease Control and Prevention. Advantages and disadvantages of different types of FDA-approved HIV immunoassays used for screening by generation and platform. Available at: www.cdc.gov/hiv/pdf/testing_Advantages&Disadvantages.pdf. Accessed January 24, 2014
8. Kowalczyk Mullins TL, Braverman PK, Dorn LD, Kollar LM, Kahn JA. Adolescent preferences for human immunodeficiency virus testing methods and impact of rapid tests on receipt of results. *J Adolesc Health.* 2010;46(2):162-168
9. Mullins TL, Kollar LM, Lehmann C, Kahn JA. Changes in human immunodeficiency virus testing rates among urban adolescents after introduction of routine and rapid testing. *Arch Pediatr Adolesc Med.* 2010;164(9):870-874
10. Hack CM, Scarfi CA, Sivitz AB, Rosen MD. Implementing routine HIV screening in an urban pediatric emergency department. *Pediatr Emerg Care.* 2013;29(3):319-323
11. Haines CJ, Uwazuoke K, Zussman B, Parrino T, Laguerre R, Foster J. Pediatric emergency department-based rapid HIV testing: adolescent attitudes and preferences. *Pediatr Emerg Care.* 2011;27(1):13-16

12. Stekler JD, O'Neal JD, Lane A, et al. Relative accuracy of serum, whole blood, and oral fluid HIV tests among Seattle men who have sex with men. *J Clin Virol.* 2013;58(Suppl 1):e119-e122
13. Centers for Disease Control and Prevention. Rapid HIV tests suitable for use in non-clinical settings (CLIA-waived). Available at: www.cdc.gov/hiv/pdf/testing_nonclinical_clia-waived-tests.pdf. Accessed January 30, 2014
14. Centers for Disease Control and Prevention. Notice to readers: protocols for confirmation of reactive rapid HIV tests. *MMWR Morb Mortal Wkly Rep.* 2004;53(10):221-222
15. Centers for Disease Control and Prevention. HIV/AIDS: Home tests. Available at: www.cdc.gov/hiv/testing/lab/hometests.html. Accessed January 27, 2014
16. Ibitoye M, Frasca T, Giguere R, Carballo-Dieguez A. Home testing past, present and future: lessons learned and implications for HIV home tests. *AIDS Behav.* 2014;18(5):933-949
17. Carballo-Diéguez A, Frasca T, Balan I, Ibitoye M, Dolezal C. Use of a rapid HIV home test prevents HIV exposure in a high risk sample of men who have sex with men. *AIDS Behav.* 2012;16(7):1753-1760
18. Frasca T, Balan I, Ibitoye M, Valladares J, Dolezal C, Carballo-Dieguez A. Attitude and behavior changes among gay and bisexual men after use of rapid home HIV tests to screen sexual partners. *AIDS Behav.* 2014;18(5):950-957
19. Workowski KA, Berman S; Centers for Disease Control and Prevention. Sexually transmitted diseases treatment guidelines, 2010. *MMWR Morb Mortal Wkly Rep.* 2010;59(RR-12):1-110
20. Centers for Disease Control and Prevention. Draft recommendations: diagnostic laboratory testing for HIV infection in the United States. Available at: www.cdc.gov/hiv/pdf/policies_Draft_HIV_Testing_Alg_Rec_508.2.pdf. Accessed January 9, 2014
21. Centers for Disease Control and Prevention. Detection of acute HIV infection in two evaluations of a new HIV diagnostic testing algorithm—United States, 2011-2013. *MMWR Morb Mortal Wkly Rep.* 2013;62(24):489-494
22. Masciotra S, Smith AJ, Youngpairoj AS, et al. Evaluation of the CDC proposed laboratory HIV testing algorithm among men who have sex with men (MSM) from five US metropolitan statistical areas using specimens collected in 2011. *J Clin Virol.* 2013;58(Suppl 1):e8-e12
23. Panel on Antiretroviral Guidelines for Adults and Adolescents. Guidelines for the use of antiretroviral agents in HIV-1-infected adults and adolescents. Department of Health and Human Services. December 1, 2009. Available at: www.aidsinfo.nih.gov/guidelines/archive/adult-and-adolescent-guidelines. Accessed January 25, 2014
24. Panel on Antiretroviral Guidelines for Adults and Adolescents. Guidelines for the use of antiretroviral agents in HIV-1-infected adults and adolescents. Department of Health and Human Services. March 28, 2012; updated. Available at: aidsinfo.nih.gov/contentfiles/lvguidelines/adultandadolescentgl.pdf. Accessed May 1, 2014
25. Viani RM, Peralta L, Aldrovandi G, et al. Prevalence of primary HIV-1 drug resistance among recently infected adolescents: a multicenter Adolescent Medicine Trials Network for HIV/AIDS Interventions study. *J Infect Dis.* 2006;194(11):1505-1509
26. Patel K, Williams PL, Seeger JD, et al. Long-term effectiveness of highly active antiretroviral therapy on the survival of children and adolescents with HIV infection: a 10-year follow-up study. *Clin Infect Dis.* 2008;46(4):507-515
27. El-Ibiary SY, Cocohoba JM. Effects of HIV antiretrovirals on the pharmacokinetics of hormonal contraceptives. *Eur J Contracept Reprod Health Care.* 2008;13(2):123-132
28. Robinson JA, Jamshidi R, Burke AE. Contraception for the HIV-positive woman: a review of interactions between hormonal contraception and antiretroviral therapy. *Infect Dis Obstet Gynecol.* 2012;2012:890160
29. Leticee N, Viard JP, Yamgnane A, Karmochkine M, Benachi A. Contraceptive failure of etonogestrel implant in patients treated with antiretrovirals including efavirenz. *Contraception.* 2012;85(4):425-427
30. Centers for Disease Control and Prevention. Update to CDC's U.S. medical eligibility criteria for contraceptive use, 2010: revised recommendations for the use of hormonal contraception among women at high risk for HIV infection or infected with HIV. *MMWR Morb Mortal Wkly Rep.* 2012;61(24):449-452

31. World Health Organization. Hormonal contraception and HIV: technical statement. 2012. Available at: whqlibdoc.who.int/hq/2012/WHO_RHR_12.08_eng.pdf. Accessed January 27, 2014
32. American Academy of Pediatrics Committee on Pediatric AIDS. Transitioning HIV-infected youth into adult health care. *Pediatrics.* 2013;132(1):192-197
33. Dowshen N, D'Angelo L. Health care transition for youth living with HIV/AIDS. *Pediatrics.* 2011;128(4):762-771
34. Sohn AH, Hazra R. The changing epidemiology of the global paediatric HIV epidemic: keeping track of perinatally HIV-infected adolescents. *J Int AIDS Soc.* 2013;16:18555
35. Laughton B, Cornell M, Boivin M, Van Rie A. Neurodevelopment in perinatally HIV-infected children: a concern for adolescence. *J Int AIDS Soc.* 2013;16:18603
36. Mellins CA, Malee KM. Understanding the mental health of youth living with perinatal HIV infection: lessons learned and current challenges. *J Int AIDS Soc.* 2013;16:18593
37. Lipshultz SE, Miller TL, Wilkinson JD, et al. Cardiac effects in perinatally HIV-infected and HIV-exposed but uninfected children and adolescents: a view from the United States of America. *J Int AIDS Soc.* 2013;16:18597
38. Puthanakit T, Siberry GK. Bone health in children and adolescents with perinatal HIV infection. *J Int AIDS Soc.* 2013;16:18575
39. Auvert B, Taljaard D, Lagarde E, Sobngwi-Tambekou J, Sitta R, Puren A. Randomized, controlled intervention trial of male circumcision for reduction of HIV infection risk: the ANRS 1265 Trial. *PLoS Med.* 2005;2(11):e298
40. Bailey RC, Moses S, Parker CB, et al. Male circumcision for HIV prevention in young men in Kisumu, Kenya: a randomised controlled trial. *Lancet.* 2007;369(9562):643-656
41. Gray RH, Kigozi G, Serwadda D, et al. Male circumcision for HIV prevention in men in Rakai, Uganda: a randomised trial. *Lancet.* 2007;369(9562):657-666
42. Gray R, Kigozi G, Kong X, et al. The effectiveness of male circumcision for HIV prevention and effects on risk behaviors in a posttrial follow-up study. *AIDS.* 2012;26(5):609-615
43. Mehta SD, Moses S, Agot K, et al. The long term efficacy of medical male circumcision against HIV acquisition. *AIDS.* 2013;27:2899-2907
44. Baeten JM, Donnell D, Kapiga SH, et al. Male circumcision and risk of male-to-female HIV-1 transmission: a multinational prospective study in African HIV-1-serodiscordant couples. *AIDS.* 2010;24(5):737-744
45. Wawer MJ, Makumbi F, Kigozi G, et al. Circumcision in HIV-infected men and its effect on HIV transmission to female partners in Rakai, Uganda: a randomised controlled trial. *Lancet.* 2009;374(9685):229-237
46. Smith DK, Taylor A, Kilmarx PH, et al. Male circumcision in the United States for the prevention of HIV infection and other adverse health outcomes: report from a CDC consultation. *Public Health Rep.* 2010;125(Suppl 1):72-82
47. Rodriguez AE, Castel AD, Parish CL, et al. HIV medical providers' perceptions of the use of antiretroviral therapy as nonoccupational postexposure prophylaxis in 2 major metropolitan areas. *J Acquir Immune Defic Syndr.* 2013;64(Suppl 1):S68-S79
48. Donnell D, Mimiaga MJ, Mayer K, et al. Use of non-occupational post-exposure prophylaxis does not lead to an increase in high risk sex behaviors in men who have sex with men participating in the EXPLORE trial. *AIDS Behav.* 2010;14(5):1182-1189
49. Mehta SA, Silvera R, Bernstein K, Holzman RS, Aberg JA, Daskalakis DC. Awareness of post-exposure HIV prophylaxis in high-risk men who have sex with men in New York City. *Sex Transm Infect.* 2011;87(4):344-348
50. Oldenburg CE, Barnighausen T, Harling G, Mimiaga MJ, Mayer KH. Adherence to post-exposure prophylaxis for non-forcible sexual exposure to HIV: a systematic review and meta-analysis. *AIDS Behav.* 2014;18(2):217-225
51. Martin JN, Roland ME, Neilands TB, et al. Use of postexposure prophylaxis against HIV infection following sexual exposure does not lead to increases in high-risk behavior. *AIDS.* 2004;18(5):787-792
52. Smith DK, Grohskopf LA, Black RJ, et al. Antiretroviral postexposure prophylaxis after sexual, injection-drug use, or other nonoccupational exposure to HIV in the United States: recommenda-

tions from the U.S. Department of Health and Human Services. *MMWR Morb Mortal Wkly Rep.* 2005;54(RR-2):1-20

53. Grant RM, Lama JR, Anderson PL, et al. Preexposure chemoprophylaxis for HIV prevention in men who have sex with men. *N Engl J Med.* 2010;363(27):2587-2599
54. Baeten JM, Donnell D, Ndase P, et al. Antiretroviral prophylaxis for HIV prevention in heterosexual men and women. *N Engl J Med.* 2012;367(5):399-410
55. Thigpen MC, Kebaabetswe PM, Paxton LA, et al. Antiretroviral preexposure prophylaxis for heterosexual HIV transmission in Botswana. *N Engl J Med.* 2012;367(5):423-434
56. Choopanya K, Martin M, Suntharasamai P, et al. Antiretroviral prophylaxis for HIV infection in injecting drug users in Bangkok, Thailand (the Bangkok Tenofovir Study): a randomised, double-blind, placebo-controlled phase 3 trial. *Lancet.* 2013;381(9883):2083-2090
57. Tellalian D, Maznavi K, Bredeek UF, Hardy WD. Pre-exposure prophylaxis (PrEP) for HIV infection: results of a survey of HIV healthcare providers evaluating their knowledge, attitudes, and prescribing practices. *AIDS Patient Care STDS.* 2013;27(10):553-559
58. US Public Health Service. Preexposure Prophylaxis for the Prevention of HIV Infection in the United States – 2014: A Clinical Practice Guideline. May 14, 2014. Available at: www.cdc.gov/hiv/pdf/PrEPguidelines2014.pdf. Accessed May 20, 2014
59. Smith DK, Toledo L, Smith DJ, Adams MA, Rothenberg R. Attitudes and program preferences of African-American urban young adults about pre-exposure prophylaxis (PrEP). *AIDS Educ Prev.* 2012;24(5):408-421
60. Al-Tayyib AA, Thrun MW, Haukoos JS, Walls NE. Knowledge of pre-exposure prophylaxis (PrEP) for HIV prevention among men who have sex with men in Denver, Colorado. *AIDS Behav.* 2014;18(Suppl 3):340-347
61. Rucinski KB, Mensah NP, Sepkowitz KA, Cutler BH, Sweeney MM, Myers JE. Knowledge and use of pre-exposure prophylaxis among an online sample of young men who have sex with men in New York City. *AIDS Behav.* 2013;17(6):2180-2184
62. Golub SA, Gamarel KE, Rendina HJ, Surace A, Lelutiu-Weinberger CL. From efficacy to effectiveness: facilitators and barriers to PrEP acceptability and motivations for adherence among MSM and transgender women in New York City. *AIDS Patient Care STDS.* 2013;27(4):248-254
63. Mugwanya KK, Donnell D, Celum C, et al. Sexual behaviour of heterosexual men and women receiving antiretroviral pre-exposure prophylaxis for HIV prevention: a longitudinal analysis. *Lancet Infect Dis.* 2013;13(12):1021-1028
64. Hosek SG, Siberry G, Bell M, et al. The acceptability and feasibility of an HIV preexposure prophylaxis (PrEP) trial with young men who have sex with men. *J Acquir Immune Defic Syndr.* 2013;62(4):447-456
65. White JM, Mimiaga MJ, Krakower DS, Mayer KH. Evolution of Massachusetts physician attitudes, knowledge, and experience regarding the use of antiretrovirals for HIV prevention. *AIDS Patient Care STDS.* 2012;26(7):395-405
66. Wilson DP. HIV treatment as prevention: natural experiments highlight limits of antiretroviral treatment as HIV prevention. *PLoS Med.* 2012;9(7):e1001231
67. Centers for Disease Control and Prevention. HIV in the United States: the stages of care—CDC fact sheet. 2012. Available at: www.cdc.gov/hiv/pdf/research–mmp–StagesofCare.pdf. Accessed June 23, 2014
68. Gardner EM, McLees MP, Steiner JF, Del Rio C, Burman WJ. The spectrum of engagement in HIV care and its relevance to test-and-treat strategies for prevention of HIV infection. *Clin Infect Dis.* 2011;52(6):793-800

Adolesc Med 025 (2014) 279–293

Bariatric Surgery for Adolescents

Linda M. Kollar, RN, CNP, CBN[a*];
Thomas H. Inge, MD, PhD[a]

[a]*Division of Pediatric Surgery, Cincinnati Children's Hospital Medical Center, Cincinnati, Ohio*

Recent data show a deceleration in the rate with which obesity is increasing among children and adolescents, with encouraging signs that the incidence may even have begun to plateau.[1] However, the fastest growing subcategory of pediatric obesity is severe obesity, and this category has not shown any signs of decreasing. Severe obesity affects 4% to 6% of youth in the United States and has serious immediate and long-term health consequences.[2-4] Medical treatment programs, including those that provide intensive behavioral and diet interventions for adolescents, have demonstrated minimal long-term efficacy for severe obesity and reversal of comorbid conditions. The lack of medical treatment and the seriousness of the comorbidities associated with obesity, such as type 2 diabetes mellitus, hypertension, obstructive sleep apnea, and reduced quality of life, have led to the introduction of bariatric surgery as a treatment option for severe obesity. The first bariatric procedures were performed on adults in the early 1960s, and most of the data about effectiveness of bariatric surgery have focused on adult outcomes. Recent literature has improved our understanding of the effectiveness and safety of bariatric procedures in the adolescent population, and ongoing longitudinal studies will add to this knowledge.

The most common bariatric procedures performed for both adults and adolescents are Roux-en-Y gastric bypass (RYGB), sleeve gastrectomy (SG), and adjustable gastric banding (AGB). All of the procedures now are most commonly performed using laparoscopic techniques. Although it has been used off label in teenagers, AGB is not approved by the US Food and Drug Administration (FDA) for use in adolescents younger than 18 years. Bariatric procedures, although highly effective, are associated with risks, which differ by procedure. This article will review the current data about weight loss surgery (WLS) in the adolescent population.

---

*Corresponding author:
E-mail address: linda.kollar@cchmc.org

 ISSN 1934-4287

BARIATRIC PROCEDURES

The AGB facilitates weight loss purely through restriction. A synthetic band with an inflatable and adjustable inner tube is placed around the proximal stomach just below the esophagogastric junction. This creates a small pouch that restricts the passage of food and delays the emptying of food into the stomach. The band can be inflated and deflated over time through a subcutaneous injection port. The band can be removed with minimal change to the overall anatomy. Problems specific to the band include port infections (5.9%), erosion of the band into the stomach (0.8%), and enlargement of the gastric "pouch" that forms above the band (<1%-6.4%).[5,6] O'Brien et al[5] conducted a randomized controlled trial comparing 50 adolescents, 25 of whom received lifestyle modification and 25 of whom received the AGB. The outcomes for weight loss were encouraging, with 25% to 30% body mass index (BMI) reduction and significantly improved comorbidity and metabolic parameters over 2 years. However, there was a higher reoperation rate than would have been expected in adults. Thirty-three percent of the surgical patients required a revision for proximal pouch dilation or tubing/port complications during the 2-year study period.[7] In a smaller but longer-term study, 4 of 8 pediatric AGB patients required a subsequent RYGB surgery because of insufficient initial weight loss or significant weight regain.[8] The AGB requires absolute commitment from the patient to return for adjustments of the band, especially in the first 6 months after placement because the balloon is slowly inflated over time.

The increasing popularity of SG offers another surgical option for adolescents. In this irreversible procedure, about 85% of the stomach is removed, leaving the remainder in the shape of a tube or sleeve. Although many have considered the procedure primarily restrictive, evidence from clinical studies as well as preclinical models are demonstrating that the mechanisms may be more biologic than previously recognized. Insulin resistance improves significantly after SG, with a rapid improvement in glycemic control before any significant weight loss occurs.[9] Resection of the gastric fundus, which is a primary site for production of the orexigenic hormone ghrelin, could be partly responsible for appetite suppression and earlier satiety following the procedure. In addition, early satiety after this procedure may well be linked to the early postprandial increases in hindgut satiety hormones such as glucagon-like peptide-1 (GLP-1) and peptide YY (PYY).[9] SG avoids both intestinal bypass and foreign body placement while improving weight loss over AGB, with fewer complications and reoperations compared to RYGB.[10]

Laparoscopic RYGB is performed through 3 basic steps. A 15- to 30-mL gastric pouch is created just beyond the gastroesophageal junction. A roux limb of jejunum is anastomosed to the gastric pouch, bypassing the remaining stomach, duodenum, and a small portion of jejunum. The biliopancreatic limb is attached to the distal jejunum. The RYGB limits food intake and results in some micronutrient malabsorption, although most believe that the amount of macronutrient malabsorption is not significant.[11-13] It is considered an appropriate procedure for both adults and adolescents, and it has particularly important antidiabetic actions.[14] In fact, RYGB is associated with significant β-cell rescue in people with type 2 diabetes[15] and thus results in more durable glycemic control.[16]

INDICATIONS FOR BARIATRIC SURGERY

Consideration for surgery in the adolescent has traditionally been driven by BMI and the presence of serious comorbidities, which are consistent with the recommendations for adult bariatric surgery.[17] The BMI recommendations include a cutoff of 35 kg/m^2 or more with the presence of 1 or more serious comorbidities such as type 2 diabetes mellitus, severe steatohepatitis, pseudotumor cerebri, or moderate-to-severe sleep apnea (eg, apnea hypopnea index scores of at least 15). At a BMI of 40 kg/m^2 or more, adolescents with less severe comorbidities, which include psychosocial impairments such as poor quality of life, cardiovascular risk factors, or mild sleep apnea, are considered surgical candidates.[18] Other suggested criteria for surgical consideration for adolescents include evidence of physical maturity as determined by a sexual maturity rating of Tanner IV or higher or a bone age of at least 13 for females and 15 years for males, a stable psychosocial environment, the ability to give informed assent, and a demonstrated commitment to lifestyle change.[19-21]

These criteria are widely accepted by pediatric bariatric surgeons, but pediatric and family practice physicians are less comfortable referring adolescents for bariatric surgery, with many endorsing a minimum age of 18 years for referral. Other concerns in addition to age include potentially serious perioperative complications, unknown long-term effects, poor social support, lack of an existing pediatric bariatric program, and belief that medical therapy is superior.[22,23] A delay in referral is not in the best interest of the adolescent with severe obesity whose weight is most likely to continue to climb. In fact, when we examined 51 non–treatment-seeking severely obese (BMI $\geq$40 kg/m^2) 5th- to 12th-grade students enrolled in the Princeton School District Study, over the course of 5 years of follow-up, only 6.3% decreased to BMI less than 40 kg/m^2. However, 83% experienced progressive increase in BMI (1.1 kg/m^2 per year) and waist circumference (2.5 cm per year) over the study period (P <.001 for both; unpublished results). Similarly, a treatment-seeking group of 12 severely obese adolescents with BMI of 47 kg/m^2 who participated for at least 1 year in a comprehensive pediatric weight management program were only able to decrease their mean BMI by 1.2 kg/m^2.[24] Notably, in 2012, Danielsson et al[25] examined 3-year outcomes of behavioral treatment of 643 children. Severely obese adolescents did not experience any beneficial change in BMI, but more promising results were seen in young children.[25] Also underscoring the importance of timing of surgical intervention, we have shown that RYGB results in a 37% decrease in BMI over the first year, irrespective of starting BMI. Therefore, those with an initial BMI between 40 and 54.9 kg/m^2 can reach a nadir BMI of 31 kg/m^2, but patients with an initial BMI between 65 to 95 kg/m^2 only reached a nadir BMI of 47 kg/m^2. When surgery was delayed, most patients were not able to obtain nonobese status after surgery.[26,27]

Contraindications to adolescent bariatric surgery include a medically correctable cause of obesity, current substance abuse problem, inability to adhere to postoperative treatment recommendations, current or planning pregnancy within 18 months or breastfeeding, untreated psychiatric disorder, and lack of decisional capacity to provide informed assent. Careful evaluation of the adolescent is an ongoing process, and a multidisciplinary team approach is helpful for identifying these issues before offering surgery.

Consent for surgery in a minor is obtained from the legal guardian; assent from the adolescent should be obtained and documented. The adolescent patient should demonstrate understanding of the benefits and risks of surgical and medical treatment options, the possible complications, and the long-term dietary and behavioral changes necessary for optimal outcomes, including the long-term follow-up schedule.

SAFETY OF BARIATRIC SURGERY IN ADOLESCENTS

Part of the controversy about bariatric surgery for adolescents has been the question of the immediate risks of surgery. Particularly problematic, however, is the general lack of uniform reporting of negative outcomes in the published bariatric literature. For instance, most reports that describe complications of adolescent bariatric surgery do not provide sufficient methodologic details to discern what events qualified for inclusion and what events did not reach a level of significance to trigger inclusion in the data reported. In contrast, our approach has been to err on the side of more detail rather than less, even if more detail means counting and reporting more events, resulting in higher estimates of adverse event rates compared to other complication data in the literature. In our single-center study of perioperative (<90 days from operation) complications of 77 severely obese adolescents (mean BMI 59.4 kg/m^2) undergoing laparoscopic RYGB, no mortality or conversion to open surgery was observed, and intraoperative complications were uncommon (3%). No anesthetic complications or blood transfusions occurred, and median hospital stay was 3 days. Complications occurred in 22% from discharge to 30 days, and 13% experienced a complication between 31 and 90 days. The common types of postoperative complications included gastrojejunal anastomotic stricture (17%), leak (7%), dehydration (7%), and small bowel obstruction (5%). Reoperation was required in 12%.[28] The largest and most detailed reporting of perioperative complications (within 30 days of surgery) was recently published from the NIH funded multicenter Teen-Longitudinal Assessment of Bariatric Surgery (Teen-LABS) study. The most common surgical procedure was RYGB (66.5%), followed by SG (27.7%) and AGB (5.8%). The adolescents were severely obese with a median BMI of 50.5 kg/m^2 and significant comorbidities. The most common comorbidities were dyslipidemia, sleep apnea, back and joint pain, hypertension, and fatty liver disease.[29] Perioperative complications were classified as major (life-threatening events) or minor (non–life-threatening but unplanned). Within 30 days of surgery, among 242 adolescents enrolled at 5 centers, 92% experienced no major complications, and no deaths occurred. A total of 19 subjects (7.9%) experienced 20 major complications, and 36 (14.9%) experienced 47 minor complications. Most of the complications occurred while the adolescent was still in the hospital. The length of hospital stay was 3 days for RYGB and SG and 1 day for AGB. Although this study was neither designed nor powered to compare procedures and scientifically discern differences, procedure-specific rates of complications were calculated. Major complications within 30 days of operation were as follows: RYGB 9.3%, VSG 4.5%, and AGB 7.1%. Comparable rates for minor events were RYGB 16.8%, VSG 11.9%, and AGB 7.1%. Of the events that required readmission after initial postoperative discharge, only 4 occurred in SG subjects and 21 occurred in RYGB patients.[29]

WEIGHT LOSS OUTCOMES OF BARIATRIC SURGERY

Adolescents achieve comparable weight loss to that seen in adults after RYGB, with an average of 50% to 60% of excess weight lost in the first year and up to 75% of excess weight lost by the end of year 2.[30-32] Although this excess weight loss metric has been overwhelmingly used to report adult outcomes, it is not recommended for adolescent age groups. Larger studies of RYGB weight loss outcome, such as the Swedish Nationwide Study (AMOS), have reported a significant mean BMI decrease in 81 adolescents, from 45.5 to 30.2 kg/m^2, similar to the magnitude of change in a matched adult group (43.5 to 29.7 kg/m^2) over 2 years after surgery.[33] Adult studies show similar weight reduction in SG compared to RYGB. Comparative results between RYGB and SG are limited in adolescents because SG has only recently been introduced as a surgical option. One small study evaluated surgical outcomes of 18 adolescents 55 months after RYGB and SG and found no statistically significant difference in maximum weight loss between the 2 groups.[34]

Weight loss typically is slower with AGB, but with 28% BMI reduction over 2 years in an Australian study, it is superior to lifestyle modification.[7]

COMORBID CONDITIONS

The improvement and resolution of comorbidities demonstrate the ability of WLS to treat not only obesity but also the significant health issues that develop in those with obesity. Results that directly compare the resolution of comorbidities between the 3 surgical options in adolescents are not yet available.

Improved cardiovascular health is a significant outcome of bariatric surgery, with tremendous potential to decrease cardiac morbidity and mortality in adulthood. It can be postulated that resolution of hypertension may be more likely among adolescents after WLS than among adults, presumably related to earlier intervention. In fact, in 1 small study of AGB in adolescents, only 19% of adolescents with preoperative diagnosis of hypertension required continued treatment for hypertension after operation compared to 41.3% of adults.[35] Regardless of initial BMI, both systolic and diastolic blood pressures are improved after RYGB in adolescents by 1 year after surgery.[7,36,37] These improvements in blood pressure seem to persist for at least 2 years as noted in 74 adolescents enrolled in the Adolescent Morbid Obesity Surgery (AMOS) study, who demonstrated an average systolic blood pressure of 125 mmHg at baseline, which decreased to 117 at 2-year follow-up ($P < .001$). Similar improvements in diastolic values were seen with a mean 77 mm Hg decreasing to 74 ($P < .001$).[33] Other indices of cardiac health also show significant improvement for adolescents after RYGB, including significant reductions in left ventricular hypertrophy as demonstrated echocardiographically,[38] cholesterol, low-density lipoprotein (LDL), and triglyceride levels, with improved high-density lipoprotein (HDL) levels.[33,36,37] Results comparing the cardiac effects of SG with RYGB for adolescents are not available at this time.

Another effect of bariatric surgery is the reversal of metabolic disorders, including type 2 diabetes and insulin resistance. The Treatment Options for Type Two Diabetes in Adolescents and Youth (TODAY) study has demonstrated that type 2 diabetes may have a much more aggressive course in youth with early and rapid deterioration of beta-cell function compared to adults with newly diagnosed type 2 diabetes. Over the course of 1 year, 22% of pediatric patients advanced to insulin therapy, and 37% required insulin therapy by 2 years.[39] These data and other studies of young people with type 2 diabetes suggest an urgency to intervene in youth.[40-42] When examining the results of surgery, glucose homeostasis seems to improve very soon after surgery, preceding weight loss. Preoperative BMI and weight loss do not predict improvement in hyperglycemia after RYGB and SG procedures.[43,44] A recent meta-analysis comparing treatment outcomes of bariatric surgery versus conventional medical therapy for type 2 diabetes reviewed 16 studies with a total of 6131 adult patients. They found that bariatric surgery was significantly more effective for weight loss, reducing hemoglobin A_{1c} levels, fasting glucose, and diabetes remission. The diabetes remission rate with surgery was 63.5% versus 15.6% for conventional therapy.[45] Smaller studies with adolescent patients have shown equally encouraging results for those with insulin resistance or type 2 diabetes. At 1 year after RYGB, insulin levels and fasting glucose levels were within normal limits for all the adolescent patients.[24,26]

FEMALE REPRODUCTIVE HEALTH

NHANES data show that the prevalence of obesity is increasing among 12- to 19-year-old females, with rates as high as 24.8% among non-Hispanic black girls.[1] Obesity for girls entering their reproductive years has significant effects on menstrual function, fertility, contraceptive options, and pregnancy outcomes.[46] Menstrual dysfunction occurs frequently among adolescents and young women with obesity, with nearly 40% experiencing irregular cycles, amenorrhea, oligomenorrhea, and menorrhagia.[46] Although the exact mechanism is not clear, regular menstrual cycles resume for most women after bariatric surgery.[7,47-49]

Polycystic ovary syndrome (PCOS) is a complex medical condition that is associated with insulin resistance and serious other metabolic implications and reproductive health concerns for young women. The constellation of symptoms that defines PCOS includes androgen excess (eg, excessive body hair growth, male pattern baldness, acne), menstrual irregularities (eg, oligomenorrhea or amenorrhea), and 25 or more follicles per ovary.[50] The prevalence of PCOS is increased among women with obesity compared to lean women. The exact prevalence among adolescents is not really known because of variable diagnostic criteria and delays in diagnosis.[51] Symptoms of PCOS manifest during adolescence, making this a critical time for recognition and intervention to prevent the chronic health concerns associated with PCOS, including infertility, endometrial cancer, and metabolic syndrome.[51-54] First-line treatment is weight loss to decrease adiposity through dietary changes and increased exercise. Women with PCOS do not find lifestyle changes any less difficult to achieve and maintain than those with obesity. Bariatric surgery has been shown to improve the manifestations of PCOS. Although most of the studies are in adult women, the research shows improvement in hirsutism, androgen levels, resumption of regular menstrual cycles, and restoration of fertility.[55-57] It is unclear how much weight loss is necessary to achieve the improvements in menstrual function; however, when you consider the long-term risks of PCOS, including metabolic syndrome and infertility, some experts advocate including WLS as part of the treatment arsenal for PCOS.[57-59]

Special consideration and education regarding reproductive health is essential for adolescents considering surgical weight loss. Young women need to understand the long-term effects of both obesity and bariatric surgery on their reproductive system. The prevention of pregnancy is an important consideration after bariatric surgery, particularly for adolescent girls who before surgery may have had oligo-ovulatory or anovulatory cycles. One study found a pregnancy rate of 12.8% among adolescent girls after RYGB surgery. The reason for the increased rate is unclear and most likely multifactorial, but it emphasizes the importance of ongoing contraception counseling.[60] Placement of a levonorgestrel-releasing intrauterine device (IUD) at the time of bariatric surgery has been found to be an acceptable option for adolescents.[61]

Obesity and higher BMI are documented to place both the mother and fetus at increased risk for serious complications, including preeclampsia, gestational diabetes, miscarriage, hypertension, congenital malformations, macrosomia, intrauterine fetal demise, and higher rates of cesarean section.[46,62-64] Multiple studies have looked at the safety of pregnancy after bariatric surgery; the results show that pregnancy is less risky after surgery and is not likely to affect the weight loss outcomes for the women. Lower rates of hypertension, gestational diabetes, and macrosomic newborns are found in women who have had WLS compared to the risk in obese women, and the findings hold true for subsequent pregnancies.[65-69] Women who have had RYGB may be at increased risk for internal hernia as a result of increased intraabdominal pressure during pregnancy.[66,69,70]

A recent study reviewed the pregnancies of 2534 women with a history of RYGB, vertical banded gastroplasty, or gastric banding. The researchers matched at a 5:1 ratio of women who had not had surgery with those who had bariatric surgery. The women were matched at their first prenatal visit for age, parity, and BMI, as well as for smoking status, educational level, and year of delivery. They determined that the women who had surgery had a statistically higher rate of preterm birth (delivery before 37 weeks) (9.7% vs. 6.1%) and a greater incidence of small-for-gestational-age (SGA) infants (5.2% vs. 3.0%). The surgical patients were less likely to have large-for-gestational-age infants than the nonsurgical group. There was no significant difference in rate of miscarriage or neonatal death.[71]

Adolescents undergoing bariatric procedures need to understand they are at lifelong risk for nutritional deficiencies and that careful monitoring of vitamin levels during and before pregnancy are essential for best outcomes for mother and baby. We do not yet have data permitting procedure-specific distinctions of greater and lesser risks for adolescents. Most experts agree that pregnancy should be delayed by 12 to 18 months after bariatric surgery, to prevent pregnancy during the period of most rapid weight loss. However, pregnancies that occur earlier than 1 year after surgery may just require careful monitoring of intrauterine growth.[46,66,72-75]

NUTRITIONAL OUTCOMES

The intake of both macronutrients and micronutrients is diminished after WLS because of a decrease in the volume of food consumed and the absorption of nutrients. Dietary advancement protocols are used to assure adequate intake of nutrients and fluids. Adolescents are encouraged to consume 60 grams of protein and drink 80 to 90 ounces of sugar-free fluids daily.[12] We compared the nutritional content of the diet of adolescents 1 month before RYGB surgery and at 1 year after surgery. There was a 35% reduction in calories at 1 year, and fiber intake was markedly reduced, but the proportion of carbohydrate, fat, and protein was unchanged.[76]

Lifelong supplementation and medical monitoring are essential for the prevention of nutritional complications. The recommendations for supplementation following bariatric surgery are based on expert opinion and observational research. An excellent and authoritative clinical practice guideline for perioperative management including supplement recommendations was cosponsored by the American Association of Clinical Endocrinologists, the Obesity Society, and the American Society for Metabolic & Bariatric Surgery.[77] Specific recommendations are based on the surgical procedure that was performed. The risk for nutritional deficiencies is lowest for AGB and then SG, and is greatest with RYGB. Macronutrient deficiencies are uncommon with these surgical techniques, which do not interfere with macronutrient absorption. Table 1 lists recommended medical monitoring after WLS.

Preoperative nutritional status is one of the determinants of risk for postoperative nutritional deficiencies. Many studies have shown that despite their high caloric intake, people with obesity suffer from nutritional deficiencies, especially iron and iron deficiency anemia, vitamin D and vitamin B_{12} deficiencies.[78-80]

Poor adherence to supplementation recommendations has been demonstrated for adults[81] and adolescents after bariatric surgery.[82] Adolescents have traditionally been found to be at higher risk for nonadherence according to the medical literature.[83] To get insights into adherence, we used a combination of self-report and state-of-the-art electronically monitored medication caps and found very poor adherence to vitamin supplementation among adolescent bariatric patients. Forty-one adolescents were followed for 6 months after WLS; adherence to supplement recommendations was only 37% at 1 month and fell to 27% at 6 months.

Table 1
Medical management after bariatric surgery

Item (*visit frequency every 3 months first year, every 6 months second year and annual*)	AGB	SG	RYGB
Monitor weight loss progress, 3–5 pounds/week for first 6 months, then 1–2 pounds/week	X	X	X
Nadir weight loss 12–18 months			
Complete blood count (CBC), metabolic panel with each visit	X	X	X
Lipid evaluation every 6–12 months based on risk	X	X	X
Bone density (dual X-ray absorptiometry [DXA]) at 2 years	X	X	X
Vitamin B_{12} annually, then every 3–6 months if abnormal	X	X	X
Folic acid, iron studies, 25-vitamin D, parathyroid hormone (PTH) annually			X
Thiamine every 6 months for 2 years, then annually	X	X	X
Assess psychotropic medications closely with initial rapid weight loss	X	X	X
Assess blood pressure and need for antihypertensive medications at each visit	X	X	X
Repeat sleep study if history of moderate-to-severe sleep apnea at 3 months	X	X	X

Adapted from Mechanick JI, Youdim A, Jones DB, et al. Clinical practice guidelines for the perioperative nutritional, metabolic, and nonsurgical support of the bariatric surgery patient—2013 update: cosponsored by American Association of Clinical Endocrinologists, The Obesity Society, and American Society for Metabolic & Bariatric Surgery. *Obesity.* 2013;21(Suppl 1):S1-S27.

On 66% of days, participants took none of their supplements. The reasons for nonadherence given by the adolescents were forgetting and difficulty swallowing pills.[82] The lack of immediate consequences of missing prescribed supplements makes encouraging adolescents to adhere to recommendations even more challenging.

Iron deficiency may result from altered eating patterns as well as bypass of the duodenum in the case of RYGB. Many people also develop intolerance to red meat after RYGB and SG. This occurs because red meats have high levels of meat fibers that are difficult to digest when the meat is not cut up or chewed into small enough bits. A decrease in hydrochloric acid secretion in the stomach after RYGB and SG limits the absorption of nonheme iron from plant sources. RYGB results in bypass of the duodenum, which is the primary site of iron absorption. Iron deficiency and anemia are the most common and often the earliest findings, especially for menstruating females.[13,78,84]

Adolescents are at risk for vitamin B_{12} deficiency as well, especially following RYGB.[11] Because the body is able to store vitamin B_{12}, this deficiency may not be manifest for many years. The absorption of vitamin B_{12} is dependent on the presence of intrinsic factor produced in stomach parietal cells. Hydrochloric acid is needed as well for cleaving vitamin B_{12} from food sources. Supplementation is needed at higher rates than the recommended daily allowance of 2.4 mcg/day.[11] Parenteral B_{12} is better absorbed than the oral form; however, it is difficult to adhere to appointments for monthly injections. Recent recommendations for 3000 mcg given IM *annually* may assist with adherence.[77] Deficiencies in vitamin B_{12} can lead to folate deficiencies because B_{12} is needed to convert folate to the active form for absorption. Because folate is absorbed along the entire length of the small intestine, deficiencies in folate probably are related to poor adherence with multivitamin recommendations.

Thiamin deficiency is a risk after RYGB as a result of decreased acidification of food and impaired absorption. Severe deficiencies are most often seen in the first 6 weeks to 3 months after surgery.[11,12] Those with excessive vomiting and nonadherence to supplements are at greatest risk. We reported several cases of dry beriberi following adolescent RYGB, a finding that prompted us to recommend daily additional supplementation with B_1 beyond that obtained in a multivitamin.[85] We recommend this additional dedicated B_1 supplement during the first 6 months following surgery.

Vitamin D deficiency can result from bypass of the proximal small intestine, which is the site of absorption, as well as minimal milk intake because of lactose intolerance that often develops after RYGB.[79] Vitamin D and calcium deficiencies are of particular concern in the adolescent population because the surgery occurs at the time they should be reaching peak bone mass. Whole-body bone mineral content as measured through dual X-ray absorptiometry (DXA) scan was found to be above average before surgery in a retrospective review of 61 adolescent patients followed before and after RYGB. The bone mineral content decreased by 5.2% at 1 year and 7.4% at 2 years, but it did not go below the expected norms for gender and age.[86] Careful monitoring and additional research are needed in this area. Vitamin D deficiency may activate a metabolic cascade that can result in secondary hyperparathyroidism, osteoporosis, and osteomalacia.[13,87]

ADOLESCENT BARIATRIC MULTIDISCIPLINARY TEAM

Adolescent bariatric procedures in the United States are most often performed in adult hospitals. A recent study queried inpatient admissions for children age 20 years or younger undergoing bariatric surgery for obesity in 2009 found that only 21% were performed in a children's hospital.[88] Whatever the setting, the team caring for the adolescent patient must combine expertise in the medical and psychosocial care of pediatric and adolescent obesity with knowledge and skill in bariatric surgery. The multidisciplinary care team should include, at a minimum, an experienced bariatric surgeon, medical director with pediatric expertise, clinical care coordinator, dietitian, and mental health professional.[19] A support group that meets on a regular basis will provide additional peer interaction and education.

A key piece of the assessment of the adolescent is provided by a psychologist or psychiatrist. Expertise in pediatric obesity, eating disorders, and adolescent mental health issues is essential to provide a comprehensive assessment of the adolescent and family. The initial assessment by the psychologist should include an assessment of current mental health status, substance use, health-related quality of life, cognitive function, adherence to current medical regimens, desire for change, as well as social and family functioning.[89]

Developing a relationship with pediatric/adolescent consultation services will assist with timely referral and evaluation for bariatric patients. These services include anesthesiology, pulmonary, cardiology, and endocrinology. A relationship with adolescent medicine or gynecology is beneficial to assist with menstrual disorders, reproductive health care concerns, and reliable contraception in the initial postoperative years.

CONCLUSIONS

Adolescents are a unique patient population, and those with severe obesity present significant challenges to the health care team. Medical treatment modalities have not been shown to be effective in treating severe obesity or reversing the comorbid conditions in this patient population. Bariatric surgery has been shown to be safe and effective in adults and to improve or eliminate obesity-related illnesses, and data for WLS in adolescents, although limited, seem to indicate similar or better results. Performing these surgeries in centers prepared to meet the educational, surgical, and long-term needs of the adolescent and the family is essential for decreasing risk and maximizing outcomes. Ongoing research is essential to guide the care of adolescent surgical candidates in the future.

References

1. Ogden CL, Carroll MD, Kit BK, Flegal KM. Prevalence of obesity and trends in body mass index among US children and adolescents, 1999-2010. *JAMA.* 2012;307(5):483-490
2. Kelly AS, Barlow SE, Rao G, et al. Severe obesity in children and adolescents: identification, associated health risks, and treatment approaches: a scientific statement from the American Heart Association. *Circulation.* 2013;128(15):1689-1712
3. Wang YC, Gortmaker SL, Taveras EM. Trends and racial/ethnic disparities in severe obesity among US children and adolescents, 1976-2006. *Int J Pediatr Obes.* 2011;6(1):12-20
4. Koebnick C, Smith N, Coleman KJ, et al. Prevalence of extreme obesity in a multiethnic cohort of children and adolescents. *J Pediatr.* 2010;157(1):26-31.e22
5. O'Brien PE, MacDonald L, Anderson M, Brennan L, Brown WA. Long-term outcomes after bariatric surgery: fifteen-year follow-up of adjustable gastric banding and a systematic review of the bariatric surgical literature. *Ann Surg.* 2013;257(1):87-94
6. Cunneen SA, Brathwaite CE, Joyce C, et al. Clinical outcomes of the Realize Adjustable Gastric Band-C at 2 years in a United States population. *Surg Obes Relat Dis.* 2013;9(6):885-893
7. O'Brien PE, Sawyer SM, Laurie C, et al. Laparoscopic adjustable gastric banding in severely obese adolescents: a randomized trial. *JAMA.* 2010;303(6):519-526
8. Widhalm K, Fritsch M, Widhalm H, et al. Bariatric surgery in morbidly obese adolescents: long-term follow-up. *Int J Pediatr Obes.* 2011;6(Suppl 1):65-69
9. Peterli R, Wolnerhanssen B, Peters T, et al. Improvement in glucose metabolism after bariatric surgery: comparison of laparoscopic Roux-en-Y gastric bypass and laparoscopic sleeve gastrectomy: a prospective randomized trial. *Ann Surg.* 2009;250(2):234-241
10. Hutter MM, Schirmer BD, Jones DB, et al. First report from the American College of Surgeons Bariatric Surgery Center Network: laparoscopic sleeve gastrectomy has morbidity and effectiveness positioned between the band and the bypass. *Ann Surg.* 2011;254(3):410-420; discussion 420-412
11. Allied Health Sciences Section Ad Hoc Nutrition Committee, Aills L, Blankenship J, Buffington C, Furtado M, Parrott J. ASMBS Allied Health Nutritional Guidelines for the Surgical Weight Loss Patient. *Surg Obes Relat Dis.* 2008;4(5 Suppl):S73-S108
12. Fullmer MA, Abrams SH, Hrovat K, et al. Nutritional strategy for adolescents undergoing bariatric surgery: report of a working group of the Nutrition Committee of NASPGHAN/NACHRI. *J Pediatr Gastroenterol Nutr.* 2012;54(1):125-135
13. Koch TR, Finelli FC. Postoperative metabolic and nutritional complications of bariatric surgery. *Gastroenterol Clin North Am.* 2010;39(1):109-124
14. Schauer PR, Kashyap SR, Wolski K, et al. Bariatric surgery versus intensive medical therapy in obese patients with diabetes. *N Engl J Med.* 2012;366(17):1567-1576
15. Kashyap SR, Bhatt DL, Wolski K, et al. Metabolic effects of bariatric surgery in patients with moderate obesity and type 2 diabetes: analysis of a randomized control trial comparing surgery with intensive medical treatment. *Diabetes Care.* 2013;36(8):2175-2182
16. Malin SK, Samat A, Wolski K, et al. Improved acylated ghrelin suppression at 2 years in obese patients with type 2 diabetes: effects of bariatric surgery vs standard medical therapy. *Int J Obes (Lond).* 2014;38(3):364-370
17. International Pediatric Endosurgery Group. IPEG guidelines for surgical treatment of extremely obese adolescents. *J Laparoendosc Adv Surg Tech A.* 2009;19(Suppl 1):xiv-xvi
18. Pratt JS, Lenders CM, Dionne EA, et al. Best practice updates for pediatric/adolescent weight loss surgery. *Obesity.* 2009;17(5):901-910

19. Michalsky M, Kramer RE, Fullmer MA, et al. Developing criteria for pediatric/adolescent bariatric surgery programs. *Pediatrics.* 2011;128(Suppl 2):S65-S70
20. Inge TH, Krebs NF, Garcia VF, et al. Bariatric surgery for severely overweight adolescents: concerns and recommendations. *Pediatrics.* 2004;114(1):217-223
21. Daniels SR, Arnett DK, Eckel RH, et al. Overweight in children and adolescents: pathophysiology, consequences, prevention, and treatment. *Circulation.* 2005;111(15):1999-2012
22. Iqbal CW, Kumar S, Iqbal AD, Ishitani MB. Perspectives on pediatric bariatric surgery: identifying barriers to referral. *Surg Obes Relat Dis.* 2009;5(1):88-93
23. Woolford SJ, Clark SJ, Gebremariam A, Davis MM, Freed GL. To cut or not to cut: physicians' perspectives on referring adolescents for bariatric surgery. *Obes Surg.* 2010;20(7):937-942
24. Lawson ML, Kirk S, Mitchell T, et al. One-year outcomes of Roux-en-Y gastric bypass for morbidly obese adolescents: a multicenter study from the Pediatric Bariatric Study Group. *J Pediatr Surg.* 2006;41(1):137-143; discussion 137-143
25. Danielsson P, Svensson V, Kowalski J, et al. Importance of age for 3-year continuous behavioral obesity treatment success and dropout rate. *Obesity Facts.* 2012;5(1):34-44
26. Inge TH, Jenkins TM, Zeller M, et al. Baseline BMI is a strong predictor of nadir BMI after adolescent gastric bypass. *J Pediatr.* 2010;156(1):03-108.e101
27. Hatoum IJ, Stein HK, Merrifield BF, Kaplan LM. Capacity for physical activity predicts weight loss after Roux-en-Y gastric bypass. *Obesity.* 2009;17(1):92-99
28. Miyano G, Jenkins TM, Xanthakos SA, Garcia VF, Inge TH. Perioperative outcome of laparoscopic Roux-en-Y gastric bypass: a children's hospital experience. *J Pediatr Surg.* 2013;48(10):2092-2098
29. Inge TH, Zeller MH, Jenkins TM, et al. Perioperative outcomes of adolescents undergoing bariatric surgery: the Teen-Longitudinal Assessment of Bariatric Surgery (Teen-LABS) Study. *JAMA Pediatr.* 2014;168(1):47-53
30. Stanford A, Glascock JM, Eid GM, et al. Laparoscopic Roux-en-Y gastric bypass in morbidly obese adolescents. *J Pediatr Surg.* 2003;38(3):430-433
31. Frank P, Crookes PF. Short- and long-term surgical follow-up of the postbariatric surgery patient. *Gastroenterol Clin North Am.* 2010;39(1):135-146
32. Strauss RS, Bradley LJ, Brolin RE. Gastric bypass surgery in adolescents with morbid obesity. *J Pediatr.* 2001;138(4):499-504
33. Olbers T, Gronowitz E, Werling M, et al. Two-year outcome of laparoscopic Roux-en-Y gastric bypass in adolescents with severe obesity: results from a Swedish Nationwide Study (AMOS). *Int J Obes (Lond).* 2012;36(11):1388-1395
34. Cozacov Y, Roy M, Moon S, et al. Mid-term results of laparoscopic sleeve gastrectomy and roux-en-Y gastric bypass in adolescent patients. *Obes Surg.* 2014;24(5):747-752
35. Zitsman JL, Fennoy I, Witt MA, et al. Laparoscopic adjustable gastric banding in adolescents: short-term results. *J Pediatr Surg.* 2011;46(1):157-162
36. Inge TH, Miyano G, Bean J, et al. Reversal of type 2 diabetes mellitus and improvements in cardiovascular risk factors after surgical weight loss in adolescents. *Pediatrics.* 2009;123(1):214-222
37. Treadwell JR, Sun F, Schoelles K. Systematic review and meta-analysis of bariatric surgery for pediatric obesity. *Ann Surg.* 2008;248(5):763-776
38. Ippisch HM, Inge TH, Daniels SR, et al. Reversibility of cardiac abnormalities in morbidly obese adolescents. *J Am Coll Cardiol.* 2008;51(14):1342-1348
39. Group TS, Zeitler P, Hirst K, et al. A clinical trial to maintain glycemic control in youth with type 2 diabetes. *N Engl J Med.* 2012;366(24):2247-2256
40. Group TS. Rapid rise in hypertension and nephropathy in youth with type 2 diabetes: the TODAY clinical trial. *Diabetes Care.* 2013;36(6):1735-1741
41. Group TS. Effects of metformin, metformin plus rosiglitazone, and metformin plus lifestyle on insulin sensitivity and beta-cell function in TODAY. *Diabetes Care.* 2013;36(6):1749-1757
42. Dart AB, Sellers EA, Martens PJ, et al. High burden of kidney disease in youth-onset type 2 diabetes. *Diabetes Care.* 2012;35(6):1265-1271
43. Mingrone G, Panunzi S, De Gaetano A, et al. Bariatric surgery versus conventional medical therapy for type 2 diabetes. *N Engl J Med.* 2012;366(17):1577-1585

44. Peterli R, Borbely Y, Kern B, et al. Early results of the Swiss Multicentre Bypass or Sleeve Study (SM-BOSS): a prospective randomized trial comparing laparoscopic sleeve gastrectomy and Roux-en-Y gastric bypass. *Ann Surg.* 2013;258(5):690-694; discussion 695
45. Ribaric G, Buchwald JN, McGlennon TW. Diabetes and weight in comparative studies of bariatric surgery vs conventional medical therapy: a systematic review and meta-analysis. *Obes Surg.* 2014;24(3):437-455
46. Bandealy A, Stahl C. Obesity, reproductive health, and bariatric surgery in adolescents and young adults. *J Pediatr Adolesc Gynecol.* 2012;25(4):277-279
47. Rochester D, Jain A, Polotsky AJ, et al. Partial recovery of luteal function after bariatric surgery in obese women. *Fertil Steril.* 2009;92(4):1410-1415
48. Motta AB. The role of obesity in the development of polycystic ovary syndrome. *Curr Pharm Des.* 2012;18(17):2482-2491
49. Gomez-Meade CA, Lopez-Mitnik G, Messiah SE, et al. Cardiometabolic health among gastric bypass surgery patients with polycystic ovarian syndrome. *World J Diabetes.* 2013;4(3):64-69
50. Dewailly D, Lujan ME, Carmina E, et al. Definition and significance of polycystic ovarian morphology: a task force report from the Androgen Excess and Polycystic Ovary Syndrome Society. *Hum Reprod Update.* 2014;20(3):334-352
51. Christensen SB, Black MH, Smith N, et al. Prevalence of polycystic ovary syndrome in adolescents. *Fertil Steril.* 2013;100(2):470-477
52. Bates GW, Legro RS. Longterm management of polycystic ovarian syndrome (PCOS). *Mol Cell Endocrinol.* 2013;373(1-2):91-97
53. Escobar-Morreale HF. Polycystic ovary syndrome: treatment strategies and management. *Expert Opin Pharmacother.* 2008;9(17):2995-3008
54. Rahmanpour H, Jamal L, Mousavinasab SN, Esmailzadeh A, Azarkhish K. Association between polycystic ovarian syndrome, overweight, and metabolic syndrome in adolescents. *J Pediatr Adolesc Gynecol.* 2012;25(3):208-212
55. Eid GM, Cottam DR, Velcu LM, et al. Effective treatment of polycystic ovarian syndrome with Roux-en-Y gastric bypass. *Surg Obes Relat Dis.* 2005;1(2):77-80
56. Jamal M, Gunay Y, Capper A, et al. Roux-en-Y gastric bypass ameliorates polycystic ovary syndrome and dramatically improves conception rates: a 9-year analysis. *Surg Obes Relat Dis.* 2012;8(4):440-444
57. Legro RS, Dodson WC, Gnatuk CL, et al. Effects of gastric bypass surgery on female reproductive function. *J Clin Endocrinol Metab.* 2012;97(12):4540-4548
58. Malik SM, Traub ML. Defining the role of bariatric surgery in polycystic ovarian syndrome patients. *World J Diabetes.* 2012;3(4):71-79
59. Willis K, Sheiner E. Bariatric surgery and pregnancy: the magical solution? *J Perinat Med.* 2013;41(2):133-140
60. Roehrig HR, Xanthakos SA, Sweeney J, Zeller MH, Inge TH. Pregnancy after gastric bypass surgery in adolescents. *Obes Surg.* 2007;17(7):873-877
61. Hillman JB, Miller RJ, Inge TH. Menstrual concerns and intrauterine contraception among adolescent bariatric surgery patients. *J Womens Health (Larchmt).* 2011;20(4):533-538
62. Castro LC, Avina RL. Maternal obesity and pregnancy outcomes. *Curr Opin Obstet Gynecol.* 2002;14(6):601-606
63. Jacobsen BK, Knutsen SF, Oda K, Fraser GE. Obesity at age 20 and the risk of miscarriages, irregular periods and reported problems of becoming pregnant: the Adventist Health Study-2. *Eur J Epidemiol.* 2012;27(12):923-931
64. Kominiarek MA. Pregnancy after bariatric surgery. *Obstet Gynecol Clin North Am.* 2010;37(2):305-320
65. Maggard MA, Yermilov I, Li Z, et al. Pregnancy and fertility following bariatric surgery: a systematic review. *JAMA.* 2008;300(19):2286-2296
66. Bebber FE, Rizzolli J, Casagrande DS, et al. Pregnancy after bariatric surgery: 39 pregnancies follow-up in a multidisciplinary team. *Obes Surg.* 2011;21(10):1546-1551
67. Alatishe A, Ammori BJ, New JP, Syed AA. Bariatric surgery in women of childbearing age. *QJM.* 2013;106(8):717-720

68. Amsalem D, Aricha-Tamir B, Levi I, Shai D, Sheiner E. Obstetric outcomes after restrictive bariatric surgery: what happens after 2 consecutive pregnancies? *Surg Obes Relat Dis.* 2013;S1550-7289(13)00295-5.
69. Aricha-Tamir B, Weintraub AY, Levi I, Sheiner E. Downsizing pregnancy complications: a study of paired pregnancy outcomes before and after bariatric surgery. *Surg Obes Relat Dis.* 2012;8(4):434-439
70. Conrad K, Russell AC, Keister KJ. Bariatric surgery and its impact on childbearing. *Nurs Womens Health.* 2011;15(3):226-233, quiz 234
71. Roos N, Neovius M, Cnattingius S, et al. Perinatal outcomes after bariatric surgery: nationwide population based matched cohort study. *BMJ.* 2013;347:f6460
72. Burke AE, Bennett WL, Jamshidi RM, et al. Reduced incidence of gestational diabetes with bariatric surgery. *J Am Coll Surg.* 2010;211(2):169-175
73. Iavazzo C, Ntziora F, Rousos I, Paschalinopoulos D. Complications in pregnancy after bariatric surgery. *Arch Gynecol Obstet.* 2010;282(2):225-227
74. Kominiarek MA. Preparing for and managing a pregnancy after bariatric surgery. *Semin Perinatol.* 2011;35(6):356-361
75. Sheiner E, Edri A, Balaban E, Levi I, Aricha-Tamir B. Pregnancy outcome of patients who conceive during or after the first year following bariatric surgery. *Am J Obstet Gynecol.* 2011;204(1):50 e51-56
76. Jeffreys RM, Hrovat K, Woo JG, et al. Dietary assessment of adolescents undergoing laparoscopic Roux-en-Y gastric bypass surgery: macro- and micronutrient, fiber, and supplement intake. *Surg Obes Relat Dis.* 2012;8(3):331-336
77. Mechanick JI, Youdim A, Jones DB, et al. Clinical practice guidelines for the perioperative nutritional, metabolic, and nonsurgical support of the bariatric surgery patient—2013 update: cosponsored by American Association of Clinical Endocrinologists, The Obesity Society, and American Society for Metabolic & Bariatric Surgery. *Obesity.* 2013;21(Suppl 1):S1-S27
78. Schweiger C, Weiss R, Berry E, Keidar A. Nutritional deficiencies in bariatric surgery candidates. *Obes Surg.* 2010;20(2):193-197
79. Vasconcelos RS, Viegas M, Marques TF, et al. Factors associated with secondary hyperparathyroidism in premenopausal women undergoing Roux-en-Y gastric bypass for the treatment of obesity. *Arq Bras Endocrinol Metabol.* 2010;54(2):233-238
80. Xanthakos SA. Nutritional deficiencies in obesity and after bariatric surgery. *Pediatr Clin North Am.* 2009;56(5):1105-1121
81. Cooper PL, Brearley LK, Jamieson AC, Ball MJ. Nutritional consequences of modified vertical gastroplasty in obese subjects. *Int J Obes Relat Metab Disord.* 1999;23:382-388
82. Modi AC, Zeller MH, Xanthakos SA, Jenkins TM, Inge TH. Adherence to vitamin supplementation following adolescent bariatric surgery. *Obesity.* 2013;21(3):E190-E195
83. Rapoff M. *Adherence to Pediatric Medical Regimens.* 2nd ed. New York: Springer Science+Business Media; 2010
84. von Drygalski A, Andris DA. Anemia after bariatric surgery: more than just iron deficiency. *Nutr Clin Pract.* 2009;24(2):217-226
85. Towbin A, Inge TH, Garcia VF, et al. Beriberi after gastric bypass surgery in adolescence. *J Pediatr.* 2004;145(2):263-267
86. Kaulfers AM, Bean JA, Inge TH, Dolan LM, Kalkwarf HJ. Bone loss in adolescents after bariatric surgery. *Pediatrics.* 2011;127(4):e956-e961
87. Bhan A, Rao AD, Rao DS. Osteomalacia as a result of vitamin D deficiency. *Endocrinol Metab Clin North Am.* 2010;39(2):321-331, table of contents
88. Zwintscher NP, Azarow KS, Horton JD, Newton CR, Martin MJ. The increasing incidence of adolescent bariatric surgery. *J Pediatr Surg.* 2013;48(12):2401-2407
89. Austin H, Smith K, Ward WL. Psychological assessment of the adolescent bariatric surgery candidate. *Surg Obes Relat Dis.* 2013;9(3):474-480

Adolesc Med 025 (2014) 294–315

Update on the Diagnosis of Sexually Transmitted Infections

Sherine Patterson-Rose, MD, MPH[a*]; Paula K. Braverman, MD[b]

[a]*Assistant Professor of Pediatrics, Cincinnati Children's Hospital Medical Center, Cincinnati, Ohio;*
[b]*Professor of Pediatrics, Cincinnati Children's Hospital Medical Center, Cincinnati, Ohio*

INTRODUCTION

According to the Centers for Disease Control and Prevention (CDC), an estimated 20 million new sexually transmitted infections (STIs) occur every year, with about half of these infections occurring in the 15- to 24-year-old age group.[1] In the United States in 2012, among the 1,422,976 reported cases of chlamydia, 30% occurred in 15- to 19-year-olds and 39% occurred in 20- to 24-year-olds. Similarly in 2012, among the 334,826 reported cases of gonorrhea, 24% occurred in 15- to 19-year-olds and 34% occurred in 20- to 24-year-olds.[1] Of the 15,667 cases of primary and secondary syphilis reported nationally, 6% occurred in 15- to 19-year-olds and 21% occurred in 20- to 24-year-olds.[2]

STIs can lead to many short- and long-term complications, including pelvic inflammatory disease, infertility, anogenital cancers, reactive arthritis, endocarditis, meningitis, epididymitis and ectopic pregnancies,[3] yet many cases continue to go undiagnosed and unreported. Routine STI screening is 1 method to combat this problem. This article will address recommendations for STI screening and provide an overview of the US Food and Drug Administration (FDA)-approved STI tests currently available for *Chlamydia trachomatis* (CT), *Neisseria gonorrhoeae* (GC), *Trichomonas vaginalis* (TV), herpes simplex virus (HSV), and syphilis. Human immunodeficiency virus (HIV) testing is covered in another article in this AMSTARs issue. Testing for vulvovaginal candidiasis (VVC) and bacterial vaginosis (BV) will also be briefly addressed because these disease entities are part of the differential diagnosis in symptomatic patients.

*Corresponding author:
E-mail address: Sherine.Patterson-Rose@cchmc.org

 ISSN 1934-4287

Practical recommendations related to incorporating STI testing in the office setting are also included.

STI SCREENING RECOMMENDATIONS

Both the CDC and the US Preventive Services Task Force (USPSTF) provide STI screening guidelines (see Table 1 for further details).[4-6] Although these guidelines provide general recommendations, it is important to understand the inci-

Table 1
STI screening guidelines from the CDC and USPSTF

STI	CDC screening guidelines[4,5]	USPSTF guidelines[6]
Chlamydia	**General Population** • Annual screening of all sexually active females ≤25 years • Consider screening in males seen in high-prevalence clinical settings[a]	**General Population** • Screen sexually active women ≤24 yrs and older women who are at increased risk[b]; optimal screening interval unknown • Evidence is insufficient to assess screening men
	Pregnant Women • Test at first prenatal visit and again during the third trimester if new or >1 partner	**Pregnant Women** • Test all pregnant women ≤24 years and older pregnant women who are at increased risk[b]
	MSM • Annual screening, including screening for rectal infections in men who have had receptive anal intercourse; more frequent screening is recommended for those at increased risk[c]	**MSM** • No recommendations
Gonorrhea	**General Population** • Annual screening of all sexually active women at risk for infection[d] • Consider screening for males at increased risk per USPSTF	**General Population** • Screen all sexually active women if they are at increased risk[e] • Insufficient evidence to recommend for or against routine screening in men; physicians should consider local gonorrhea epidemiology and other risk factors when making screening decisions
	Pregnant Women • Women at high risk[d] or living in an area of high prevalence should be screened	**Pregnant Women** • All pregnant women if they are at increased risk[e]
	MSM • Annual screening, including a test for rectal infections in men who have had receptive anal intercourse and a test for pharyngeal infection in men who have had receptive oral intercourse; more frequent screening is recommended for those at increased risk[c]	**MSM** • Consider screening because defined as a population at risk

Table 1
STI screening guidelines from the CDC and USPSTF (continued)

STI	CDC screening guidelines[4,5]	USPSTF guidelines[6]
Syphilis	**General Population** • Routine screening is not recommended; however, screen those at high risk[f] or those living in areas with high prevalence of syphilis **Pregnant Women** • Should be tested at first prenatal visit; if at high risk, should also be tested in the third trimester **MSM** • Annual screening; more frequent screening is recommended for those at increased risk[c]	**General Population** • Screen individuals at increased risk[g] for syphilis infection **Pregnant Women** • Screen all pregnant women **MSM** • Consider screening because defined as a population at risk
HSV	**General Population** • Routine screening is not recommended **Pregnant Women** • Routine screening is not recommended	**General Population** • Routine screening is not recommended **Pregnant Women** • Routine screening is not recommended
HPV	**General Population** • Routine HPV screening is not recommended[h]	**General Population** • HPV testing only recommended in conjunction with cervical cancer screening in women >30 years[h]
Tricho-monas	**General Population** • Screen HIV-positive females annually • Consider screening females at high risk[i] **Pregnant Women** • Routine screening not recommended	**General Population** • No recommendations **Pregnant Women** • No recommendations

CDC, Centers for Disease Control and Prevention; HIV, human immunodeficiency virus; HPV, human papillomavirus; USPSTF, US Preventive Services Task Force.
[a]High-prevalence clinic settings include sexually transmitted infection (STI) clinics, correctional facilities, and adolescent clinics.
[b]An increased risk of infection for chlamydia includes a history of chlamydial or other sexually transmitted infection, new or multiple sexual partners, inconsistent condom use, and exchanging sex for money or drugs.
[c]More frequent STI screening (ie, at 3- to 6-month intervals) is indicated for men who have sex with men (MSM) who have multiple or anonymous partners, those who have sex in conjunction with illicit drug use (particularly methamphetamine use), or those whose sex partners participate in illicit drug activities.
[d]An increased risk of infection for gonorrhea includes age <25 years, previous gonorrhea infection, presence of other STIs, new or multiple sex partners, inconsistent condom use, commercial sex work, correctional facilities, and drug use.
[e]An increased risk of infection for gonorrhea includes women and men <25 years, history of previous gonorrhea infection, other STIs, new or multiple sexual partners, inconsistent condom use, commercial sex work, and drug use.
[f]An increased risk of infection for syphilis includes members of an at-risk subpopulation (ie, persons in correctional facilities and MSM); those who describe sexual behaviors that put them at risk for STIs (ie, having unprotected vaginal, anal, or oral sexual contact; having multiple sexual partners; using drugs and alcohol, and engaging in commercial or coerced sex); those have partner(s) who have tested positive for syphilis.
[g]An increased risk of infection for syphilis includes MSM who engage in high-risk sexual behavior, commercial sex workers, persons who exchange sex for drugs, and those in adult correctional facilities.
[h]Screen immunocompetent women ≥21 years for cervical dysplasia with Pap smear.
[i]High risk for trichomonas infection includes women who have new or multiple partners, have a history of STIs, exchange sex for payment, and use injection drugs.

dence of STIs in your patient population to aid in screening decisions based on local epidemiology. It is important to discuss sexual practices with your patient not only to determine which STI tests to conduct but also which anatomic sites to test. The guidelines primarily address heterosexual females and men who have sex with men (MSM). There is a paucity of evidence for heterosexual males and no specific guidelines for women who have sex with women (WSW). It is believed that more than half of WSW have had sex with men in the past, and some may continue to do so in the future. In addition to acquisition of STIs from previous male partners, studies suggest that there is also a risk of transmission of STIs between WSW couples.[4] The CDC recommends that this population be screened according to the guidelines for the general female populations.

OVERVIEW OF STI TESTING METHODS

Culture was the traditional gold standard for STI testing for the common pathogens GC, CT, TV, and HSV. Culture for GC remains an important testing method because it is essential for conducting antibiotic susceptibility testing and guiding treatment decisions with the rise in antibiotic resistance. Although cultures have the advantage of providing a definitive diagnosis when the results are positive, they may produce false-negative results because of technical difficulties in the culture process and the fastidious nature of some the organisms, which may not survive during transport to the laboratory. For example, CT culture will miss approximately 15% of CT infections. In addition, growing the organism in culture can take several days and delay the time to diagnosis and treatment.[7]

Various nonculture tests have been developed during the past 2 decades, starting with enzyme-linked immunoassays (EIAs) and direct fluorescent antibody (DFA) tests and progressing to nonamplified and amplified nucleic acid molecular tests. The nonamplified tests are hybridization assays using a nucleic acid probe that binds with sequences in the organism's gene fragments. The nucleic acid amplification tests (NAATs) currently available in the United States use polymerase chain reaction (PCR), transcription-mediated amplification (TMA), and strand displacement amplification (SDA) to amplify nucleic acid in the organism before hybridization with a nucleic acid probe, increasing sensitivity. The EIA and DFA tests are no longer used for CT or GC diagnosis because they have inferior sensitivities. NAATs are now preferred over both culture and other nonculture tests because of their superior sensitivities.[7] Because NAATs can be used on urine and vaginal swab specimens, STI screening is facilitated by eliminating invasive urethral testing in males and the need for speculum examinations in females. Screening in nontraditional venues outside of the office setting with NAATs has become a reality.[8]

Having a high sensitivity is not the only consideration when choosing a testing modality. In populations with a low prevalence of disease, the positive predictive value of a test is much lower than in high-prevalence populations. It is important to note that nonculture tests generally have lower specificity than cultures because of the potential for false-positive results. In some cases, such as abuse evaluations, some courts still request culture results because this eliminates the possibility of false-positive results.[7] However, for the purposes of screening and testing in sexually active individuals, NAATs are currently considered the optimal tests for GC and CT.[3]

Part of the challenge of addressing the STI epidemic is the delay in diagnosing infection and promptly treating the index patient and their partners to prevent further spread of the disease and potential complications. Even NAAT results may take several days because of time for transport of samples to the laboratory and reporting results back to the physician. In many cases, physicians will provide presumptive treatment, particularly to symptomatic patients, while awaiting STI testing results. There has been substantial research on point-of-care tests (POCTs) as a way to accurately diagnose STIs in the office setting. POCT typically provide test results in minutes, allowing physicians to provide immediate treatment and education to patients as well as expedite partner treatment. In 1990, the World Health Organization launched an initiative to improve the detection of CT, GC, and syphilis.[9] The initiative promoted the development of diagnostic tests that met the criteria of ASSURED (Affordable, Sensitive, Specific, User-friendly, Rapid and Robust, Equipment Free and Delivered). The ASSURED criteria blend well with the requirements of POCTs. Although the rapid tests currently available on the market may take only 1 to 2 hours rather than days to perform in the laboratory, they are not truly POCTs because of the need for specialized equipment and the extended wait time for results, making them less practical in the busy clinical setting.

In a comprehensive review of the scientific literature, several rapid tests for CT and GC were reported.[10] Tests for CT have sensitivities ranging from 25% to 95% and specificities ranging from 97.2% to 100%. Tests for GC have sensitivities of 60% to 98.3% and specificities of 89.9% to 98.2%. Cepheid GeneXpert for GC and CT is the only rapid test currently FDA-approved and available in the United States. It has a sensitivity of 97.4% to 98.7% and specificity of more than 99.4% for CT and sensitivity of 95.6% to 100% and specificity of more than 99.8% for GC. However, the test requires a specific instrument and 90 minutes to perform.[11] None of the rapid tests for GC or CT are Clinical Laboratory Improvement Amendments (CLIA) waived, making them less practical in a busy clinical setting. Similarly for syphilis, many rapid and point-of-care tests have been studied, with sensitivities ranging from 75% to 90% and specificities ranging 94% to 99%.[12-14] Although extremely useful in resource-poor settings, the syphilis POCT is less sensitive than standard treponemal tests and has the disadvantage of not distinguishing current from past infection. There are currently no FDA-approved POCT CLIA waived tests for syphilis in the United States. For trichomoniasis, there is 1 FDA-cleared CLIA waived POCT, the OSOM Trichomonas Rapid Test (Sekisui Diagnostics, Framingham, MA), which has excellent sensitivity and specificity and can easily be performed in the office setting in 10 minutes without specialized equipment (Table 2).

Table 2
Comparison of sensitivity and specificity of commonly used trichomonas tests from package insert data[34-37]

Diagnostic test	Technique	Specimen	Sensitivity	Specificity	Time to test
OSOM trichomonas rapid test (Sekisui Diagnostics)	Immunochromatographic assay	Vaginal swabs	83%[a]	99%[a]	10 minutes
Affirm VPIII microbial identification test (Becton Dickinson)	DNA probe test	Vaginal swabs[c]	89.6%[b]	99.9%[b]	<1 hour
APTIMA *Trichomonas vaginalis* assay (Gen-Probe)	Transcription-mediated amplification (TMA)	Female urine	95.2%[a]	98.9%[a]	Hours
		Physician-collected vaginal	100%[a]	99.0%[a]	
		Endocervical swab	100%[a]	99.4%[a]	
		PreservCyt solution liquid Pap	100%[a]	99.6%[a]	
ProbeTec Trichomonas Vaginalis QX (Becton Dickinson)	Strand displacement amplification	Female urine	95.5%[a,b]	98.7%[a,b]	Hours
		Cervical	96.3%[a,b]	99.4%[a,b]	
		Self vaginal swab	98.3%[a,b]	99.0%[a,b]	

[a]Compared to wet mount and culture.
[b]Compared to culture.
Tests approved for both asymptomatic and symptomatic patients except as noted below:
[c]Only approved for symptomatic patients.

Chlamydia trachomatis

Chlamydia trachomatis is a gram-negative, obligate intracellular genital pathogen. It commonly causes asymptomatic infections but also is responsible for a variety of clinical presentations, including urethritis, epididymitis, and proctitis in males and urethritis, cervicitis, salpingitis, and perihepatitis in females.[15] CT also can cause conjunctivitis and reactive arthritis (Reiter syndrome).

NAATs have become the gold standard for CT testing and are recommended for detection of infection in symptomatic and asymptomatic males and females (Table 3).[16-21] When using NAATs, first-catch urine is the optimal specimen for males, with sensitivities equivalent to urethral specimens. Vaginal swabs are preferred for females; they have been shown to be equivalent or superior to endocervical specimens and urine.[22] Urethral swabs in males, and endocervical swabs and urine in females can also be used for testing, although first-void urine in females may have reduced performance compared to genital samples.[22] Recent evidence has also shown that liquid-based cytology specimens used for Pap smears can be acceptable for NAATs, and certain NAATs are FDA-approved for testing using theses specimens. Sensitivities for liquid-based Pap specimens range from 77% to 97%, and specificities range from 98% to 100%.[23-25] In addition, studies have shown that both self-collected and physician-collected vaginal swabs are as sensitive as cervical swabs for testing,[26] so pelvic examinations may not be warranted for screening of asymptomatic patients. Other nonculture tests, such as DNA probe assays, are available for CT testing using endocervical swabs for females and urethral swabs for males. However, as mentioned earlier, these tests have lower sensitivity than NAATs, which therefore are preferred when available.[22]

For those who engage in receptive anal and oral sex, CT testing should be recommended. Of note, although the CDC does not recommend routine screening for asymptomatic pharyngeal CT, if the patient is symptomatic, testing should be conducted.[4] Although there are no FDA-approved nonculture CT tests for oropharyngeal or rectal infections, NAATs are recommended for these locations. Compared to CT cultures, rectal CT testing with the currently available NAATs showed sensitivity of 80.7% to 100% and specificity ranging from 95.6% to 98.5%.[27] Laboratories must ensure CLIA adherence by validating specimens in their own facilities before using oropharyngeal or rectal NAAT results clinically.[22] Physicians should check with the laboratories they utilize because many academic centers as well as major commercial laboratories (eg, Quest, LabCorp) have already validated this process. If NAATs are not available, CT cultures should be conducted.

Tests of cure are not currently recommended for CT if first-line recommended treatments have been used, but because of the risk of reinfection from an untreated partner or a new partner, the CDC currently recommends that repeat

Table 3
Comparison of sensitivity and specificity of FDA-approved chlamydia tests from package insert data[16-21]

Test (manufacturer)	Type of test	Specimen	Sensitivity	Specificity
Cobas CT/NG v2.0 (Roche Molecular Diagnostics)	Polymerase chain reaction	Female urine	94.0%	99.6%
		Cervical	94.9%	99.4%
		Self vaginal swab	97.6%	99.3%
		Physician-collected vaginal swab	98.2%	99.1%
		PreservCyt liquid-based Pap specimen	93.7%-94.2%	99.5%-99.7%
		Male urine	98.4%	99.2%
APTIMA Combo2 (Gen-Probe)	Transcription-mediated amplification	Female urine	94.7%	98.9%
		Cervical	94.2%	97.6%
		Self vaginal swab[a]	98.4%	96.8%
		Physician-collected vaginal swab	96.6%	96.8%
		PreservCyt liquid-based Pap specimen	96.7%	99.2%
		Male urine	97.9%	98.5%
		Urethral	95.9%	97.5%
ProbeTec QX CT (Becton Dickinson)	Strand displacement amplification	Female urine	91.4%-93.1%	99%
		Cervical	91.3%	98.3%
		Self vaginal swab	96.5%	99.2%
		PreservCyt Pap specimen	94.1%	99.8%
		BD SurePath Pap specimens	95%	99.7%
		Male urine	97%	97.4%-99.5%
		Urethral	92.1%	98.4%
ProbTec ET CT/GC (Becton Dickinson)	Strand displacement amplification	Female urine	83%	97.1%
		Cervical	95.1%	96.7%
		Male urine	94.6%	89%
		Urethral	94.7%	91.7%
Abbott RealTime CT/NG (Abbott Molecular Inc.)	Polymerase chain reaction	Female urine	91.3%-93.5%	99.7%
		Cervical[b]	93.8%	99.8%
		Self vaginal swab	97.3%-98.4%	98.9%-99.1%
		Physician-collected vaginal swab	97.2%-98.4%	99.3%-100%
		Male urine	95.5%-96.6%	99.1%-99.3%
		Urethral[b]	93.4%	98.3%

FDA, Food and Drug Administration.
Tests approved for both asymptomatic and symptomatic patients except as noted below:
[a]Only approved for asymptomatic patients.
[b]Only approved for symptomatic patients.

testing be conducted 3 months after treatment of a person with a positive test result.[4] NAATs conducted less than 3 weeks after completion of therapy in persons who were treated successfully could yield false-positive results because of the continued presence of nonviable organisms.[4]

Neisseria gonorrhoeae

Neisseria gonorrhoeae is a gram-negative diplococcus that causes asymptomatic and symptomatic genitourinary infections, including urethritis, cervicitis, proctitis, pharyngitis, and conjuncitivitis.[28] Complications include salpingitis, epididymitis, and disseminated infection with septic arthritis, tenosynovitis, skin lesions, endocarditis, and meningitis.

Multiple modalities are available for the detection of GC; however, as with CT, NAATs have become the gold standard for testing in both males and females. For females, vaginal swabs for NAAT are the optimal specimen type.[22] Other modalities include culture and nucleic acid hybridization tests, which both require an endocervical specimen. NAATs allow for more variety in specimen types, including endocervical swabs as well as the less invasive vaginal swabs and urine,[4] which do not require a speculum examination in females.

In males, a positive gram stain demonstrating polymorphonuclear leukocytes with intracellular gram-negative diplococci can be considered diagnostic, but many clinical settings do not have the ability to perform this testing on site. Furthermore, because a negative gram stain cannot rule out infection, it still would be necessary to conduct more sensitive testing for gonorrhea. The NAAT remains the current test of choice in males using either urethral swabs or urine.[22] Because there are no significant differences between the sensitivity and specificity of urine versus urethral swabs for testing in males, noninvasive first-catch urine is preferred.[29]

Although nonculture testing for GC has become the standard of care in both men and women, these tests do not provide antimicrobial sensitivity results. If there is a suspicion of antibiotic-resistant gonorrhea in a particular patient, it is important to work with your local laboratory or health department to determine the need for gonorrhea culture[4] (see Antimicrobial Resistance in *Neisseria gonorrhoeae* for more information).

For those who engage in receptive anal and oral sex, gonorrhea testing of the pharynx and rectum is recommended both for screening of asymptomatic individuals as well as for testing of those who are symptomatic. The anatomic location tested is based on the reported sexual practices. Although there are no FDA-approved nonculture tests for gonorrhea, NAATs are recommended for detection of oropharyngeal and rectal gonorrheal infections. Compared to gonorrhea cultures, currently available NAATs showed sensitivity of 91.4% to 100% and specificity ranging from

98.3% to 98.8% for rectal specimens,[24] whereas for oropharyngeal infections, NAATs have a sensitivity ranging from 80.3% to 93.2% and a specificity ranging from 73% to 98.6% compared to culture.[30] As discussed for CT, many academic centers and commercial laboratories have performed CLIA adherence for validation of rectal and oropharyngeal specimens. Physicians should verify with their laboratories that they have completed this process before using results clinically.[22] If NAATs are not available, gonorrhea culture should be conducted.

Similar to CT, tests of cure are not currently recommended for GC if first-line recommended treatments have been used. However, because of the risk of reinfection from an untreated partner or a new partner, the CDC currently recommends that repeat testing be conducted 3 months after treatment of a person with a positive test result.[3] NAATs conducted less than 3 weeks after completion of therapy in persons who were treated successfully could yield false-positive results because of the continued presence of nonviable organisms.[4] It is important to check the package insert for the particular NAAT being used because not all tests are approved for all specimen types (Table 4).

Trichomonas vaginalis

Trichomonas vaginalis is a protozoan parasite that causes vaginitis in women and urethritis in men, and it can cause premature rupture of membranes in pregnancy.[31] Immediate light microscopic evaluation of vaginal secretions with a wet mount is commonly used to diagnose TV because this method can be quick and inexpensive; however, training is required to perform the test. Furthermore, because the organism typically lyses in an acidic environment, the sensitivity of this method only approaches 51% to 65%,[32] and many cases of TV can be missed (see Table 2 for a list of FDA-approved tests for TV).

Culture is the gold standard for TV testing in females using a variety of liquid and semisolid media.[31] Several culture media and culture systems are available. The InPouch TV culture system (BioMed Diagnostics, San Jose, CA) allows for direct inoculation, culture, and microscopic examination, and can be used to transport the specimen.[32] However, because of the need to incubate vaginal secretions for 3 to 5 days, the variable culture sensitivity of 75% to 96%,[32] as well as the availability of newer diagnostic methods, TV culture is not typically used in the clinical setting.[33]

Several FDA-approved rapid tests currently available for TV testing in females are more sensitive than wet mount and have high specificity. The OSOM Trichomonas Rapid Test (Sekisui Diagnostics) uses an immunochromatographic assay to detect antigen directly from the vaginal swab.[34] This test is considered CLIA complexity waived, and results typically are available in 10 minutes without the need for special equipment, making it practical for the office setting. Affirm VPIII (Becton Dickinson, Franklin Lakes, NJ) uses a DNA hybridization probe

Table 4
Comparison of sensitivity and specificity of FDA-approved gonorrhea tests from package insert data[16-21]

Test (manufacturer)	Type of test	Specimen	Sensitivity	Specificity
Cobas CT/NG v2.0 (Roche Molecular Diagnostics)	Polymerase chain reaction	Female urine	95.6%	99.7%
		Cervical	96.6%	99.9%
		Self vaginal Swab	96.7%	100%
		Physician-collected vaginal swab	100%	99.7%
		PreservCyt liquid-based Pap specimen	95.6%-96.7%	99.7%-99.8%
		Male urine	100%	99.3%
Aptima Combo2 (Gen-Probe)	Transcription-mediated amplification	Female urine	91.3%	99.3%
		Cervical	99.2%	98.7%
		Self vaginal swab[a]	100%	99.5%
		Physician-collected vaginal swab	96%	99.2%
		PreservCyt Pap liquid-based Pap specimen	92.3%	99.8%
		Male urine	98.5%	99.6%
		Urethra	99.1%	97.8%
ProbeTec QX GC (Becton Dickinson)	Strand displacement amplification	Female urine	93%	99.2%-99.4%
		Cervical	98.5%	99.7%
		Self vaginal swab	100%	99.1%
		PreservCyt Pap specimen	95.3%	99.95%
		BD SurePath Pap specimens	100%	99.9%
		Male urine	98%	98.1%-99.2%
		Urethral	100%	99.1%
ProbTec ET GC/CT (Becton Dickinson)	Strand displacement amplification	Female urine	86.3%	99.1%
		Cervical	96.4%	99.0%
		Male urine	98.1%	97.9%
		Urethra	98.1%	97.9%
Abbott RealTime CT/NG (Abbott Molecular Inc.)	Polymerase chain reaction	Female urine	91.3%-93.5%	99.5%-99.6%
		Cervical[b]	88%	99.8%
		Self vaginal swab	96.2%-100%	99.6%-100%
		Physician-collected vaginal swab	96.3%-100%	100%
		Male urine	98.7%-100%	99.2%-100%
		Urethral[b]	99.5%	99%

FDA, Food and Drug Administration.
Tests approved for both asymptomatic and symptomatic patients except as noted below:
[a]Only approved for asymptomatic patients.
[b]Only approved for symptomatic patients.

test to evaluate for TV, *Gardnerella vaginalis*, and *Candida albicans* via a vaginal swab.[35] This test is considered CLIA moderate complexity, it requires special laboratory equipment, and results are available in less than an hour.

Current FDA-approved NAATs for TV include APTIMA (Gen-Probe, San Diego, CA) and ProbeTec *Trichomonas vaginalis* (TV) Q*x* Amplified DNA Assay (Becton Dickinson).[36,37] These tests can be conducted on various female specimens (see Table 2 for more details). Although not FDA-approved at this time, the Amplicor PCR assay (Roche Diagnostic Corp.) used to detect gonorrhea and CT has been evaluated for detecting TV. This test has been modified for TV testing using vaginal and endocervical swabs or urine in females. Sensitivity was 88% to 95% and specificity 98% to 99% compared to microscopy.[38]

In males, TV culture using urine, semen, or urethral swab is also considered the gold standard.[31] However, as mentioned earlier, it can be time intensive. Light microscopy is not an option in males because of poor sensitivity. Neither antigen nor DNA hybridization test for TV (OSOM or Affirm VPIII) can be used for urethral swabs or urine.[32] However, although there are no currently FDA-approved nonculture TV tests, studies have evaluated NAATs for TV in males. APTIMA was studied using male urethral swabs and urine specimens and showed a sensitivity of 92% and 92% and specificity of 87% and 92% compared to culture.[39] The Amplicor test was found to be 96% sensitive and 99.2% specific compared to culture using first-catch urine samples in males.[38]

Syphilis

Syphilis is caused by the spirochete *Treponema pallidum*. The disease manifestation progresses in stages over time from a chancre (primary infection) to diffuse rash, mucosal lesions, as well as numerous others systemic symptoms (secondary infection), followed by a latent phase and then cardiac, neurologic, or bone lesions (tertiary infection). During the course of this illness, patients may be completely asymptomatic.[40] Although dark-field examinations of specimens from syphilis lesions can be used to detect *T pallidum*, most laboratories do not have this diagnostic capability. Other available direct detection tests, such as PCR and DFA test for *T pallidum*, are not routinely used in the clinical setting.[41] Because direct tests require an actual lesion, which may not be clinically apparent, blood serologic tests remain the standard of diagnosis.[4] Guidelines recommend the use of 2 types of serologic tests, nontreponemal and treponemal, to confirm the diagnosis of syphilis. Nontreponemal tests include Venereal Disease Research Laboratory (VDRL), rapid plasma reagin (RPR), toluidine red unheated serum test (TRUST), and complement fixation test–Wasserman reaction. Treponemal tests include fluorescent treponemal antibody absorption (FTA-ABS), *Treponema pallidum* hemagglutination assay (TPHA), chemiluminescence immunoassay (CIA), and EIA.[42] The use of only one serologic test (ie, only a treponemal or nontreponemal test) is insufficient for diagnosis.

Nontreponemal tests traditionally have been used to screen patients, followed by confirmation of positive results by a treponemal test. With this algorithm, one can detect active disease; however, there is a high rate of false-positives with nontreponemal tests in conditions such as pregnancy, systemic lupus erythematosus, and mononucleosis, and false-negatives can occur in early primary disease.[42] Recently, some laboratories have moved to using the treponemal test for screening (reverse sequence testing). This algorithm can better detect early primary disease, has a higher sensitivity and specificity, and removes operator biases; however, there is the inability to distinguish between active and previously treated disease[42] because the treponemal test usually remains positive for life. For reverse sequence testing, the CDC recommends starting with either EIA or CIA.[41] Interpretation of results can be somewhat confusing. The CDC currently recommends that a positive treponemal screening test be confirmed by a standard nontreponemal test (RPR or VDRL). If the confirmatory nontreponemal test is negative, then a second, different treponemal test should be performed to confirm the results of the initial test. If the second treponemal test is positive, patients with a history of previous treatment would require no further management unless there is a strong likelihood of re-exposure. Patients without a history of syphilis should be offered treatment. If the second treponemal test is negative, no further evaluation is warranted[4] (see Figure 1 for syphilis serologic screening algorithms).

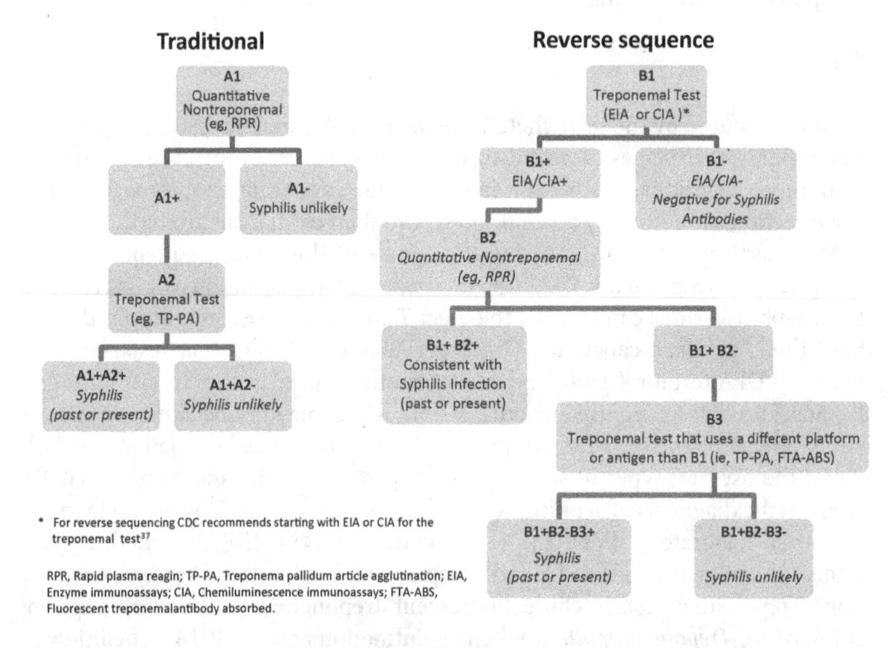

Adapted from CDC Reverse Sequence Syphilis Screening Webinar : http://www.cdc.gov/std/syphilis/Syphilis-Webinar.htm; Association of Public Health Laboratories and CDC. Laboratory diagnostic testing for Treponema pallidum Expert consultation meeting summary report.

Fig 1. Algorithm for traditional and reverse sequence syphilis serologic screening.

For patients diagnosed with syphilis, nontreponemal tests titers are used to determine disease activity and monitor for cure after antibiotic therapy. A 4-fold change in titer is necessary to confirm a clinically significant difference between 2 test results. Sequential tests should be performed using the same nontreponemal tests, ideally performed at the same laboratory, because results for different nontreponemal tests cannot be directly compared.[4]

For neurosyphilis, there is no single laboratory test to confirm the diagnosis. A positive VDRL in uncontaminated cerebrospinal fluid (CSF) is considered diagnostic; however, this test is highly specific but insensitive. Sensitivity and specificity of all other tests when used in CSF is and should be interpreted based on clinical findings and other test results, such as CSF cell count or protein.[4]

Herpes

Genital herpes is caused by the herpes simplex virus (HSV). It can present with vesicles, painful genital ulcers, dysuria, fever, and tender local inguinal lymphadenopathy.[43] In some cases, the diagnosis is missed because there may be an atypical presentation, such as a painful fissure rather than a vesicle or ulcer. After the initial infection, the virus can be found in the nerve root ganglion and may be associated with a recurrence of clinical symptoms as well as subclinical shedding, which can lead to transmission to a sexual partner.[43] HSV is associated with an increased risk of HIV transmission and can be passed perinatally, leading to increased infant morbidity and mortality, and is considered a public health concern.[44] Although HSV-2 is typically associated with genital herpes, there has been an increased prevalence of genital infection caused by HSV-1.[44,45] Because those infected with HSV-1 tend to have fewer occurrences and less clinical shedding, knowledge of virus type can be beneficial for patient education.[46,47]

Although viral cultures are still considered the gold standard for diagnosis of herpes in symptomatic patients, because of the culture's poor sensitivity (as low as 54%),[48] nucleic acid amplification assays are becoming increasingly popular. The poor sensitivity of culture results in part because of the difficulty in obtaining an adequate sample when the lesions have begun to heal. There are currently only 3 FDA-approved NAAT molecular tests available for HSV, with sensitivity ranging 92.4% to 97.1% and specificity ranging from 93.4% to 98.3%.[48] Each of these tests has different limitations for use (eg, patient age, gender, specimen type, inability to distinguish HSV-1 from HSV-2) (Table 5). In addition to the FDA-approved tests, many laboratories have developed their own molecular diagnostic tests, commonly using PCR, which has also been recommended for testing anogenital lesions.[4,49] The molecular tests have the advantage of detecting virus from lesions that have passed the vesicular or pustular stage. Some also provide viral typing, which can assist in counseling about potential recurrences. Physicians should check with their laboratories about the available commercial or laboratory-developed molecular tests in their area.

Table 5
Comparison of sensitivity and specificity of FDA-approved HSV tests from package insert data[62-64]

Diagnostic test	Technique	Specimen	Sensitivity (compared to culture)	Specificity (compared to culture)	Limitations
MultiCode®-RTx HSV1&2 kit (Luminex)	PCR molecular detection	Vaginal swab for HSV-1	92.4%	98.3%	Only vaginal swab samples of symptomatic females >10 years
		Vaginal swab for HSV-2	95.2%	93.6%	
ProbeTec HSV Qx test (Becton Dickinson)	Strand displacement amplification	Anogenital swab for HSV-1	96.8/96.7%[a]	97.6/95.1%[a]	Not intended to be used for prenatal screening or for females <17 years
		Anogenital swab for HSV-2	98.4%	83.7/80.6%[a]	
IsoAmp HSV assay (Biohelix)	Isothermal helicase-dependent amplification	Genital sample	97.1%	93.4%	Can be used in males and females but unable to distinguish between HSV-1 and HSV-2
		Oral sample	93.8%	87.4%	

FDA, Food and Drug Administration; HSV, herpes simplex virus; PCR, polymerase chain reaction.
[a]Sensitivity and specificity varied by type of specimen collection kit.

In general, screening for HSV infection with serology is not recommended, and direct testing from a genital lesion is the best way to confirm a clinical diagnosis. However, in instances of a recurrent/atypical genital symptom with a negative direct herpes or PCR test, a clinical diagnosis of herpes without confirmatory tests, a herpes discordant sexual partner, MSM with unknown HSV status, or a person with HIV infection and unknown HSV status,[4] type-specific HSV serology can be considered. Testing in these instances would be of value in counseling patients regarding treatment, including suppressive therapy to reduce recurrences or transmission to an HSV-negative partner. Serologic tests are based on the recognition of envelope protein gG-1 (HSV-1) and gG-2 (HSV-2). It is important to request serologic gG-based type specific assays by name[50] because some commercial tests available on the market do not use this method of serotyping, and a positive result from another type of assay could reflect a past oral HSV-1 infection and not a current or past genital HSV infection. Sensitivities for G-type specific serologic assay range from 80% to 98%, and specificities are more than 96%.[3]

Human Papilloma Virus

Human papilloma virus (HPV) is the most common STI in the United States; it affects more than 50% of sexually active persons.[51] HPV types 6 and 11 are associated with genital warts, and HPV types 16 and 18, as well as other oncogenic strains, are associated with cervical, anal, vulvar, vaginal, penile, and oropharyngeal cancers.[52] Because HPV infection is generally self-limited, screening for the virus as a part of routine STI testing is not recommended. In females, Pap smear screening is recommended starting at age 21 years to screen for HPV-related cancers and precancerous lesions.[4,6] There are currently 4 FDA-approved HPV tests available for screening in conjunction with Pap smears; however, the CDC and USPSTF recommend HPV testing during cervical cancer screening only in females older than 30 years.[4,6]

Vulvovaginal Candidiasis

Vulvovaginal candidiasis occurs from an overgrowth of *Candida* spp. It typically presents in females with vaginal itching; white, cottage cheese–like discharge; dyspareunia; irritation; and soreness.[53] Although it is not an STI, VVC has a high incidence in women; 70% to 75% of women have an infection during their lifetime.[53] Because it can present with symptoms similar to other STIs, VVC should be considered in the differential diagnosis of women presenting with genital symptoms.

Diagnosis of VVC is typically made using a wet prep with 10% KOH or Gram stain of vaginal discharge. Either specimen may reveal yeast, hyphae, or pseudo-hyphae. Vaginal cultures for *Candida* usually are not utilized or recommended because the organism can be part of the normal flora. However, cultures can be considered when evaluating cases of suspected recurrent infection or those not responsive to usual treatment, suggesting infection with a non–*C albicans* species. The only FDA-approved rapid tests to diagnose *Candida* is the Affirm VPIII (Becton Diagnostics), a DNA probe that can provide results for TV, VVC, and BV in less than 1 hour. Sensitivity and specificity are 81% and 98.2%, respectively.[35]

Bacterial Vaginosis

Bacterial vaginosis is one of the most common lower genitourinary tract infections in females. It represents a change in normal vaginal flora because of a lack of hydrogen-producing lactobacilli and a prominence of gram-variable coccobacilli, including *G vaginalis*.[54] Women typically present with a complaint of a vaginal discharge with a fishy odor, although they also can be asymptomatic. Lack of diagnosis and treatment can result in an increased risk for pelvic infection after gynecologic surgery, pelvic inflammatory disease, and an increased susceptibility to other STIs. In pregnant women, BV can be associated with prematurity and chorioamnionitis.[54]

BV can be diagnosed by Gram stain using the Nugent or Hay/Ison criteria.[54,55] Because access to Gram stain can be limited, the Amsel diagnostic criteria is commonly used in the clinical setting. According to the Amsel criteria, a diagnosis of BV requires 3 of the following signs and symptoms[4]:

- Homogeneous, thin, white discharge
- Presence at least 20% of epithelial cells resembling clue cells on microscopic examination
- pH of vaginal fluid more than 4.5
- A fishy odor of vaginal discharge before or after addition of 10% KOH (whiff test)

Commercial tests for BV are available and can be used when microscopy is not available. They include Affirm VPIII, an automated DNA probe assay for detecting G. vaginalis[35]; OSOM BVBlue (Sekisui Diagnostics), a 10-minute CLIA waived chromogenic diagnostic test based on the presence of elevated sialidase enzyme activity, which is produced by bacterial pathogens including Gardnerella[56]; and Pip Activity TestCard (Quidel Corporation), a proline-aminopeptidase that detects proline iminopeptidase (PIP) activity found with *G vaginalis* and *Mobiluncus* spp.[57] Sensitivities and specificities for these tests are 95% and 100%, 90.3% and 96.6%, and 91.6% and 97.67%, respectively, compared to Gram stain or the Amsel criteria.[35,56,57]

INCORPORATING STI TESTING INTO THE OFFICE SETTING

All 50 states and the District of Columbia allow minors to consent for their own health services for STIs, although 11 states require that a minor be of a certain age (generally 12 or 14 years).[58] Physicians should become familiar with their own state laws and keep in mind that it is still necessary to abide by state laws for reporting of suspected abuse in minors. Although STI testing is recommended by many professional organizations, it is not always easy to incorporate into everyday office practices. Here are some useful tips to ensure a smoother process.

With adolescents and young adults, it is important to **incorporate an annual sexual history**[59] to determine the need for testing. Information can be gathered using forms/computer applications completed before the visit that the physician can review or through questions asked during the examination. The sexual history should be obtained confidentially to optimize responses. The key is to develop a rapport with your patient and to ask questions in a neutral, nonjudgmental manner. For further reference, see the Chlamydia Coalition Monograph, "Why Screen for Chlamydia? An Implementation Guide for Healthcare Providers" for more tips and resources.[59]

Attempt to keep services confidential.[59] Most states allow minors to receive confidential reproductive health services starting between ages 12 and 14 years.[58] The availability of confidential testing could make the difference between teenagers getting tested or not. Although the law allows for confidential testing, you should always disclose to the adolescents the reasons why you may have to breach confidentiality, including instances of abuse. Also, although you as a physician may not disclose testing, the explanation of benefits (EOBs), typically mailed to the health insurance policy holder, may include a list of services provided at the visit. Other ways to ensure confidentiality include allowing adolescents to pay cash for services, referring the patient to a Title X or public health clinic that can provide free or low-cost confidential services, or working with the insurance company to arrange for protection of confidential services.[59] Specific information on these strategies is available from the Chlamydia Coalition Web site (http://ncc.prevent.org/).

Make your office teen friendly.[59] There are many ways to make your office more teen friendly including:

- Offer hours that are convenient for teenagers
- Provide written information in areas where a teen would feel comfortable
- Provide free condoms
- Make brochures, condom packages small enough to fit into a pocket or purse
- Obtain a confidential phone number where the teen can be contacted directly
- Make it a policy that adolescents will be seen for a part of their visit without their parent or guardian present

Develop an STI testing and notification protocol for your office setting.[59] Having a standard protocol in place for STI testing can ensure that the office provides coordinated STI related care. The protocol should include the specific testing methods, including utilization of POCTs; methods for patient notification of positive or negative results; treatment options; partner notification and treatment guidelines; and positive STI follow-up protocols. Expedited partner therapy (EPT), permissible in 35 states and potentially allowable in 9 states, allows physicians to treat sex partners of patients positive for GC or CT without examination.[60] For more details about EPT, please refer to the position statement from the Society of Adolescent Health and Medicine and the American Academy of Pediatrics[61] as well as the CDC.[4] Once the protocols are developed, it is important to make sure that everyone in the practice, starting with the individual making the patient appointments, is on board and to have a plan to offer continuing education for physicians to ensure that the latest guidelines are being followed.[59]

References

1. Centers for Disease Control and Prevention. CDC Fact Sheet. Reported STDs in the United States. 2012 National data for chlamydia, gonorrhea, and syphilis. 2014. Available at: www.cdc.gov/nchhstp/newsroom/docs/STD-Trends-508.pdf. Accessed January 28, 2014
2. Centers for Disease Control and Prevention. *Sexually Transmitted Disease Surveillance 2012*. Atlanta, GA: US Department of Health and Human Services; 2012
3. Holmes K, Sparling PF, Stamm W, et al, ed. *Sexually Transmitted Diseases*. 4th ed. New York: McGraw-Hill Companies; 2008
4. Workowski KA, Berman S. Sexually transmitted diseases treatment guidelines, 2010. *MMWR Recomm Rep*. 2010;59(RR-12):1-110
5. Centers for Disease Control and Prevention. Sexually transmitted diseases. Syphilis—CDC fact sheet. Available at: www.cdc.gov/std/syphilis/STDFact-Syphilis-detailed.htm. Accessed January 28, 2014
6. US Preventive Services Task Force (USPSTF). A-Z topic guide. Available at: www.uspreventiveservicestaskforce.org/uspstf/uspstopics.htm. Accessed January 28, 2014
7. Kuypers J, Gaydos CA, Peeling RW. Principles of laboratory diagnosis of STIs. In: Holmes K, Sparling PF, Stamm W, et al, eds. *Sexually Transmitted Diseases*. 4th ed. New York: McGraw-Hill Companies; 2008:938-957
8. Cohen DA, Kanouse DE, Iguchi MY, Bluthenthal RN, Galvan FH, Bing EG. Screening for sexually transmitted diseases in non-traditional settings: a personal view. *Int J STD AIDS*. 2005;16(8):521-527
9. World Health Organization. From bench to bedside: setting a path for the translation of improved sexually transmitted infections diagnostics into health care delivery in the developing world Sexually transmitted diseases diagnostics initiative 2001. Available at: www.who.int/std_diagnostics/about_SDI/priorities.htm; 2009. Accessed January 28, 2014
10. Huppert J, Hesse H, Gaydos CA. What's the point? How point-of-care STI tests can impact infected patients. *Point Care*. 2010;9(1):36-46
11. Gaydos CA, van der Pol B, Jett-Goheen M, et al. Performance of the Cepheid CT/NG Xpert Rapid PCR Test for detection of *Chlamydia trachomatis* and *Neisseria gonorrhoeae*. *J Clin Microbiol*. 2013;51(6):1666-1672
12. Jafari Y, Peeling RW, Shivkumar S, et al. Are *Treponema pallidum* specific rapid and point-of-care tests for syphilis accurate enough for screening in resource limited settings? Evidence from a meta-analysis. *PLoS One*. 2013;8(2):e54695
13. Castro AR, Esfandiari J, Kumar S, et al. Novel point-of-care test for simultaneous detection of nontreponemal and treponemal antibodies in patients with syphilis. *J Clin Microbiol*. 2010;48(12):4615-4619

14. Guinard J, Prazuck T, Péré H, et al. Usefulness in clinical practice of a point-of-care rapid test for simultaneous detection of nontreponemal and *Treponema pallidum*-specific antibodies in patients suffering from documented syphilis. *Int J STD AIDS*. 2013;24(12):944-950
15. Stamm W. *Chlamydia trachomatis:* infections of the adult. In: Holmes K, Sparling PF, Stamm W, et al, eds. *Sexually Transmitted Diseases*. 4th ed. New York: McGraw-Hill Companies; 2008:575-593
16. Roche Molecular Diagnostics. Cobas® CT/NG v2.0 Test. Product insert
17. Gen-Probe. APTIMA Combo 2 Assay. Product insert. Available at: www.gen-probe.com/pdfs/pi/502446-IFU-PI__001_01.pdf. Accessed January 28, 2014
18. Becton Dickinson. ProbTec ET *Chlamydia trachomatis* and *Neisseria gonorrhoeae* Amplified Assays. Product insert
19. Becton Dickinson. ProbeTec *Neisseria gonorrhoeae* (GC) Qx Amplified DNA Assay. Product insert. Available at: http://moleculardiagnostics.bd.com/product/viperxtr/
20. Becton Dickinson. ProbeTec *Chlamydia trachomatis* (CT) Qx Amplified DNA Assay. Product insert. Available at: http://moleculardiagnostics.bd.com/product/viperxtr/
21. Abbott Molecular. Abbott RealTime CT/NG. Product insert. Available at: www.abbottmolecular.com/static/cms_workspace/pdfs/US/CTNG_8L07-91_US_FINAL.pdf. Accessed January 28, 2014
22. Papp J, Schachter J, Gaydos, C, VenDer Pol B. Recommendations for the laboratory-based detection of *Chlamydia trachomatis* and *Neisseria gonorrhoeae*–2014. *MMWR Morb Mortal Wkly Rep*. 2014;63(RR02):1-19
23. Chernesky M, Freund GG, Hook E III, et al. Detection of *Chlamydia trachomatis* and *Neisseria gonorrhoeae* infections in North American women by testing SurePath liquid-based Pap specimens in APTIMA assays. *J Clin Microbiol.* 2007;45:2434-2438
24. Chernesky M, Jang D, Portillo E, et al. *Comparison of three assays for detection of Chlamydia trachomatis* and *Neisseria gonorrhoeae* in SurePath Pap samples and the role of pre- and postcytology testing. *J Clin Microbiol.* 2012;50(4):1281-1284
25. Khader SN, Schlesinger K, Grossman J, Henry RI, Suhrland M, Fox AS. APTIMA assay on SurePath liquid-based cervical samples compared to endocervical swab samples facilitated by a real time database. *CytoJournal*. 2010;7:11
26. Hobbs MM, van der Pol B, Totten P, et al. From the NIH: proceedings of a workshop on the importance of self-obtained vaginal specimens for detection of sexually transmitted infections. *Sex Transm Dis*. 2008;35:8-13
27. Bachmann LH, Johnson RE, Cheng H, et al. Nucleic acid amplification tests for diagnosis of *Neisseria gonorrhoeae* and *Chlamydia trachomatis* rectal infections. *J Clin Microbiol.* 2010;48(5):1827-1832
28. Hook EW III, Handsfield HH. Gonococcal infections in the adult. In: Holmes K, Sparling PF, Stamm W, et al, eds. *Sexually Transmitted Diseases*. 4th ed. New York: McGraw-Hill Companies; 2008:627-646
29. Chernesky MA, Martin DH, Hook EW, et al. Ability of new APTIMA CT and APTIMA GC assays to detect *Chlamydia trachomatis* and *Neisseria gonorrhoeae* in male urine and urethral swabs. *J Clin Microbiol.* 2005;43(1):127-131
30. Bachmann LH, Johnson RE, Cheng H, et al. Nucleic acid amplification tests for diagnosis of *Neisseria gonorrhoeae* oropharyngeal infections. *J Clin Microbiol.* 2009;47:902-907
31. Hobbs MM, Sena AC, Swygard H, Schwebke JR. *Trichomonas vaginalis* and trichomoniasis. In: Holmes K, Sparling PF, Stamm W, et al, eds. *Sexually Transmitted Diseases*. 4th ed. New York: McGraw-Hill Companies; 2008:771-794
32. Association of Public Health Laboratories. Advances in laboratory detection of trichomonas vaginalis. Issues in brief: laboratory detection of trichomonas. August 2013. Available at: www.aphl.org/AboutAPHL/publications/Documents/ID_2013August_Advances-in-Laboratory-Detection-of-Trichomonas-vaginalis.pdf. Accessed January 28, 2014
33. Coleman JS, Gaydos CA, Witter F. *Trichomonas vaginalis* vaginitis in obstetrics and gynecology practice: new concepts and controversies. *Obstet Gynecol Surv*. 2013;68(1):43-50
34. Sekisui Diagnostics. OSOM trichomonas rapid test. Product insert. Available at: www.sekisuidiagnostics.com/pdf/OSOM_Trich_181_PI.pdf. Accessed January 28, 2014

35. Becton Dickinson. Affirm VPIII Microbial identification test. Package insert. Available at: www.bd.com/ds/technicalCenter/inserts/670160 JAA(201008).pdf. Accessed January 28, 2014
36. Gen-Probe. APTIMA trichomonas vaginalis assay. Package insert. Available at: www.gen-probe.com/pdfs/pi/503684-EN-RevA.pdf. Accessed January 28, 2014
37. Becton Dickinson. ProbeTec *Trichomonas vaginalis* (TV) Q*x* amplified DNA assay. Product insert. Available at: http://moleculardiagnostics.bd.com/product/viperxtr/
38. van der Pol B, Kraft CS, Williams JA. Use of an adaptation of a commercially available PCR assay aimed at diagnosis of chlamydia and gonorrhea to detect *Trichomonas vaginalis* in urogenital specimens. *J Clin Microbiol.* 2006;44(2):366-373
39. Nye MB, Schwebke JR, Body BA. Comparison of APTIMA *Trichomonas vaginalis* transcription-mediated amplification to wet mount microscopy, culture, and polymerase chain reaction for diagnosis of trichomoniasis in men and women. *Am J Obstet Gynecol.* 2009;200(2):188.e1-7
40. Sparling PF, Swartz MN, Musher DM, Healy BP. Clinical manifestations of syphilis. In: Holmes K, Sparling PF, Stamm W, et al, eds. *Sexually Transmitted Diseases.* 4th ed. New York: McGraw-Hill Companies; 2008:661-684
41. Centers for Disease Control and Prevention. Reverse sequence syphilis screening, an overview by the CDC. Available at: www.cdc.gov/std/syphilis/Syphilis-Webinar.htm. Accessed January 16, 2014
42. Association of Public Health Laboratories and CDC. Laboratory diagnostic testing for *Treponema pallidum*: expert consultation meeting summary report. January 13-15, 2009. Available at: www.aphl.org/aphlprograms/infectious/std/Documents/ID_2009Jan_Laboratory-Guidelines-Treponema-pallidum-Meeting-Report.pdf. Accessed January 28, 2014
43. Corey L, Wald A. Genital herpes. In: Holmes K, Sparling PF, Stamm W, et al, eds. *Sexually Transmitted Diseases.* 4th ed. New York: McGraw-Hill Companies; 2008:399-438
44. Gardella C. Herpes simplex virus genital infections: current concepts. *Curr Infect Dis Rep.* 2011;13(6):588-594
45. Ryder N, Jin F, McNulty AM, Grulich AE, Donovan B. Increasing role of herpes simplex virus type 1 in first-episode anogenital herpes in heterosexual women and younger men who have sex with men, 1992-2006. *Sex Transm Infect.* 2009;85(6):416-419
46. Benedetti J, Corey L, Ashley R. Recurrence rates in genital herpes after symptomatic first-episode infection. *Ann Intern Med.* 1994;121(11):847-854
47. Engelberg R, Carrell D, Krantz E, Corey L, Wald A. Natural history of genital herpes simplex virus type 1 infection. *Sex Transm Dis.* 2003;30(2):174-177
48. Anderson NW, Buchan BW, Ledeboer NA. Light microscopy, culture, molecular, and serologic methods for detection of herpes simplex virus. *J Clin Microbiol.* 2014;52(1):2-8
49. Wald A, Huang ML, Carrell D, Selke S, Corey L. Polymerase chain reaction for detection of herpes simplex virus (HSV) DNA on mucosal surfaces: comparison with HSV isolation in cell culture. *J Infect Dis.* 2003;188(9):1345-1351
50. Morrow RA, Friedrich D. Inaccuracy of certain commercial enzyme immunoassays in diagnosing genital infections with herpes simplex virus types 1 or 2. *Am J Clin Pathol.* 2003;120(6):839-844
51. Myers ER, McCrory DC, Nanda K, et al. Mathematical model for the natural history of human papillomavirus infection and cervical carcinogenesis. *Am J Epidemiol.* 2000;151:1158-1171
52. Centers for Disease Control and Prevention. Human papillomavirus-associated cancers—United States, 2004–2008. *MMWR Morb Mortal Wkly Rep.* 2012;61:258
53. Sobel JD. Vulvovaginal candidiasis. In: Holmes K, Sparling PF, Stamm W, et al, eds. *Sexually Transmitted Diseases.* 4th ed. New York: McGraw-Hill Companies; 2008:823-838
54. Hillier SL, Marrazzo JM, Holmes KK. Bacterial vaginosis. In: Holmes K, Sparling PF, Stamm W, et al, eds. *Sexually Transmitted Diseases.* 4th ed. New York: McGraw-Hill Companies; 2008:737-768
55. Ison CA, Hay PE. Validation of a simplified grading of Gram stained vaginal smears for use in genitourinary medicine clinics. *Sex Transm Infect.* 2002;78:413
56. Sekisui Diagnostics. OSOM BVBlue Test. Product insert
57. Quidel Corporation. QuickVue Advance *G. vaginalis* test. Product insert

58. Guttmacher Institute. State policies in brief: minors' access to STI services. Available at: www.guttmacher.org/statecenter/spibs/spib_ MASS.pdf. Accessed January 20, 2014
59. Partnership for Prevention. *Why Screen for Chlamydia? An Implementation Guide for Health Care Providers.* 2nd ed. Washington, DC: Partnership for Prevention; 2012. Available at: ncc.prevent.org/body/WhyScreen-2012-update.pdf. Accessed January 20, 2014
60. Centers for Disease Control and Prevention. Sexually transmitted diseases. Legal status of expedited partner therapy (EPT). Available at: www.cdc.gov/std/ept/legal/default.htm. Accessed January 20, 2014
61. Burstein GR, Eliscu A, Ford K, et al. Expedited partner therapy for adolescents diagnosed with chlamydia or gonorrhea: a position paper of the Society for Adolescent Medicine. *J Adolesc Health.* 2009;45(3):303-309
62. Luminex Molecular Technology. MultiCode®-RTx HSV 1&2 kit. Product insert
63. Becton Dickinson. BD ProbeTec™ herpes simplex viruses (HSV 1 & 2) Q*x* amplified DNA assays. Product insert
64. BioHelix. IsoAmp® HSV assay. Product insert

Adolesc Med 025 (2014) 316–331

Antimicrobial Resistance in *Neisseria gonorrhoeae*

Sarah Kidd, MD, MPH[a*]; Robert D. Kirkcaldy, MD, MPH[a]; Gale R. Burstein, MD, MPH[b]

[a]*Division of STD Prevention, National Center for HIV/AIDS, Viral Hepatitis, STD and TB Prevention, Centers for Disease Control and Prevention, Atlanta, Georgia;* [b]*Erie County Department of Health, Buffalo, New York, and Department of Pediatrics, SUNY at Buffalo School of Medicine and Biomedical Sciences, Buffalo, New York*

INTRODUCTION

Gonorrhea is the second most commonly reported notifiable disease in the United States. In 2012, a total of 334,826 gonorrhea cases were reported nationwide to the Centers for Disease Control and Prevention (CDC).[1] However, case detection and case reporting are known to be incomplete, and it is estimated that the true number of new gonococcal infections in the United States exceeds 800,000 per year.[2] Adolescents aged 15 to 19 years and young adults aged 20 to 24 years are disproportionately affected by gonorrhea; they accounted for 58.7% of all gonorrhea cases reported in the United States in 2012. As in previous years, the 2012 gonorrhea rates among adolescents (376.8 cases per 100,000 population) and young adults (520.1 cases per 100,000 population) were significantly greater than the overall national rate (107.5 cases per 100,000 population).

Neisseria gonorrhoeae can infect the urogenital tract, rectum, oropharynx, and conjunctivae, and it is transmitted almost exclusively through sexual contact or perinatally.[3] Urogenital infection may be associated with dysuria and urethral discharge in males or cervical discharge in females, but most urogenital infections in females and a substantial minority in males are asymptomatic.[3-5] Rectal infection most often is asymptomatic but may be associated with rectal pain, discharge, bleeding, or tenesmus.[3] Similarly, pharyngeal infection most often is

*Corresponding author:
E-mail address: skidd@cdc.gov

 ISSN 1934-4287

asymptomatic but may be associated with sore throat or pharyngeal exudate.[3] Disseminated gonorrhea is rare, occurring in less than 3% of untreated acute gonococcal infections, but it can be life threatening when complicated by endocarditis or meningitis.[3] More common complications of gonococcal infection include pelvic inflammatory disease, tubal infertility, and ectopic pregnancy, as well as facilitated transmission and acquisition of human immunodeficiency virus (HIV).[3,6]

The timely administration of effective treatment for infected patients and their partners, preferably in the form of a single-dose regimen, has been a critical tool for gonorrhea control efforts. Timely and effective treatment limits the duration of infection in affected individuals, thereby minimizing transmission to others and risk of complications within the infected individual. For these reasons, CDC has historically recommended only treatment regimens that are at least 95% effective against *N gonorrhoeae* infection.[7] However, the number of highly effective treatment options for gonorrhea is diminishing because *N gonorrhoeae* has proven to be adept at developing antimicrobial resistance. *N gonorrhoeae* has progressively acquired resistance to each of the antimicrobials previously recommended as first-line treatment of gonorrhea, leaving only 1 regimen that is currently recommended by CDC: dual treatment with ceftriaxone 250 mg intramuscularly plus azithromycin 1 g orally.[8] As gonococcal susceptibility to cephalosporins has declined over the last decade, the emergence of gonococcal resistance to cephalosporins, including ceftriaxone, seems inevitable. Antimicrobial-resistant *N gonorrhoeae* has been declared an urgent public health threat, and experts are warning that an era of "untreatable" gonorrhea may be on the horizon.[9,10] This article refers to the management of adolescents by physicians, physician assistants, nurse practitioners, and other health care providers, hereinafter referred to as "clinicians." Clinicians and public health officials should be aware of the threat of cephalosporin-resistant gonorrhea and should take action now to mitigate its effect on patients and public health.

HISTORY OF GONOCOCCAL ANTIMICROBIAL RESISTANCE IN THE UNITED STATES

Resistance to Sulfonamides, Penicillin, and Tetracycline

Gonorrhea treatment and control have been complicated by antimicrobial resistance ever since the introduction and widespread use of antimicrobials in the 1930s. The first class of antimicrobials to be introduced, the sulfonamides, revolutionized the management of patients with gonorrhea, but treatment failures were common.[11] By 1944, it was reported that approximately 30% of patients with uncomplicated gonorrhea failed to respond to the standard 5- to 7-day course of sulfonamide therapy, and 15% to 20% also failed a second course of therapy.[12] When penicillin became available in the 1940s, it quickly replaced the sulfonamides as the drug of choice for treatment of gonorrhea.[12,13] However, gonococcal susceptibility to penicillin gradually declined from 1945 to 1969 as the result of the accumulation of multiple chromosomal mutations.[14-16] This decline in penicillin susceptibility prompted progressive increases in the recommended therapeutic dose, from a total dose of 50,000 to 200,000 units in the mid-1940s to 4.8 million units in 1972.[12,13,17-20] The addition of probenecid, to be coadministered with penicillin, was recommended by the early 1970s to maintain penicillin's efficacy against *N gonorrhoeae*.[20,21] High-level penicillin resistance, conferred by plasma-mediated production of penicillinase and resistance to even the highest doses of penicillin, was first reported in 1976 in the United States in 2 patients who acquired gonococcal urethritis in the Philippines.[22,23] In the same year, a different strain of penicillinase-producing *N gonorrhoeae* (PPNG), linked to West Africa, was reported from the United Kingdom.[24-26] Within a few years, PPNG had been identified throughout the world, and multiple outbreaks had been reported in the United States.[27,28] By 1989, resistance to penicillin, both PPNG and chromosomally mediated *N gonorrhoeae*, was widespread throughout the United States, and penicillin was no longer recommended for treatment of gonorrhea.[29] In the meantime, tetracycline had become available and was added as a recommended regimen for gonorrhea treatment in 1978.[30] However, gonococcal resistance to tetracycline increased alongside resistance to penicillin, and high-level tetracycline resistance was soon detected in the United States.[31-33] By 1985, tetracycline was no longer recommended as a first-line gonorrhea treatment regimen.[34] Ceftriaxone was added as a first-line regimen in 1985, and when penicillin was no longer recommended in 1989, ceftriaxone became the only recommended treatment of gonorrhea.[29,34] Oral fluoroquinolones (ciprofloxacin and ofloxacin) and cefixime (an oral third-generation cephalosporin) were first added as recommended first-line regimens in 1993.[35]

The US Gonococcal Isolate Surveillance Project

As concerns about antimicrobial-resistant gonorrhea grew in the 1980s, in 1986 the CDC established a national sentinel surveillance system to monitor gonococcal resistance in the United States, the Gonococcal Isolate Surveillance Project (GISP).[36] GISP collects approximately 5000 to 6000 urethral isolates per year from symptomatic men attending sexually transmitted infection clinics in 25 to 30 cities throughout the United States. GISP has monitored trends in gonococcal susceptibility to penicillin, tetracycline, ciprofloxacin, and other antimicrobials over time (Figure 1) and has provided a rational basis for determining which treatment regimens the CDC should recommend.

Fluoroquinolone Resistance

GISP data, in conjunction with supplemental susceptibility data provided by state and local health departments, were instrumental in detecting and documenting the emergence of fluoroquinolone resistance in the United States. In the early 1990s, fluoroquinolone resistance was emerging in Asia and the Western

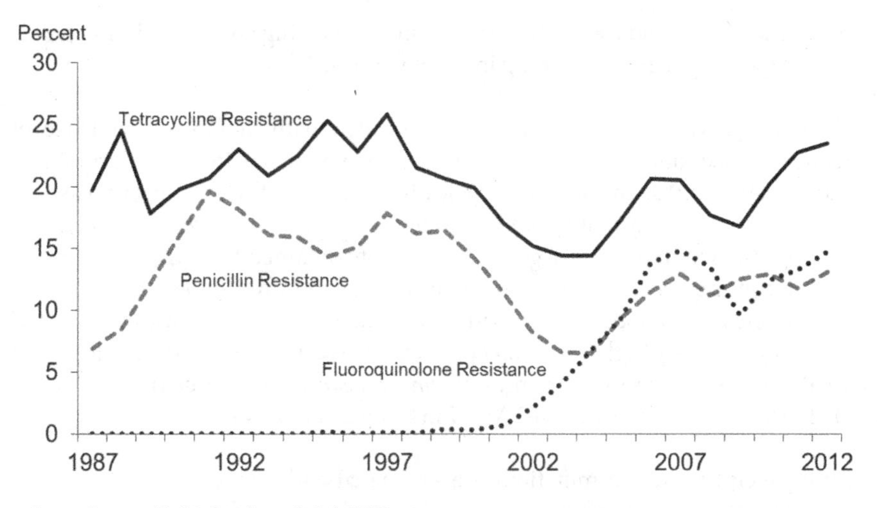

Fig 1. Prevalence of penicillin, tetracycline, and fluoroquinolone resistance in urethral *Neisseria gonorrhoeae* isolates in the United States, 1987-2012.

Pacific and had already been detected in Hawaii in patients who had recently traveled to or whose sex partners had recently traveled to Southeast Asia.[37-39] Sporadic cases of fluoroquinolone resistance were detected in the United States throughout the 1990s, and gradually became more common, primarily in Hawaii and on the West Coast.[40-42] By 1999, 14.3% of GISP isolates from Honolulu exhibited resistance to fluoroquinolones, compared with 0.2% of isolates obtained from the continental United States and Alaska, and in 2000 fluoroquinolones were no longer recommended for gonorrhea treatment in Hawaii.[42,43] Shortly after, similar increases were observed in California, and fluoroquinolones were no longer advised in California in 2002.[44,45] Over the next few years, fluoroquinolone resistance became widespread throughout the United States, first among men who have sex with men (MSM) and then among heterosexuals,[46,47] so in 2007 fluoroquinolones were no longer recommended for treatment of gonorrhea anywhere in the United States. This again left the third-generation cephalosporins (intramuscular [IM] ceftriaxone or oral cefixime) as the only remaining class of drugs recommended for treatment of gonorrhea.[47]

DECLINING GONOCOCCAL SUSCEPTIBILITY TO CEPHALOSPORINS

Worryingly, there is evidence that *N gonorrhoeae* is beginning to develop resistance to cephalosporins. Although the in vitro susceptibility breakpoint that correlates with clinically significant cephalosporin resistance has not yet been defined, at the population level, the minimum inhibitory concentrations (MICs) of cephalosporins required to inhibit *N gonorrhoeae* growth in the laboratory have been increasing in Asia for more than a decade and more recently in Australia, Europe, Canada, and the United States, indicating gonococcal susceptibility to cephalosporins is declining in these regions.[48-52]

Cases of cefixime treatment failures associated with laboratory evidence of reduced susceptibility have been detected in Asia since 1999, in Europe and Canada since 2010, and in South Africa in 2012.[53-61] Of most concern, cases of ceftriaxone treatment failure and resistance have now been reported in Japan, France, and Spain. In 2009, a gonococcal isolate obtained from the pharynx of a female commercial sex worker in Japan who failed to respond to a 1-g dose of ceftriaxone intravenously was found to have an MIC of 2 to 4 mcg/mL, an MIC that is significantly higher than any previously described ceftriaxone MIC.[62,63] In 2010 and 2011, a second strain of *N gonorrhoeae* with high ceftriaxone MICs (1-2 mcg/mL) was detected in 3 MSM in France and Spain.[59,64]

Multiple chromosomal mutations are associated with reduced susceptibility to cephalosporins, including mutations in *penA*, which encodes penicillin-binding protein 2, the primary target for the cephalosporins; *mtrR*, which alters expression of an efflux pump and affects efflux of antimicrobials from the bacterial cell; *penB*, which encodes an outer membrane protein channel that affects drug entry; and at least 1 other unknown determinant, termed "factor X."[65] High-level cephalosporin resistance seems to result from the combined effect of these mutations, the most important of which is *penA*. Many strains of *N gonorrhoeae* with reduced susceptibility to cephalosporins contain regions of *penA* genes (mosaic *penA*) apparently acquired from commensal *Neisseria* species commonly residing in the oropharynx, suggesting that pharyngeal gonococcal infections may provide the opportunity for horizontal transfer of DNA and resistance mutations between *Neisseria* species.

Although no cefixime or ceftriaxone treatment failures have been documented in the United States, the proportion of GISP isolates with elevated cefixime and ceftriaxone MICs increased during 2000 to 2011. The proportion of GISP isolates with elevated cefixime MICs (MIC ≥0.25 mcg/mL) was stable at 0.1% to 0.2% during 2000 to 2006 but increased to 1.4% in 2010 and 2011 (Figure 2).[1,52] The proportion of GISP isolates with elevated ceftriaxone MICs (MIC ≥0.125) has remained low but increased from 0.1% in 2000 to 0.3% in 2010 and to 0.4% in 2011 (Figure 2).[1,52] As was seen with the emergence of fluoroquinolone resistance, during 2000 to 2010 the greatest increases in cefixime MICs were seen in the West and among MSM.[52] In the West, the proportion of isolates with elevated cefixime MICs increased from 0% in 2000 to 3.3% in 2010 but remained 0.5% or less in other regions of the country. Among MSM, the proportion of isolates with elevated cefixime MICs increased from 0% in 2000 to 4.0% in 2010. In comparison, among men who have sex exclusively with women (MSW), the proportion of isolates with elevated MICs remained less than 0.5%. The greatest increases in MICs were observed among MSM in the West and Midwest.

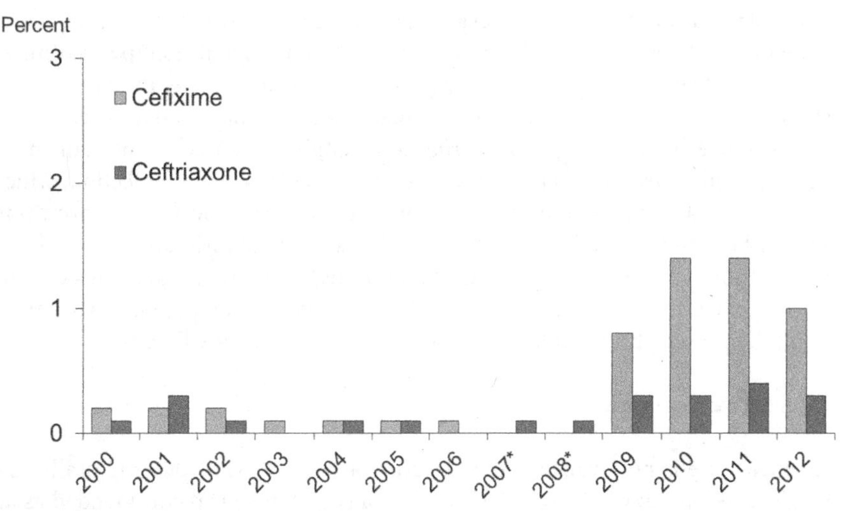

Fig 2. Prevalence of urethral *Neisseria gonorrhoeae* isolates with elevated cefixime minimum inhibitory concentrations (MICs) (MIC ≥0.25 mcg/mL) and elevated ceftriaxone MICs (MIC ≥0.125 mcg/mL) in the United States, 2000-2012.

Because of the observed declines in susceptibility to cephalosporins, particularly cefixime, globally and in the United States in the previous decade, the CDC began recommending dual therapy (either ceftriaxone or cefixime plus either azithromycin or doxycycline) for all cases of gonorrhea in 2010.[66] In 2012, recommendations were revised once again, and cefixime was no longer recommended as a first-line regimen for treatment of gonorrhea.[67]

In 2012, the most recent year for which complete GISP data are available, the proportion of GISP isolates with elevated cephalosporin MICs decreased slightly compared with 2011 (Figure 2): 1.0% had elevated cefixime MICs, and 0.3% had elevated ceftriaxone MICs.[1] Although it is encouraging that cephalosporin MICs did not continue to increase in 2012, it will be important to monitor gonococcal susceptibility to cephalosporins closely in the coming years.

RECOMMENDED TREATMENT OF UNCOMPLICATED GONOCOCCAL INFECTION

Recommended Regimen

As of 2014, the only recommended first-line treatment regimen for uncomplicated gonococcal infection in adolescents and adults is dual therapy with ceftriaxone 250 mg in a single IM dose plus azithromycin 1 g orally in a single dose.[8] Because of the high prevalence of tetracycline resistance among GISP isolates, particularly among those with elevated cefixime MICs, azithromycin is now preferred over doxycycline as the second antimicrobial. Dual therapy minimizes the risk of transmission of resistant *N gonorrhoeae* as long as the organism is susceptible to at least 1 of the antimicrobials used and may hinder development of resistance by targeting *N gonorrhoeae* through more than 1 mechanism of action. Azithromycin also provides coverage for chlamydial coinfection, which is common among patients with gonorrhea.[68] Ceftriaxone and azithromycin should be administered together, preferably simultaneously and under direct observation. For clinical settings that do not dispense oral medications on site, prescriptions for azithromycin should be accompanied by patient instructions to fill the prescription and take azithromycin as soon as possible.

Alternative Regimen

If ceftriaxone is not available, dual treatment with cefixime 400 mg orally as a single dose plus azithromycin 1 g orally as a single dose is recommended as an alternative regimen for patients with uncomplicated urogenital or rectal gonorrhea. Pharyngeal infections are more difficult to eradicate, and ceftriaxone is clearly more effective than cefixime for treatment of gonococcal infection of the pharynx, with a 99% cure rate (95% confidence interval [CI] 94.4%-100%) for ceftriaxone compared with a 92.3% cure rate (95% CI 74.9%-99.1%) for cefixime.[69] Therefore, cefixime or cefixime-based regimens are not recommended for treatment of pharyngeal gonorrhea.

A recent clinical trial of patients aged 15 to 60 years demonstrated the effectiveness of 2 new dual-therapy regimens for urogenital gonococcal infection: gemifloxacin 320 mg orally plus azithromycin 2 g orally (99.5% cure rate, lower 1-sided 95% CI bound = 97.5%), and gentamicin 240 mg intramuscularly plus azithromycin 2 g orally (100% cure rate, lower 1-sided 95% CI bound = 98.5%).[70] These regimens may be considered as additional alternative regimens for treatment of uncomplicated urogenital gonorrhea if ceftriaxone is not available. Both regimens cured the small numbers of rectal and pharyngeal infections included in the trial, but the trial was not powered to estimate the efficacy of these regimens for extragenital infections. Additionally, the gastrointestinal side effects associated with these regimens may limit their use in many settings. Overall, 7.7% of patients treated with gemifloxacin plus azithromycin and 3.3% of patients treated with gentamicin and azithromycin vomited within 1 hour and required retreatment with a different regimen.

Other Antimicrobials

Higher-dose azithromycin (2 g) is effective as monotherapy against uncomplicated urogenital and rectal *N gonorrhoeae* infection. The proportion of GISP isolates with elevated azithromycin MICs has remained less than 1%, with no apparent temporal trend.[1,71,72] However, azithromycin monotherapy is not recommended because of the ease with which *N gonorrhoeae* develops resistance to macrolide antimicrobials, and because high-level azithromycin resistance has already been detected on multiple continents, including North America.[73-77] Because resistance to penicillin, tetracycline, and ciprofloxacin has persisted in the United States, returning to empiric use of any of these previously recommended antimicrobials as a first-line treatment regimen is not an option. In 2012, 13.1% of GISP isolates were resistant to penicillin, 23.5% were resistant to tetracycline, and 14.7% were resistant to ciprofloxacin.[1] Spectinomycin is effective for treatment of urogenital and rectal infections, but it does not reliably cure pharyngeal infections and is not currently available in the United States, and resistance has emerged rapidly when it has been widely used in the past.[69,78] Monotherapy with gentamicin has been considered as a potential treatment option, but a recent meta-analysis demonstrated a pooled cure rate of 91.5% (95% CI 88.1%-94.0%) for urogenital gonorrhea and therefore was not sufficiently effective to be recommended on its own.[79]

Management of Sex Partners

Clinical management of a patient with gonorrhea must include appropriate treatment of the patient's recent sex partners (any partners within the 60 days preceding a patient's onset of symptoms or diagnosis of gonorrhea) in order to prevent reinfection of the index patient and to prevent further transmission in the community. Ideally, sex partners would be evaluated in a clinic-based setting and treated with the recommended regimen of ceftriaxone plus azithromycin. However, in states where expedited partner therapy (EPT) for gonorrhea is permissible and if prompt evaluation and treatment cannot be assured, EPT with the alternative regimen (cefixime plus azithromycin), delivered to the partner by the patient, disease investigation specialist, or collaborating pharmacy, should be offered to females and heterosexual males. EPT is not recommended as a routine partner management strategy for partners of MSM because of the high risk of undiagnosed sexually transmitted infection or HIV coinfection. Legal status of EPT by state is available at www.cdc.gov/std/ept/legal.

DETECTION AND DIAGNOSIS OF ANTIMICROBIAL-RESISTANT GONORRHEA

Detection of antimicrobial resistant gonorrhea begins with detection of gonorrhea. Patients with genitourinary symptoms or physical examination findings consistent with urethritis/cervicitis, and those who report having had sexual contact with a person recently diagnosed with gonorrhea, should be tested for *N gonorrhoeae* infection at the anatomic site(s) of exposure (urogenital tract, rectum, and/or pharynx). Because urogenital gonococcal infection in females frequently is asymptomatic, the CDC, the US Preventive Services Task Force, and the American Academy of Pediatrics (AAP) recommend annual screening for gonococcal infection for all sexually active females who are at increased risk for infection.[8,80,81] Females younger than 25 years, including sexually active adolescents, are at highest risk for gonococcal infection.[1] Other risk factors for gonococcal infection include previous history of gonococcal infection, other sexually transmitted infections, new or multiple sex partners, inconsistent condom use, commercial sex work, and drug use.[8,80] The CDC also recommends screening MSM at least annually for gonococcal infection at all anatomic sites of exposure.[8]

Nucleic acid amplification tests (NAATs) have largely replaced gonococcal culture for gonorrhea diagnosis in most clinical settings.[82] NAATs are more sensitive than culture for detecting *N gonorrhoeae*, have comparable specificity, and can be performed on a wider variety of specimen types, including urine.[83-88] In addition, compared with gonococcal culture, NAATs have less stringent storage and transport requirements. Although NAATs have not been cleared by the US Food and Drug Administration (FDA) for use at pharyngeal and rectal sites, some public and commercial laboratories, including laboratories such as Quest and LabCorp, have conducted verification studies, allowing use of these tests for clinical management. Unfortunately, at present, antimicrobial susceptibility testing cannot be conducted on NAAT specimens. As a result, the increased use of NAATs, accompanied by diminished access to gonococcal culture, has complicated detection and confirmation of antimicrobial resistance in *N gonorrhoeae*.

Few clinical settings continue to use culture for the routine diagnosis of gonorrhea, and antimicrobial susceptibility testing is generally not routinely conducted outside of surveillance programs. Therefore, in order to detect cephalosporin-resistant gonorrhea, clinicians must be vigilant for possible cephalosporin treatment failures. Clinicians should suspect gonorrhea treatment failure and resistance in patients who have persistent or recurrent symptoms and who report no re-exposure following treatment with the recommended regimen. For patients who report their partners have been treated, clinicians should take a careful history that includes timing of patient and partner treatment and resumption of sexual activity. Detection of treatment failure or resistance in patients with asymptomatic infection requires a test of cure. Routine test of cure currently is not recommended for patients who receive the recommended first-line regimen, but test of cure is recommended for patients with pharyngeal gonorrhea who are treated with an alternative regimen.[8] If culture is used, test of cure may be performed 7 days after treatment. The optimal timing of test of cure using a NAAT is not yet clear. If performed too soon after treatment, NAATs can detect nonviable nucleic acids that persist after eradication of infection, causing a false-positive NAAT result.[89,90] For this reason, the current CDC recommendation is to perform test of cure 14 days after treatment if a NAAT is being used.[19]

MANAGEMENT OF SUSPECTED CEPHALOSPORIN TREATMENT FAILURE OR RESISTANCE

Clinicians who suspect cephalosporin treatment failure or resistance based on clinical history or laboratory data should report these cases to the CDC through the local or state health department within 24 hours of diagnosis and should consult a specialist in infectious diseases, the local or state health department, or the CDC for advice on obtaining cultures, antimicrobial susceptibility testing, and appropriate treatment. Guidance regarding which laboratories can process clinical *N gonorrhoeae* culture specimens is best obtained from the local or state health department. Patients with suspected cephalosporin treatment failure should be retested for *N gonorrhoeae* using culture, preferably with simultaneous NAAT, at exposed anatomic sites. If gonococcal culture is positive, *N gonorrhoeae* isolates should be tested for antimicrobial susceptibility and retained for possible additional testing.

Because suspected treatment failures following treatment with the recommended regimen (dual treatment with IM ceftriaxone 250 mg plus oral azithromycin 1 g) are most likely to be reinfections, retreatment with the recommended regimen should be given in most cases. Patients with suspected treatment failure after treatment with an alternative regimen (oral cefixime 400 mg plus oral azithromycin 1 g) should be treated with IM ceftriaxone 250 mg plus oral azithromycin 2 g. For patients in whom treatment failure is likely because of cephalosporin resistance (eg, the collected isolate exhibits elevated cephalosporin MICs, the patient reports no reexposure and fails a second course of the recommended regimen, or the patient has other evidence of exposure to cephalosporin-resistant *N gonorrhoeae*), dual treatment with oral gemifloxacin 320 mg plus oral azithromycin 2 g or dual treatment with IM gentamicin 240 mg plus oral azithromycin 2 g may be considered. A test of cure should be conducted 7 to 14 days after retreatment, preferably using culture. Identifying and treating sex partners of patients with suspected treatment failure is a priority. Sex partners within the 60 days preceding the initial onset of symptoms or diagnosis of gonorrhea in the patient, as well as any sex partners since the initial diagnosis, should be evaluated for *N gonorrhoeae* infection by culture and antimicrobial susceptibility testing and treated as indicated.

PUBLIC HEALTH RESPONSE TO THE THREAT OF CEPHALOSPORIN RESISTANCE

In the absence of new treatment options, cephalosporin-resistant gonorrhea would significantly impair gonorrhea control in the United States and worldwide. A key component of the public health response to resistant gonorrhea is strengthening surveillance for gonococcal susceptibility and improving the ability to detect emerging antimicrobial resistance. To do so, local laboratory capacity for gonococcal culture and antimicrobial susceptibility testing must be rebuilt. As a national sentinel surveillance system, GISP samples approximately 2% of all gonorrhea cases reported nationally, so large gaps in surveillance exist throughout the country. Local access to gonococcal culture and antimicrobial susceptibility testing are critical not only for enhancing local surveillance but also for confirmation of resistance in suspected treatment failures and for informing treatment decisions for patients who are not successfully treated with a CDC-recommended regimen. Health departments are encouraged to assess which local laboratories perform gonococcal culture and antimicrobial susceptibility testing and to facilitate linkages between these laboratories and clinics, either through referral systems or through increased availability of the appropriate culture plates or transport media.

A second component of the public health response is increasing general gonorrhea prevention and control activities that reduce the overall gonorrhea disease burden. Clinicians play an important role in this strategy, which includes screening high-risk populations, such as females younger than 25 years and MSM, to identify new infections; assuring that patients are treated quickly with the most effective regimen available; evaluating and treating patients' sex partners; and providing risk-reduction counseling. When cases of suspected cephalosporin treatment failure or cephalosporin resistance are identified, health departments should prioritize these cases for investigation, report them to the CDC, and work with clinicians to facilitate evaluation and appropriate treatment of the sex partners of these cases.

In the long run, successful gonorrhea control will require new antimicrobials or antimicrobial combinations that are effective against *N gonorrhoeae*. Unfortunately, the number of new antimicrobials developed and approved has decreased significantly over the last 30 years, and few new antimicrobials are in the development pipeline.[9] Just 2 new antimicrobials, solithromycin and delafloxacin, have entered clinical trials for treatment of gonorrhea.[91,92] A fluoroketolide, solithromycin has greater in vitro potency against *N gonorrhoeae* than other macrolides, including azithromycin; it also has high in vitro activity against cephalosporin-resistant and multidrug-resistant strains, and the results of early clinical trials are promising.[93] Delafloxacin, a novel fluoroquinolone, exhibits high in vitro activity against *N gonorrhoeae*, including ciprofloxacin-resistant isolates.[94] Additional treatment options are urgently needed. Promoting the development of new antimicrobials for gonorrhea must be a priority.

CONCLUSION

Given previous experience with other classes of antimicrobials, it seems inevitable that gonococcal resistance to cephalosporins, including ceftriaxone, eventually will emerge in the United States, severely limiting treatment options and impairing gonorrhea control. Because adolescents and young adults are the age groups most affected by gonorrhea, they and their clinical providers are on the frontlines of the public health battle to delay the emergence and mitigate the effect of cephalosporin resistance. It is critical that clinicians providing care for adolescents and young adults screen high-risk populations to identify gonococcal infections, treat patients infected with *N gonorrhoeae* and their partners with the most effective regimen available, maintain vigilance for cephalosporin treatment failures, and team with public health officials to assure the early detection and rapid response to suspected cephalosporin treatment failure or resistance.

References

1. Centers for Disease Control and Prevention. *Sexually Transmitted Disease Surveillance 2012.* Atlanta, GA: US Department of Health and Human Services; 2014
2. Satterwhite CL, Torrone E, Meites E, et al. Sexually transmitted infections among US women and men: prevalence and incidence estimates, 2008. *Sex Transm Dis.* 2013;40(3):187-193
3. Hook EW, Handsfield HH. Gonococcal infections in the adult. In: Holmes KK, Sparling PF, Stamm WE, et al, eds. *Sexually Transmitted Diseases.* 4th ed. New York: McGraw Hill; 2008:627-645
4. Peterman TA, Tian LH, Metcalf CA, et al. High incidence of new sexually transmitted infections in the year following a sexually transmitted infection: a case for rescreening. *Ann Intern Med.* 2006;145(8):564-572
5. Handsfield HH, Lipman TO, Harnisch JP, Tronca E, Holmes KK. Asymptomatic gonorrhea in men: diagnosis, natural course, prevalence and significance. *N Engl J Med.* 1974;290(3):117-123
6. Fleming DT, Wasserheit JN. From epidemiological synergy to public health policy and practice: the contribution of other sexually transmitted diseases to sexual transmission of HIV infection. *Sex Transm Dis.* 1999;75(1):3-17
7. Handsfield HH, McCutchan JA, Corey L, Ronald AR. Evaluation of new anti-infective drugs for the treatment of uncomplicated gonorrhea in adults and adolescents. *Clin Infect Dis.* 1992;15(Suppl 1):S123-S1130
8. Centers for Disease Control and Prevention. Sexually transmitted diseases treatment guidelines, 2014. *MMWR.* 2014;(In press)
9. Centers for Disease Control and Prevention. *Antibiotic Resistance Threats In The United States, 2013.* Atlanta, GA: US Department of Health and Human Services; 2013
10. Bolan GA, Sparling PP, Wassherheit JN. The emerging threat of untreatable gonococcal infection. *N Engl J Med.* 2012;366(6):485-487
11. Kampmeier RH. Introduction of sulfonamide therapy for gonorrhea. *Sex Transm Dis.* 1983;10(2): 81-84
12. Turner TB, Sternberg TH. Management of venereal diseases in the army. *JAMA.* 1944;124(3):133-137
13. Herrell WE, Cook EN, Thompson L. Use of penicillin in sulfonamide resistant gonorrheal infections. *JAMA.* 1943;122(5):289-292
14. Garson W, Barton GD. Problems in the diagnosis and treatment of gonorrhea. *Public Health Rep.* 1960;75(2):119-123
15. Martin JE, Lester A, Price EV, Schmale JD. Comparative study of gonococcal susceptibility to penicillin in the United States, 1955-1969. *J Infect Dis.* 1970;122(3):459-461
16. Ison CA. Antimicrobial agents and gonorrhoea: therapeutic choice, resistance and susceptibility testing. *Genitourin Med.* 1996;72:253-257
17. Koch RA, Haines JS, Hollingsworth WY. Evaluation of penicillin in gonorrhea treatment and control. *JAMA.* 1945;129(7):491-495
18. Sternberg TH, Turner TB. The treatment of sulfonamide resistant gonorrhea with penicillin sodium. *JAMA.* 1944;126(3):157-161
19. Doubling of dosage of penicillin in treating gonorrhea recommended. *JAMA.* 1965;193(8):23-26
20. Center for Disease Control. Recommended treatment schedules for gonorrhea. *Ann Intern Med.* 1972;76(6):991
21. Holmes KK, Karney WW, Harnisch JP, Wiesner PJ, Turck M, Pedersen AH. Single-dose aqueous procaine penicillin G therapy for gonorrhea: use of probenecid and cause of treatment failure. *J Infect Dis.* 1973;127(4):455-460
22. Center for Disease Control. Penicillinase-producing Neisseria gonorrhoeae. *MMWR.* 1976;25(33):261
23. Ashford WA, Golash RG, Hemming VG. Penicillinase-producing Neisseria gonorrhoeae. *Lancet.* 1976;ii:657-658

24. Phillips I. Beta-lactamase-producing penicillin-resistant gonococcus. *Lancet.* 1976;ii:656-657
25. Percival A, Corkill JE, Arya OP, et al. Penicillinase-producing gonococci in Liverpool. *Lancet.* 1976;ii:1379-1382
26. Perine PL, Schalla W, Siegel MS, Thornsberry C, Biddle J, Wong K. Evidence for two distinct types of penicillinase-producing Neisseria gonorrhoeae. *Lancet.* 1977;2:993-995
27. Centers for Disease Control and Prevention. Follow-up on penicillinase-producing *Neisseria gonorrhoeae*—worldwide. *MMWR.* 1977;26(19):153-154
28. Perine PL, Morton RS, Piot P, Siegel MS, Antal GM. Epidemiology and treatment of penicillinase-producing *Neisseria gonorrhoeae. Sex Transm Dis.* 1979;6(2):152-158
29. Centers for Disease Control and Prevention. 1989 Sexually transmitted diseases treatment guidelines. *MMWR.* 1989;38(S-8):1-43
30. Center for Disease Control and Prevention. Gonorrhea: Center for Disease Control recommended treatment schedules, 1979. *Ann Intern Med.* 1979;90:809-811
31. Jaffe HW, Biddle JW, Johnson SR, Wiesner PJ. Infections due to penicillinase-producing *Neisseria gonorrhoeae* in the United States: 1976–1980. *J Infect Dis.* 1981;144(2):191-197
32. Faruki H, Kohmescher RN, McKinney WP, Sparling PF. A community-based outbreak of infection with penicillin-resistant Neisseria gonorrhoeae not producing penicillinase (chromosomally mediated resistance). *N Engl J Med.* 1985;313(10):607-611
33. Centers for Disease Control and Prevention. Tetracycline-resistant Neisseria gonorrhoeae—Georgia, Pennsylvania, New Hampshire. *MMWR.* 1985;34(37):563-564, 569-570
34. Centers for Disease Control and Prevention. 1985 STD treatment guidelines. *MMWR.* 1985;34(4S): 75S-108S
35. Centers for Disease Control and Prevention. 1993 sexually transmitted diseases treatment guidelines. *MMWR.* 1993;42(RR-14):1-102
36. Centers for Disease Control and Prevention. Sentinel surveillance system for antimicrobial resistance in clinical isolates of Neisseria gonorrhoeae. *MMWR.* 1987;36(35):585-586, 591-593
37. WHO Regional Office for the Western Pacific. The Gonococcal Antimicrobial Surveillance Programme (GASP). WHO western Pacific region, 1995. *Releve epidemiologique hebdomadaire/ Section d'hygiene du Secretariat de la Societe des Nations = Weekly epidemiological record/Health Section of the Secretariat of the League of Nations.* 1997;72(5):25-27
38. Knapp JS, Ohye R, Neal SW, Parekh MC, Higa H, Rice RJ. Emerging in vitro resistance to quinolones in penicillinase-producing Neisseria gonorrhoeae strains in Hawaii. *Antimicrob Agents Chemother.* 1994;38(9):2200-2203
39. Centers for Disease Control and Prevention. Decreased susceptibility of Neisseria gonorrhoeae to fluoroquinolones—Ohio and Hawaii, 1992-1994. *MMWR.* 1994;43(18):325-327
40. Centers for Disease Control and Prevention. Fluoroquinolone resistance in Neisseria gonorrhoeae—Colorado and Washington, 1995. *MMWR.* 1995;44(41):761-764
41. Centers for Disease Control and Prevention. Fluoroquinolone-resistant Neisseria gonorrhoeae—San Diego, California, 1997. *MMWR.* 1998;47(20):405-408
42. Centers for Disease Control and Prevention. *Sexually Transmitted Diseases Surveillance 1999 Supplement: Gonococcal Isolate Surveillance Project (GISP) Annual Report*—1999. Atlanta, GA: US Department of Health and Human Services, Public Health Service; 2000
43. Centers for Disease Control and Prevention. Fluoroquinolone-resistance in *Neisseria gonorrhoeae*, Hawaii, 1999, and decreased susceptibility to azithromycin in N. gonorrhoeae, Missouri, 1999. *MMWR.* 2000;49(37):833-837
44. Centers for Disease Control and Prevention. Increases in fluoroquinolone-resistant Neisseria gonorrhoeae—Hawaii and California, 2001. *MMWR.* 2002;51:1041-1044
45. Centers for Disease Control and Prevention. Sexually transmitted diseases treatment guidelines 2002. *MMWR.* 2002;51(RR-6):1-78
46. Centers for Disease Control and Prevention. Increases in fluoroquinolone-resistant *Neisseria gonorrhoeae* among men who have sex with men—United States, 2003, and revised recommendations for treatment, 2004. *MMWR.* 2004;53:335-338
47. Centers for Disease Control and Prevention. Update to CDC's sexually transmitted diseases treatment guidelines, 2006: fluoroquinolones are no longer recommended for treatment of gonococcal infections. *MMWR.* 2007;56(14):332-336

48. Ito M, Yasuda M, Yokoi S, et al. Remarkable increase in central Japan in 2001-2002 of *Neisseria gonorrhoeae* isolates with decreased susceptibility to penicillin, tetracycline, oral cephalosporins, and fluoroquinolones. *Antimicrob Agents Chemother.* 2004;48(8):3185-3187
49. Su X, Jiang F, Quimuge, Dai X, Sun H, Ye S. Surveillance of antimicrobial susceptibilities in *Neisseria gonorrhoeae* in Nanjing, China, 1999-2006. *Sex Transm Dis.* 2007;34(12):995-999
50. Lahra MM. Annual report of the Australian Gonococcal Surveillance Programme, 2011. *Commun Dis Intell Q Rep.* 2012;36(2):E166-E173
51. European Centre for Disease Prevention and Control. *Gonococcal Antimicrobial Susceptibility Surveillance In Europe, 2011.* Stockholm, Sweden: ECDC; 2013
52. Centers for Disease Control and Prevention. Cephalosporin susceptibility among *Neisseria gonorrhoeae* isolates—United States, 2000–2010. *MMWR.* 2011;60(26):873-877
53. Deguchi T, Yasuda M, Yokoi S, et al. Treatment of uncomplicated gonococcal urethritis by double-dosing of 200 mg cefixime at a 6-h interval. *J Infect Chemother.* 2003;9:35-39
54. Yokoi S, Deguchi T, Ozawa T, et al. Threat to cefixime treatment for gonorrhea. *Emerg Infect Dis.* 2007;13(8):1275-1277
55. Unemo M, Golparian D, Syversen G, Vestrheim DF, Moi H. Two cases of verified clinical failures using internationally recommended first-line cefixime for gonorrhoea treatment, Norway, 2010. *Euro Surveill.* 2010;15(47):pii:19721
56. Ison CA, Hussey J, Sankar KN, Evans J, Alexander S. Gonorrhoea treatment failures to cefixime and azithromycin in England, 2010. *Euro Surveill.* 2011;16(14):pii:19833
57. Forsyth S, Penney P, Rooney G. Cefixime-resistant Neisseria gonorrhoeae in the UK: a time to reflect on practice and recommendations. *Int J STD AIDS.* 2011;22:296-297
58. Unemo M, Golparian D, Stary A, Eigentler A. First *Neisseria gonorrhoeae* strain with resistance to cefixime causing gonorrhoeae treatment failure in Austria, 2011. *Euro Surveill.* 2011;16(43):pii:19998
59. Unemo M, Golparian D, Nicholas R, Ohnishi M, Gallay A, Sednaoui P. High-level cefixime- and ceftriaxone-resistant Neisseria gonorrhoeae in France: novel penA mosaic allele in a successful international clone causes treatment failure. *Antimicrob Agents Chemother.* 2012;56(3):1273-1280
60. Allen VG, Mitterni L, Seah C, et al. Neisseria gonorrhoeae treatment failure and susceptibility to cefixime in Toronto, Canada. *JAMA.* 2013;309(2):163-170
61. Lewis DA, Sriruttan C, Muller EE, et al. Phenotypic and genetic characterization of the first two cases of extended-spectrum-cephalosporin-resistant Neisseria gonorrhoeae infection in South Africa and association with cefixime treatment failure. *J Antimicrob Chemother.* 2013;68(6):1267-1270
62. Ohnishi M, Saika T, Hoshina S, et al. Ceftriaxone-resistant *Neisseria gonorrhoeae,* Japan. *Emerg Infect Dis.* 2011;17:148-149
63. Ohnishi M, Golparian D, Shimuta K, et al. Is Neisseria gonorrhoeae initiating a future era of untreatable gonorrhea?: detailed characterization of the first strain with high-level resistance to ceftriaxone. *Antimicrob Agents Chemother.* 2011;55(7):3538-3545
64. Camara J, Serra J, Ayats J, et al. Molecular characterization of two high-level ceftriaxone-resistant Neisseria gonorrhoeae isolates detected in Catalonia, Spain. *J Antimicrob Chemother.* 2012;67(8):1858-1860
65. Unemo M, Nicholas RA. Emergence of multidrug-resistant, extensively drug-resistant and untreatable gonorrhea. *Fut Microbiol.* 2012;7(12):1401-1422
66. Centers for Disease Control and Prevention. Sexually transmitted diseases treatment guidelines, 2010. *MMWR.* 2010;59(RR-12):1-110
67. Centers for Disease Control and Prevention. Update to CDC's sexually transmitted diseases treatment guidelines, 2010: oral cephalosporins no longer recommended for treatment of gonococcal infections. *MMWR.* 2012;61(31):590-594
68. Lyss SB, Kamb ML, Peterman TA, et al. Chlamydia trachomatis among patients infected with and treated for Neisseria gonorrhoeae in sexually transmitted disease clinics in the United States. *Ann Intern Med.* 2003;139(3):178-185
69. Moran JS. Gonorrhoea. *Clin Evid (Online).* 2007;2007:pii:1604
70. Kirkcaldy RD. Treatment of gonorrhoea in an era of emerging cephalosporin resistance and results of a randomised trial of new potential treatment options. Paper presented at STI & AIDS World Congress 2013, Vienna, Austria

71. Newman LM, Moran JS, Workowski KA. Update on the management of gonorrhea in adults in the United States. *Clin Infect Dis*. 2007;44(Suppl 3):S84-S101
72. Kirkcaldy RD, Kidd S, Weinstock HS, Papp JR, Bolan GA. Trends in antimicrobial resistance in Neisseria gonorrhoeae in the USA: the Gonococcal Isolate Surveillance Project (GISP), January 2006-June 2012. *Sex Transm Infect*. 2013;89(Suppl 4):iv5-iv10
73. Soge OO, Harger D, Schafer S, et al. Emergence of increased azithromycin resistance during unsuccessful treatment of *Neisseria gonorrhoeae* infection with azithromycin (Portland, OR, 2011). *Sex Transm Dis*. 2012;39(11):877-879
74. Katz AR, Komeya AY, Soge OO, et al. *Neisseria gonorrhoeae* with high-level resistance to azithromycin: case report of the first isolate identified in the United States. *Clin Infect Dis*. 2012;54(6):841-843
75. Lo JY, Ho KM, Lo AC. Surveillance of gonococcal antimicrobial susceptibility resulting in early detection of emerging resistance. *J Antimicrob Chemother*. 2012;67(6):1422-1426
76. Chisholm SA, Neal TJ, Alawattegama AB, Birley HDL, Howe RA, Ison CA. Emergence of high-level azithromycin resistance in *Neisseria gonorrhoeae* in England and Wales. *J Antimicrob Chemother*. 2009;64:353-358
77. Galarza PG, Alcala B, Salcedo C, et al. Emergence of high level azithromycin-resistant Neisseria gonorrhoeae strain isolated in Argentina. *Sex Transm Dis*. 2009;36(12):787-788
78. Boslego JW, Tramont EC, Takafuji ET, et al. Effect of spectinomycin use on the prevalence of spectinomycin-resistant and of penicillinase-producing *Neisseria gonorrhoeae*. *N Engl J Med*. 1987;317:272-278
79. Dowell D, Kirkcaldy RD. Effectiveness of gentamicin for gonorrhoea treatment: systematic review and meta-analysis. *Sex Transm Infect*. 2012;88:589-594
80. US Preventive Services Task Force. Screening for gonorrhea: recommendation statement. *Ann Fam Med*. 2005;3:263-267
81. American Academy of Pediatrics. Sexually transmitted infections in adolescents and children. In: Pickering LK, Baker CJ, Kimberlin DW, Long SS, eds. *Red Book: 2012 Report of the Committee on Infectious Diseases*. 29th ed. Elk Grove Village, IL: American Academy of Pediatrics; 2012:176-185
82. Yee E, Satterwhite CL, Braxton J, Tran A, Steece R, Weinstock H. Current STD laboratory testing and volume in the United States among public health laboratories, 2007. Poster presentation at the International Society for Sexually Transmitted Diseases Research Conference, 2009, London, United Kingdom
83. Centers for Disease Control and Prevention. Screening tests to detect Chlamydia trachomatis and Neisseria gonorrhoeae infections—2002. *MMWR*. 2002;51(RR-15):1-38
84. Schachter J, Moncada J, Liska S, Shayevich C, Klausner JD. Nucleic acid amplification tests in the diagnosis of chlamydial and gonococcal infections of the oropharynx and rectum in men who have sex with men. *Sex Transm Dis*. 2008;35(7):637-642
85. Mimiaga MJ, Mayer KH, Reisner SL, et al. Asymptomatic gonorrhea and chlamydial infections detected by nucleic acid amplification tests among Boston area men who have sex with men. *Sex Transm Dis*. 2008;35(5):495-498
86. Bachmann LH, Johnson RE, Cheng H, Markowitz LE, Papp JR, Hook EW 3rd. Nucleic acid amplification tests for diagnosis of Neisseria gonorrhoeae oropharyngeal infections. *J Clin Microbiol*. 2009;47(4):902-907
87. Bachmann LH, Johnson RE, Cheng H, et al. Nucleic acid amplification tests for diagnosis of Neisseria gonorrhoeae and Chlamydia trachomatis rectal infections. *J Clin Microbiol*. 2010;48(5):1827-1832
88. Bissessor M, Tabrizi SN, Fairley CK, et al. Differing Neisseria gonorrhoeae bacterial loads in the pharynx and rectum in men who have sex with men: implications for gonococcal detection, transmission, and control. *J Clin Microbiol*. 2011;49(12):4304-4306
89. Bachmann LH, Desmond RA, Stephens J, et al. Duration of persistence of gonococcal DNA detected by ligase chain reaction in men and women following recommended therapy for uncomplicated gonorrhea. *J Clin Microbiol*. 2002;40(10):3596-3601

90. Hjelmevoll SO, Olsen ME, Sollid JU, et al. Appropriate time for test-of-cure when diagnosing gonorrhoea with a nucleic acid amplification test. *Acta Derm Venereol.* 2012;92(3):316-319
91. Hook EW, Jamieson BD, Oldach D, Harbison H, Whittington A, Fernandes P. A phase II, dose ranging study to evaluate the efficacy and safety of single-dose oral solithromycin (CEM-101) for treatment of patients with uncomplicated urogenital gonorrhoea. Paper presented at STI & AIDS World Congress 2013, Vienna, Austria
92. Golparian D, Fernandes P, Ohnishi M, Jensen JS, Unemo M. In vitro activity of the new fluoroketolide solithromycin (CEM-101) against a large collection of clinical Neisseria gonorrhoeae isolates and international reference strains, including those with high-level antimicrobial resistance: potential treatment option for gonorrhea? *Antimicrob Agents Chemother.* 2012;56(5):2739-2742
93. Comparison of delafloxacin versus ceftriaxone for the treatment of uncomplicated gonorrhea. ClinicalTrials.gov. Available at: clinicaltrials.gov/ct2/show/study/NCT02015637. Accessed July 21, 2014
94. Roberts MC, Remy JM, Longcor JD, et al. *In vitro* activity of delafloxacin against *Neisseria gonorrhoeae* clinical isolates. Poster presented at STI & AIDS World Congress 2013, Vienna, Austria

Adolesc Med 025 (2014) 332–346

Adolescents, Young Adults, and the Legalization of Marijuana

Andrea J. Hoopes, MD[a*]; Inga Manskopf, BS[b]; Leslie Walker, MD[c]

[a]Fellow, Division of Adolescent Medicine, University of Washington Department of Pediatrics, Seattle, Washington; [b]Coordinator, Prevention WINS Coalition, Division of Adolescent Medicine, Seattle Children's, Seattle, Washington; [c]Chief, Division of Adolescent Medicine, Seattle Children's, Director, University of Washington LEAH (Leadership Education in Adolescent Health), Professor, Vice Chair of Faculty Affairs, University of Washington Department of Pediatrics, Seattle, Washington

WHAT IS MARIJUANA?

Cannabis sativa is typically what is referred to as marijuana in the United States. Other Cannabis plants are also consumed. The next most commonly used plant is *Cannabis indica*. The green leafy Cannabis plants are used all over the world for medicinal, spiritual, and recreational purposes. The flowers and leaves can be dried and used to make products to smoke, but there are also oils, powders, resins, and tinctures that can be extracted or distilled to increase potency or bring out specific effects for the user. The main psychoactive ingredient is delta-9-tetrahydrocannabinol (delta-9-THC). Additionally, more than 450 different chemicals have been isolated from the plant. When ingested, THC preferentially binds to the cannabinoid (CB) receptors in the brain. These are naturally occurring receptors that normally bind endocannabinoids, chemicals in the brain that are related to brain development and function. Some areas of the brain have large concentrations of CB receptors. When THC binds at these sites instead of the endocannabinoids, effects may be observed on memory, thought, sensory and time perception, appetite, pain, concentration, and movement coordination. Given the broad range of influences on the brain, people who use marijuana report widely varying experiences.

Marijuana manufactured today can be produced with very high levels of THC, ranging from 4% to 22%. Higher percent compositions of THC often lead to

*Corresponding author
E-mail address: annie.hoopes@seattlechildrens.org

 ISSN 1934-4287

more intense and longer-lasting effects, causing reactions such as paranoia, severe depression, increased heart rate, and even increased risk for stroke.[1] The acute effects peak within 10 minutes to 1 hour, depending on whether the marijuana is inhaled or orally ingested. The inhaled drug can reach the bloodstream much faster and produce a more rapid effect.

ACUTE EFFECTS

Marijuana can cause acute physical effects, including euphoria, relaxation, a feeling of well-being, decreased nausea, and change in pain sensation. It also can cause distorted sensory perception and slowed reaction time to stimuli, hallucinations, paranoia, anxiety, psychosis, memory impairment, and excessive vomiting.[1] There is no mechanism to predict which effect a particular person will experience.

Overdose

The oils and other concentrated liquid forms that are infused into edible products or directly ingested can be significantly more potent than smoked marijuana and have the potential for unintentional overdose in inexperienced users or children who accidentally ingest edibles found in the home.[2] For toddlers in particular, the overdose can lead to hyperactivity, which may progress to a body "slowdown" and in some cases may lead to a comatose state and respiratory failure.[2] Although there are no studies or records of death directly from marijuana overdose, there is an accepted term for overdose in the using community called "greening out." This happens typically to an inexperienced user when a large amount of THC is ingested, leading to a temporary feeling of anxiety, paranoia or fear, nausea and vomiting, increased heart rate, uncontrollable shaking, hallucination, and/or disorientation. Supportive care is the only treatment currently available for overdose situations when patients present to the emergency department.[3]

The expansion of marijuana for medicinal reasons has increased adolescents' exposure to many different kinds of ingested cannabis, and for a growing number the edible and vaporized forms may now be preferred over smoking. National surveys of drug use in the adolescent age group will need to expand their questionnaires to include questions about nonsmoked forms of the drug in order to assess trends in use and potential differences in outcomes as the supply of marijuana in various forms increases across the country.

REGULAR USE AND LONG-TERM EFFECTS

Regular use of marijuana by adolescents can result in[1]

- Chronic bronchitis and impaired respiratory function in regular smokers
- Psychotic symptoms and disorders in heavy users, especially those with a history of psychotic symptoms or a family history of psychotic disorders

- Impaired educational attainment in adolescents who are regular users
- Short-term memory impairment
- Permanent cognitive impairment and loss of IQ in adolescents who begin use at an early age and continue into late adolescence[4]

Regular use is defined as use more than once every 30 days. Given the slow but progressive damage marijuana causes in a developing brain, it is sometimes mistaken for being more benign than other illicit drugs. Additionally, because it is an illegal substance for minors to use in the United States, it may lead to suspensions from school, legal problems, and potential for inequitable enforcement of the law for marginalized youth.

MARIJUANA DEPENDENCE

Marijuana is addictive and causes physical dependence and craving that can result in difficulty in abstaining from the drug even when abstinence is a desired goal by the user. Although dependence can occur in 10% of adults, adolescents who use marijuana are about 3 to 4 times more likely to develop dependence than adults.[5] In fact, in the United States, currently 1 in 10 adolescents report smoking more than 20 times a month, a frequency of use that usually is associated with dependence and functional compromise.[5] Teenagers are at higher risk for becoming dependent on marijuana because the human brain is not fully developed until about 25 years of age.[6,7] Before this age, the teen and young adult brain is still processing where to make permanent connections and where to prune parts of brain function that are not being used. Marijuana, when used during adolescence and young adulthood, affects this development and can lead to craving of marijuana weeks and months after last use.[5,7] Unlike drugs that leave the system quickly and cause strong cravings and withdrawal symptoms very proximal to last use, marijuana can stay in the system for more than 3 weeks, depending on the amount of use and the fat composition of the person using it. This leads to the incorrect yet widespread belief that there are no physical or mental withdrawal symptoms from marijuana, when, in fact, physical dependence and withdrawal symptoms occur later than with other drugs. Withdrawal symptoms include irritability, headache, depressed mood, sleep disturbance, and craving for marijuana. Although there is no pharmaceutical treatment for managing withdrawal symptoms or achieving recovery, studies currently are underway evaluating medications that may help manage cravings for marijuana when abstinence is desired.[8]

MEDICINAL USES OF MARIJUANA

A review of the literature did not yield any studies that have evaluated medicinal uses of the marijuana plant specifically for adolescents. A number of states have made provision for use of marijuana for medicinal purposes. However, marijuana is not an accepted medicine regulated by the federal Food and Drug Administration (FDA). There is no practical difference between state-approved medical marijuana and recreational marijuana. To be considered a medicine, a substance must be able to be reliably dosed for an expected effect and must be uniformly manufactured and formulated so that the user is assured that the product composition remains consistent. It also must be regulated to assure that the manufacturer's description of the content is consistent with the actual content. In addition, an FDA-approved drug must undergo scientific study to support its superior effects over placebo, with short- and long-term side effects or risks not outweighing its benefit. This has not happened for the marijuana plant.

Although a synthetic THC compound has been approved by the FDA for use in treating nausea and appetite, the marijuana plant has not been approved as a medication. The approved THC-based medications currently under FDA regulation are dronabinol and nabilone, both of which are synthetic delta-9-THC agents. These medications are approved for adults with acquired immunodeficiency syndrome (AIDS) or adults receiving chemotherapy to improve appetite and reduce nausea.[9,10] It is considered a psychoactive, controlled drug that can lead to dependence when used at high doses over prolonged periods of time. No studies in the pediatric age group have been published on this medication, and its use in this population is off-label.[9,10]

In spite of the lack of research on medicinal uses for adolescents and evidence showing contradictory effects, adolescents have anecdotally stated they use the marijuana plant to treat pain, sleep, depression, stress, concentration, and anxiety.[11,12] Given the known risks of using marijuana in adolescents, these claims of medicinal benefit need to be weighed with the currently known risks and evaluated through rigorous study.

EPIDEMIOLOGY

Marijuana is second only to alcohol among the most commonly used illicit substances by adolescents. Data from the 2013 Monitoring the Future (MTF) study indicate that adolescent marijuana use has been increasing in recent years, which is a change from previous declines in the decade prior. Use among 8th- and 10th-graders increased in 2013, with the annual prevalence (the percent using 1 or more times in the past 12 months) rising from 11% to 13% among 8th-graders and 28% to 30% among 10th-graders, although these national trends were not statistically significant. Among 12th-graders, use remained steady at 36%. Lifetime use also was examined, with 17% of 8th-graders, 36% of 10th-graders, and 46% (or almost half) of all 12th-graders reporting ever having used marijuana. Trends in daily use also have been rising steadily, with 1 in every 15 high school seniors (or about 7%) now reporting daily or near-daily marijuana use, compared to 1% of 8th-graders and 4% of 10th-graders.[13] It is important to note that marijuana use is increasing while cigarette use has declined, as noted in Figure 1, which demonstrates the percentage of 12th-graders reporting cigarette and marijuana use in the past month from 1976 to 2012. Of note, a

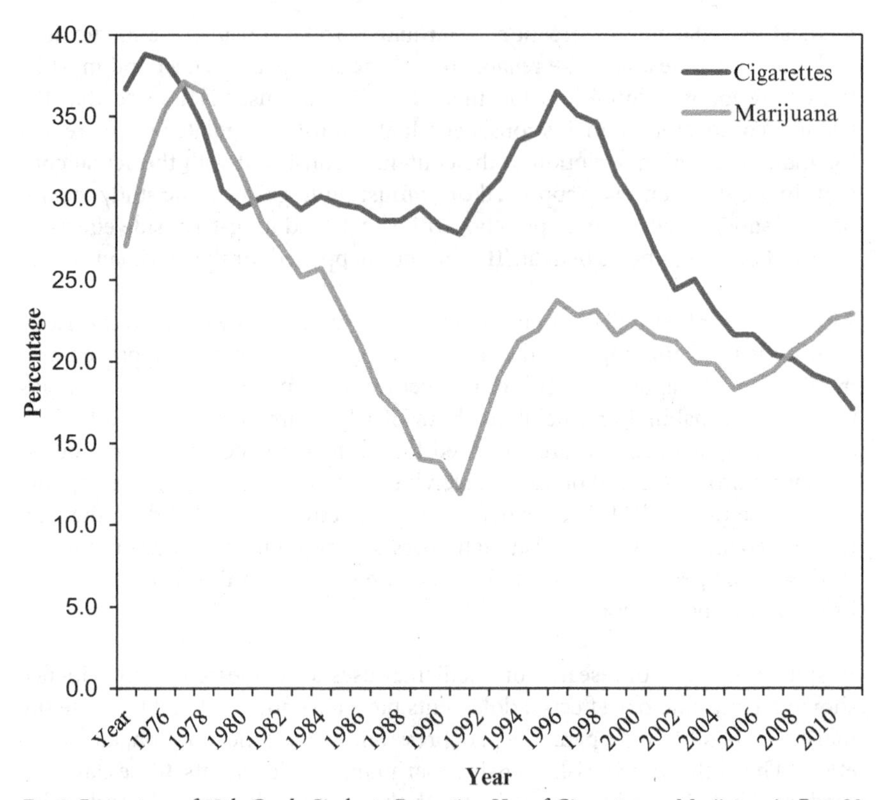

Fig 1. Percentage of 12th Grade Students Reporting Use of Cigarettes or Marijuana in Past 30 Days—United States, 1975 to 2012. (From Johnston LD, O'Malley PM, Miech RA, Bachman JG, Schulenberg JE, *Monitoring the Future national results on adolescent drug use: Overview of key findings*. Ann Arbor, MI: Institute for Social Research, The University of Michigan; 2014.)

strong relationship between alcohol and marijuana use was identified in a recent study, which found that 86% of adolescents who reported marijuana use in the past year also used alcohol within that same period.[5]

The MTF data highlight the fact that perceived risk among teenagers, which has been a strong indicator for use of both marijuana and other drugs, has continued to decrease in 2013. From 2005 to 2013, the percent of 8th-graders perceiving a great risk from regular marijuana use decreased from 74% to 61%, whereas among 10th-graders the percent decreased from 66% to 47% and among 12th-graders decreased from 58% to 40%. These significant decreases raise concerns that marijuana use among teenagers will increase in the future.[13]

The availability of marijuana has been associated with increased rates of use. A national survey of more than 78,000 youth found that adolescents who have been offered marijuana are 7 times more likely to use it than are those who have not been offered marijuana. Furthermore, adolescents who report that marijuana is “easy to get” are approximately 2.5 times more likely to use it than those who consider it “hard to get.”[14]

A study published in 2007 found that

- 88% of adolescents who used marijuana obtained it from a friend or relative.
- 59% of adolescents who used marijuana obtained it for free.
- 87% of distribution transactions occur indoors, not on the street.
- Only 6% of adolescents who use marijuana reported obtaining it from a stranger.[15]

The MTF report examined sources of marijuana among teens living in states that have medical marijuana laws. The study found that among teens who reported use within the past 12 months and resided in a state with medical marijuana laws, 34% reported that 1 of their sources of marijuana was another person's medical marijuana prescription.[13] This phenomenon, known as diversion, was investigated in a 2011 study among adolescents enrolled in a substance abuse program in Colorado, a state that has legalized marijuana for medicinal purposes.[16] The authors found that 74% of participants had diverted someone else's medical marijuana. Furthermore, the study found that adolescents who used medical marijuana had an earlier age of regular marijuana use and more marijuana abuse and dependence symptoms, as well as more conduct disorder symptoms than those who did not use medical marijuana. A review of the recent literature did not reveal any current epidemiologic data on adolescent marijuana use for medicinal purposes.

PREDICTORS, PROTECTIVE FACTORS, AND CONSEQUENCES OF MARIJUANA USE AMONG ADOLESCENTS

A number of predictors for marijuana use among adolescents have been identified, including participation in antisocial behavior, friends' marijuana use, lower perceived risk of marijuana use, and positive attitude toward marijuana use.[17] Protective factors include high commitment to school and exposure to prevention messages.[17] A recent study examining the relative influence of risk and protective factors found that the strongest protective factors against marijuana use were localized to the community domain, including high neighborhood attachment and community prosocial involvement.[18]

Adolescent marijuana use has been linked to a number of significant neuropharmacologic, cognitive, behavioral, and somatic consequences, including negative effects on short-term memory, concentration, attention span, motivation, and problem-solving. All of these effects are known to interfere with learning. A recent large prospective cohort study found that individuals who began using marijuana heavily during adolescence lower their IQ by as much as 8 points between the ages of 13 and 38 years, and that lost cognitive function was not restored in those who discontinued smoking marijuana as adults.[4]

A number of recent studies have observed an association between marijuana use and subsequent development of mental health problems. A recent review of more than 120 studies evaluating the effects of marijuana on the adolescent brain concluded that data from epidemiologic studies repeatedly show an association between cannabis use and subsequent addiction to heavy drugs, as well as psychosis, with this relationship often correlated with genetic factors, intensity of marijuana use, and age at which it first occurs, suggesting that younger age at first use may be more damaging.[7] An additional review of the preclinical evidence that focused on the relationship between marijuana use during adolescence and the risk of psychosis concluded that adolescent cannabinoid exposure in rodent models was associated with the presence of impaired social behaviors, cognitive and sensorimotor deficits, and psychotic-like signs in adult rodents. This relationship was not observed after adult rodent cannabinoid exposure. Although mental health conditions, including substance abuse and dependence, often are multifactorial in their origins, the data clearly support adolescent marijuana use as a risk factor for mental health problems later in life.

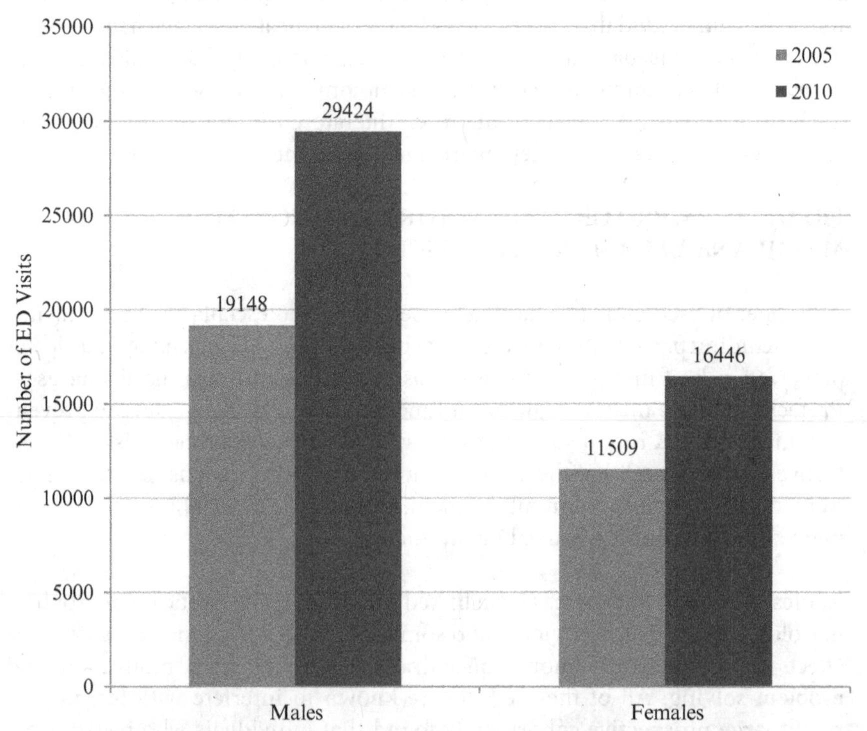

Fig 2. Marijuana-Related Emergency Department (ED) Visits Among Adolescents Aged 15 to 17, by Gender—United States, 2005 and 2010. (From Drug Abuse Warning Network. *CBHSQ Data Spotlight: Emergency Department Visits Involving Marijuana among Adolescents Aged 15 to 17: Increase from 2005 to 2010 Varied by Gender*, 2012.)

Additionally, adverse effects on coordination, judgment, reaction time, and tracking ability contribute to unintentional deaths and injuries among teens. A recent report from the Drug Abuse Warning Network highlighted the fact that emergency department visits involving marijuana among adolescents aged 15 to 17 years increased 50% from 2005 to 2010, with the increase more significant in males than in females (Figure 2).[19] Based on these data, an increase in adolescent marijuana use that may accompany legalization could have significant public safety implications.

MARIJUANA POLICY

Marijuana is classified as a controlled substance by the United Nations, and almost all countries, including the United States, have signed conventions against the trafficking of drugs, including marijuana. In Europe, national control policies vary country by country. Three general types of policies inform how nations govern marijuana production, possession, and use.

1. **Prohibition.** Marijuana remains illegal in most countries. It is illegal to produce, possess, or use the substance, and sanctions for these activities vary.
2. **Decriminalization**. The Netherlands and Portugal removed criminal sanctions for marijuana use. In the Netherlands, "coffee shops" are allowed to sell small amounts of marijuana under strict conditions, including a ban on advertising. Portugal decriminalized the use and possession of a 10-day supply of any illicit drug, including marijuana. All drug sales and manufacturing are illegal. In the United States between 2012 and 2013, voters in 5 Michigan cities and Portland, Maine, decriminalized the possession of small amounts of marijuana by adults older than 21 years. In many jurisdictions, laws regarding the possession of small amounts of marijuana are not enforced. In 2007, the city of Seattle adopted an initiative that made the enforcement of marijuana laws their lowest police priority. In Canada, Australia, and New Zealand, less than 2% of marijuana users are arrested.[20]
3. **Legalization**. Uruguay and the states of Colorado and Washington in the United States recently adopted legislation to create legal marijuana systems. In November 2013, Uruguay adopted legislation that allows the production, distribution, and use of marijuana after registering with the government. In November 2012, voters in Colorado and Washington adopted referenda that set the stage for the legal commercial production and distribution of marijuana and for the legal possession of limited amounts of the substance. Although possession and use of marijuana for people 21 years and older was quickly decriminalized after the vote, it took the states more than 1 year to establish regulatory systems for production and distribution. Marijuana retail outlets opened in Colorado on January 1, 2014, and outlets are expected to open in Washington in the summer of 2014. As of January 2014, 21 states and the District of Columbia adopted

laws allowing people to use marijuana for medicinal purposes. In what has been called "medicine by popular vote,"[21] each state has its own regulations, including how much marijuana people may possess, what medical problems qualify people to be authorized for its use, patient registries, how many plants can be grown, and how the product may be dispensed. In contrast to the conventional medical model, the patient rather than the physician determines the correct doses.[22]

Washington and Colorado: A Closer Look

In 2012, the voters of the states of Colorado and Washington both passed legislation to decriminalize the possession of small amounts of marijuana and to create commercial marketplaces for the drug. The laws in both states[23,24]

- Restrict marijuana to people 21 years and older
- Require marijuana growers, manufacturers, and retailers to obtain licenses
- Tax marijuana products
- Ban public consumption

Legislators in both states are considering bills to make changes to the new laws, which contain different rules in their respective states. For instance, Colorado's law allows people to grow up to 6 marijuana plants and to share a small amount with other adults. Washington's law does not allow people to grow their own or to share marijuana with others. Washington's law establishes a legal limit for adults driving under the influence of marijuana, whereas in Colorado it is prohibited. It is illegal for minors in both states to drive with any amount of marijuana in their systems.

Policy as Prevention

For the purposes of this article, prevention is defined as preventing the *onset* of marijuana use among adolescents. Because most high school students do not use marijuana, and health risks associated with adolescent use can be significant, the goal of no marijuana use among adolescents supports current norms and healthy adolescent development. Although most people think of school-based curricula and programs when they think of adolescent substance use prevention, a multisector approach is needed to be most effective. Public policy plays a role in whether a community supports healthy youth development.

Multiple studies indicate that policies that aim to increase the cost of alcohol and tobacco, reduce availability and accessibility, restrict where it can be used, and establish a minimum legal age for use are especially effective in reducing teen drug use.[25-29] To inform underage marijuana use prevention strategies, including policy, availability of marijuana is 1 risk factor identified by the University of Washington as being strongly associated with youth marijuana use.[30] No research has been conducted to determine if policy that is effective for preventing adolescent alcohol and tobacco use is effective for preventing and reducing adolescent marijuana use. Until such research is conducted, the best that can be done is to look at alcohol and tobacco policy and extrapolate that similar policy for marijuana will have similar outcomes.

Table 1 lists best practice policies for preventing underage drinking and tobacco use, comparing the policies to rules established for the new marijuana systems in Colorado and Washington.

Table 1
Best practice policies for preventing underage drinking and tobacco use compared to new marijuana regulations in Colorado and Washington

Best practice policy[1-4]	Washington[5]	Colorado[6]
Maintain and enforce age limits	21 years and older, minors not allowed in stores. Local jurisdictions enforce marijuana laws regarding minors according to local policy.	21 years and older, minors not allowed in stores. Local jurisdictions enforce marijuana laws regarding minors according to local policy.
Limit retail outlet density	1000-foot buffer between marijuana businesses and schools, parks, libraries, and other places frequented by children. A limited amount of retail licenses are to be issued per local jurisdiction based on population. Twenty-one retail licenses are allocated for the City of Seattle. Local jurisdictions may enact zoning and land use ordinances for marijuana businesses. Some jurisdictions have placed moratoria on the establishment of businesses to give local decision-makers time to determine local policy. Some jurisdictions ban marijuana businesses and some restrict businesses to nonresidential areas. Some communities are concerned about marijuana business density in low-income areas.	State law does not limit but "a locality may enact ordinances or regulations . . . governing the time, place, manner and number of marijuana establishment operations." Some jurisdictions do not limit outlet density and some jurisdictions ban marijuana businesses.
Taxes	A 25% excise tax is imposed on businesses that produce (grow), process, and sell marijuana. The tax is collected at all 3 business tiers. Washington sales tax: 6.5% with most local jurisdictions levying additional amounts, which can total up to 9.6%.	A 15% excise tax is imposed on marijuana sold by a cultivator to a manufacturer or to a retailer "prior to January 1, 2017 and a rate to be determined . . . thereafter." Colorado sales tax: 10% Local jurisdictions are choosing to levy additional taxes.
Limit hours of sale	8:00 a.m. to midnight	8:00 a.m. to midnight; local jurisdictions may further restrict.

Continued

Table 1
Best practice policies for preventing underage drinking and tobacco use compared to new marijuana regulations in Colorado and Washington (Continued)

Best practice policy[1-4]	Washington[5]	Colorado[6]
Restrict advertising	Advertising may not contain statements or illustrations that "depict a child or other person under legal age to consume marijuana or includes objects, such as toys, characters, or cartoon characters suggesting the presence of a child, or any other depiction designed in any manner to be especially appealing to children or other persons under legal age to consume marijuana, or is designed in any manner that would be especially appealing to" minors. The law is silent on the appearance and flavor of products that are attractive to youth, such as marijuana-infused candies, carbonated beverages, and baked goods. Advertisements banned within 1000 feet of schools, playgrounds, recreation facilities, child care centers, parks, libraries, and game arcades; on or in a public transit vehicle or shelter; on or in publicly owned property. The law is silent on Internet and social media marketing and advertising, including business Web sites, Facebook and Twitter pages, and blogs. Advertisements must contain health warnings.	Retailer may not advertise on TV, radio, print media, the Internet, or sponsor events unless they have "reliable evidence that no more than 30% of the audience is reasonably expected to be under the age of 21." Bans advertising that is "visible to the public from any street, sidewalk, park or other public place, including Advertising utilizing any of the following media: any billboard or other outdoor general Advertising device; any sign mounted on a vehicle, any hand-held or other portable sign; or any handbill, leaflet or flier" handed out in public places. Bans advertising "via marketing directed toward location-based devices, including but not limited to cellular phones" unless an app is installed by an owner who is 21 years or older. No pop-up advertising for marijuana products allowed on the Internet. Internet advertising rules do not address marijuana business Web sites, Facebook and Twitter pages, and blogs.

Marijuana Legalization: Early Concerns

In a 2004 article about marijuana policy, the American Academy of Pediatrics cited several concerns with the possible decriminalization or legalization of marijuana and the effect on youth.[31] Concerns about legalization include an increase in adolescent use; advertising campaigns targeting adolescents; poor enforcement of regulations meant to keep marijuana away from minors; an increase in parental drug use that could influence use among their children and create an in-home supply of marijuana; and a decrease in price that is associated with an increase in use among adolescents. Although it will take years to determine if these concerns play out in the legal commercial systems being established in Colorado and Washington, a few adolescent health concerns are emerging in Washington.

Access to Marijuana Sold in Dispensaries

In Seattle, Washington, 38% of Seattle high school students reporting current use of marijuana said that they had used marijuana that came from a dispensary.[32] Although the majority (68%) reported having obtained marijuana through social connections, it was not uncommon for their marijuana to have come from a retail dispensary. No data about access to marijuana from personal gardens were collected. As a RAND Corporation report about the current marijuana market in Washington State notes, "It is perhaps not surprising that such a large number of marijuana users in Seattle's public high schools report consuming marijuana that came from a dispensary; there are a lot of dispensaries in the Seattle Metro Area."[33] When marijuana stores open, it is expected that some of the recreational marijuana will be similarly obtained by adolescents. During the 2014 Washington State legislative session, legislators failed to reconcile the regulated recreational and the largely unregulated medical marijuana systems.

Potent Products Attractive to Youth

In addition to dried marijuana products, retailers sell edible products such as baked goods, carbonated beverages, juices, and candies infused with marijuana extracts. Highly concentrated and potentially very potent forms of marijuana, such as hash oil, which is consumed by vaporizing, are becoming more widely available. Although rules in Washington State limit the amount of THC that can be contained in 1 serving of marijuana, packages of marijuana products can contain up to 10 servings. In March 2014, a college student jumped to his death in Colorado after eating a marijuana-infused cookie that contained 6 servings of marijuana. "Hours after ingesting an entire marijuana cookie meant to be eaten in smaller doses, he began behaving violently, culminating with his balcony leap. The Denver coroner's office listed 'marijuana intoxication' as a contributing factor in [the student's] death," according to Reuters.[34]

Marijuana at School

Anecdotal reports suggest that, in Colorado and Washington, an increasing number of students come to school under the influence of marijuana, and they also use it during the day. "There are not hard numbers yet...But school resource officers, counselors, nurses, staff and officials with Colorado school safety and disciplinary programs are anecdotally reporting an increase in marijuana-related incidents in middle and high schools," according to a November 2013 article in *The Denver Post*.[35] Another article in *The Denver Post* reports that adolescents are increasingly using vaporizers to consume marijuana. "The tiny, odorless devices are being widely used" even at middle and high schools. The story notes "there is a strong market for vaporizers among the college-aged crowd."[36]

Adolescents Driving Under the Influence

Almost one-fourth of teenagers admit to driving under the influence of alcohol or other drugs, and of those, 75% do not believe that smoking marijuana adversely affects driving.[37] In Colorado between 2006 and 2011, traffic fatalities decreased by 16%, but fatalities involving drivers testing positive for marijuana increased 114%.[38] In Washington, the state toxicologist reported that in 2013 roughly 25% of the blood tests for suspected impaired driving showed detectable THC. Before 2013, that number was around 20%. Typically, one-fourth of those individuals confirmed positive for THC are younger than 21 years. Marijuana is the most frequently detected drug (including alcohol) in that age group.[39]

SUMMARY

Marijuana is the most common illicit drug of abuse in adolescents, nationally and globally. What is currently known about the effects of marijuana on adolescents and their lives reveals a number of concerns, ranging from acute physical effects to long-term physical, mental, and social consequences. As states begin to re-evaluate marijuana policies, it is important that the health and well-being of adolescents and young adults remain a priority. Much about marijuana and its medicinal uses is still not known, nor is there adequate data about the long-term effects of use of stronger marijuana products over the life course. Although much research is needed on marijuana and its derivatives, enough is known about its effects on adolescents to recommend an increased focus on preventing marijuana use in this stage of life.

References

1. National Institute on Drug Abuse. Drug facts: marijuana. Available at: www.drugabuse.gov/sites/default/files/marijuana_0_0.pdf. Accessed June 2, 2014
2. Wang G, Roosevelt G, Heard K. Pediatric marijuana exposures in a medical marijuana state. *JAMA Pediatr*. 2013;167(7):630-633
3. National Cannabis Prevention Information Centre. Looking after a friend on cannabis. Available at: ncpic.org.au/ncpic/publications/factsheets/pdf/looking-after-a-friend-on-cannabis. Accessed June 2, 2014
4. Meier MH, Caspi A, Ambler A, et al. Persistent cannabis users show neuropsychological decline from childhood to midlife. *Proc Natl Acad Sci U S A*. 2012;109(40):E2657-E2664
5. Partnership Attitude Tracking Study (PATS) Sponsored by MetLife Foundation. 2012. Available at: www.drugfree.org/wp-content/uploads/2013/04/PATS-2012-FULL-REPORT2.pdf. Accessed June 2, 2014
6. Casey BJ, Jones RM, Hare TA. The adolescent brain. *Ann N Y Acad Sci*. 2008;1124:111-126
7. Hurd YL, Michaelides M, Miller ML, Jutras-Aswad D. Trajectory of adolescent cannabis use on addiction vulnerability. *Neuropharmacology*. 2014;76(Pt B):416-424

8. Haney M, Cooper ZD, Bedi G, Vosburg SK, Comer SD, Foltin RW. Nabilone decreases marijuana withdrawal and a laboratory measure of marijuana relapse. *Neuropsychopharmacology*. 2013;38: 1557-1565
9. US Food and Drug Administration. Marinol (dronabinol). 2004. Available at: www.fda.gov/ohrms/dockets/dockets/05n0479/05N-0479-emc0004-04.pdf. Accessed June 2, 2014
10. US Food and Drug Administration. Cesamet (nabilone). 2009. Available at: www.fda.gov/downloads/drugs/guidancecomplianceregulatoryinformation/guidances/ucm088722.pdf. Accessed June 2, 2014
11. Bottorff JL, Johnson JL, Moffat BM, Mulvogue T. Relief-oriented use of marijuana by teens. *Subst Abuse Treat Prev Policy*. 2009;4(7):1-10
12. US National Drug Control Policy. Teen "self medication" for depression leads to more serious mental illness, new report reveals. *Sci Daily*. May 10, 2008. Available at: www.sciencedaily.com/releases/2008/05/080509105348.htm. Accessed June 2, 2014
13. Johnston LD, O'Malley PM, Miech RA, Bachman JG, Schulenberg JE. *Monitoring the Future: National Results on Adolescent Drug Use: Overview of Key Findings*. Ann Arbor, MI: Institue for Social Research, The University of Michigan; 2014
14. US Department of Health and Human Services. Substance Abuse and Mental Health Administration. *Report on the 1997 National Household Survey on Drug Abuse, 1997*. Rockville, MD: Substance Abuse and Mental Health Services Administration, Office of Applied Studies; 1997. Available at: www.samhsa.gov/data/nhsda/pe1997/toc.htm. Accessed June 20, 2014
15. Harrison LD, Erickson PG, Korf DJ, Brochu S, Benschop A. How much for a dime bag? An exploration of youth drug markets. *Drug Alcohol Depend*. 2007;90(Suppl 1):S27-S39
16. Salomonsen-Sautel S, Sakai JT, Thurstone C, Corley R, Hopfer C. Medical marijuana use among adolescents in substance abuse treatment. *J Am Acad Child Adolesc Psychiatry*. 2012;51(7):694-702
17. Wright D, Pemberton M. *Risk and protective factors for adolescent drug use: findings from the 1999 National Household Survey on Drug Abuse*. Rockville, MD: Substance Abuse and Mental Health Services Administration, Office of Applied Studies; 2004. Available at: www.samhsa.gov/data/2k13/nhsda/a-19-risk-and-protective-factors-for-adolescent-drug-use.pdf. Accessed June 20, 2014
18. Cleveland MJ, Feinberg ME, Bontempo DE, Greenberg MT. The role of risk and protective factors in substance use across adolescence. *J Adolesc Health*. 2008;43(2):157-164
19. Drug Abuse Warning Network. *CBHSQ data spotlight: emergency department visits involving marijuana among adolescents aged 15 to 17: increase from 2005 to 2010 varied by gender*. 2012. Available at: www.samhsa.gov/data/spotlight/Spot099AdolescentMarijuanaUse2012.pdf. Accessed June 2, 2014
20. Shapiro GK, Buckley-Hunter L. What every adolescent needs to know: cannabis can cause psychosis. *J Psychosom Res*. 2010;69:533-539
21. Voth E. Voth EA, Guidelines for prescribing medical marijuana. *West J Med*. 2001;175(5):305-306
22. Nierengarten M. Guidelines needed for medical use of marijuana. *Lancet Oncol*. 2007;8(11):965
23. Colorado Department of Revenue Marijuana Enforcement Division. Current retail marijuana rules. 2014. Available at: www.colorado.gov/cs/Satellite/Rev-MMJ/CBON/1251592984795. Accessed June 2, 2014
24. Washington State Liquor Control Board. Initiative 502 adopted rules. 2014. Available at: liq.wa.gov/marijuana/I-502. Accessed June 2, 2014
25. The Guide to Community Preventive Services. *Preventing Excessive Alcohol Consumption*. Available at: www.thecommunityguide.org/alcohol/index.html. Accessed June 2, 2014
26. The Guide to Community Preventive Services. *Reducing Tobacco Use and Secondhand Smoke Exposure*. Available at: www.thecommunityguide.org/tobacco/index.html. Accessed June 2, 2014
27. *National Prevention Strategy, Tobacco Free Living and Preventing Dug Abuse and Excessive Alcohol Use*. Available at: www.surgeongeneral.gov/initiatives/prevention/strategy. Accessed June 2, 2014
28. The Office of the Surgeon General, National Institute on Alcohol Abuse and Alcoholism; Substance Abuse and Mental Health Services Administration. The Surgeon General's call to action to prevent and reduce underage drinking. 2007. Available at: www.ncbi.nlm.nih.gov/books/NBK44360/. Accessed June 2, 2014

29. National Research Council, Institute of Medicine of the National Academies. *Reducing Underage Drinking: A Collective Responsibility*. Washington, DC: National Academies Press; 2004
30. Bailey J. Understanding risk and protective factors for your marijuana use is essential to effective prevention. 2013. Slides available at: adai.uw.edu/mjsymposium/agenda.htm. Accessed June 2, 2014
31. Joffe A, Yancy WS, Committee on Substance Abuse, Committee on Adolescence. American Academy of Pediatrics Technical Report. Legalization of marijuana: potential impact on youth. *Pediatrics.* 2004;113(6):e632-e638. Available at: pediatrics.aappublications.org/content/113/6/e632.short. Accessed June 2, 2014
32. Centers for Disease Control and Prevention. Seattle public schools, 2012 youth risk behavior survey report. Seattle Public Schools. (2012). 2012 Youth Risk Behavior Survey results: Seattle high school survey, summary tables, weighted data. Available at: www.seattleschools.org/modules/groups/homepagefiles/cms/1583136/File/Departmental%20Content/health%20and%20safety/healthsurveys/2012%20YRBS%20Summary%20TablesREV.pdf?sessionid=cd5519ca3a3738c5de4f4a0748bec71a. Accessed June 2, 2014
33. Kilmer J. Before the grand opening, measuring Washington State's marijuana market in the last year before legalized commercial sales, *RAND Corp Drug Policy Res Cent.* 2013. Report prepared for the Washington State Liquor Control Board/BOTEC Analysis Corporation. Available at: www.rand.org/pubs/research_reports/RR466.html. Accessed June 2, 2014.
34. Colorado tightens control on marijuana edibles, concentrates. *Reuters*. May 21, 2014. Available at: www.reuters.com/article/2014/05/22/us-marijuana-colorado-idUSBREA4L02U20140522. Accessed June 20, 2014
35. Pot problem in Colorado schools increase with legalization. *The Denver Post*. November 11, 2013. Available at: www.denverpost.com/breakingnews/ci_24501596/pot-problems-colorado-schools-increase-legalization. Accessed June 2, 2014
36. Pocket hookahs proliferate with young marijuana users, sources say. *The Denver Post*. December 6, 2013. Available at: www.denverpost.com/news/ci_24673588/pocket-hookahs-proliferate-young-marijuana-users-sources-say. Accessed June 2, 2014
37. Liberty Mutual Insurance and Students Against Destructive Decisions (SADD) press release. One in four teens admits to driving under the influence and many believe it does not impact their safety. 2013. Unpublished data from www.libertymutualgroup.com/omapps/ContentServer?fid=3237831502381&pagename=LMGroup%2FViews%2FLMG&ft=8&cid=2237833722148. Accessed June 2, 2014
38. Colorado Department of Transportation. The Legalization of Marijuana in Colorado: The Impact. Rocky Mountain HIDTA, Volume 1, August 2013
39. Couper F. Analysis of suspected impaired driving cases received at the Washington State Toxicology Laboratory. Unpublished data. February 18, 2014. Washington State Patrol Toxicology Division, Seattle, WA

Adolesc Med 025 (2014) 347–359

Long-Acting Reversible Contraceptives and Adolescents: Assessing Benefits and Overcoming Barriers

Erin R. McKnight, MD[a*]; Elise D. Berlan, MD, MPH[a,b,c]

[a]Division of Adolescent Medicine, Nationwide Children's Hospital, Columbus, Ohio; [b]Department of Pediatrics, The Ohio State University College of Medicine, Columbus, Ohio; [c]Center for Clinical and Translational Research, The Research Institute at Nationwide Children's Hospital, Columbus, Ohio

INTRODUCTION

Despite an approximately 40% decline since 1990, the United States still leads the developed world in teen pregnancy.[1,2] Pregnancy during the teenage years can have immediate and long-term negative effects on teen parents, their children, and their families; it also creates considerable social and economic costs. In its commitment to improving the nation's health, Healthy People 2020 developed a new framework of goals for public health and prevention, which includes reducing pregnancies among adolescent females.[3] The Institute of Medicine highlights reducing unintended pregnancy as one of its national priorities and identifies increasing young women's access to long-acting reversible contraceptives (LARC) as a strategy to achieve this.[4] In his 2010 keynote address at the National Center for Health Statistics conference, Dr. Thomas Frieden, Director of the Centers for Disease Control and Prevention (CDC), discussed the CDC's Winnable Battles Initiative. The "Winnable Battles" include leading causes of illness, disability, and death that have evidence-based interventions, which are cost-effective and can be implemented immediately.[5] Frieden cites teen pregnancy as a "Winnable Battle," stating that "teen pregnancy and childbirth continue existing cycles of social, economic, and educational disadvantages in our nation's communities." Along with supporting evidence-based prevention programs and increasing access to family planning services, the Winnable Battles Initiative focuses on increasing adolescents' access

---

*Corresponding author:
E-mail address: erin.mcknight@nationwidechildrens.org
The authors have no financial disclosures to report.

 ISSN 1934-4287

to and use of the most effective forms of contraception, LARC. The CDC calls for efforts to reduce obstacles to the use of LARC, including educating clinicians, increasing interest among adolescents, and reducing cost barriers.[6] (This article refers to the treatment of adolescents by adolescent medicine physicians, general pediatricians, physician assistants, nurse practitioners, and other physicians, hereinafter referred to as "clinicians.")

Despite the safety and superior effectiveness of LARC,[7-9] adolescents in the United States favor shorter-acting contraceptive methods that have higher typical-use failure rates.[10] Adolescent and young adult women also have high rates of discontinuation of short-acting hormonal methods, which put them at increased risk for unintended pregnancy.[11] On the other hand, LARC methods have been shown to have improved satisfaction and continuation rates compared with shorter-acting contraceptive methods, regardless of age.[12,13] A study published in the *New England Journal of Medicine* highlights that among adolescent and adult LARC users, rates of unintended pregnancy were similarly low. However, females younger than 21 years using shorter-acting contraceptives had twice the risk of unintended pregnancy compared with adult women using the same contraceptive methods.[14] Although LARC use is low in the United States, the uptake of these contraceptive methods has increased. From 2002 to 2009, the percentage of women, including adolescents, choosing LARC methods has more than doubled.[15,16] However, the overall use remains very low; only 4.5% of 15- to 19-year-olds who use a contraceptive choose a LARC.[15]

Concerns about the safety of LARC in adolescents have been addressed in a multitude of reviews and studies and will not be addressed here.[17-19] Rather, we will provide a brief overview of each LARC method and review challenges and solutions to adolescent LARC uptake in several domains, including patient and clinician knowledge and attitudes, cost, and postpartum/postabortion placement.

OVERVIEW OF LARC METHODS

LARC methods, which include the levonorgestrel (LNG) intrauterine device (IUD), the copper IUD, and the etonogestrel subdermal implant, have typical use failure rates of less than 1%.[7] The probability of pregnancy during the first year of typical use for the LNG IUD (0.2%), copper IUD (0.8%), and etonogestrel implant (0.05%) mirror rates of perfect use and are less than typical use failure rates of oral contraceptives (9%) and depot medroxyprogesterone acetate (6%).[20] "Counseling Pearls" for clinicians are included in Table 1.

Contraceptive Implant

Nexplanon and its predecessor, Implanon, are subdermal etonogestrel contraceptive implants that are effective for at least 3 years. The device, which consists of a single rod, secretes etonogestrel, a progestin, at an initial rate of 60 to

Table 1
Counseling pearls

Nexplanon
- Safe
- More than 99% effective
- Reversible
- High rates of satisfaction and continuation
- Does not protect against sexually transmitted infection (STI)
- Main side effect is irregular bleeding
- Placement involves a quick office procedure
- No specific follow-up is necessary

Intrauterine Device (IUD)
- Safe
- More than 99% effective
- Reversible
- High rates of satisfaction and continuation
- Does not protect against STI
- Pelvic examination is required
- Women may have irregular bleeding and cramping for several months after placement
- With Mirena, women generally have less menstrual bleeding
- With ParaGard, women may have more cramping and menstrual bleeding
- Slightly increased risk of pelvic inflammatory disease for 3 weeks after placement
- Follow-up is recommended in 4-8 weeks and annually thereafter

70 mcg/day, decreasing to 25 to 30 mcg/day by the end of the third year. Etonogestrel inhibits ovulation and induces changes in cervical mucus, making it less penetrable to sperm.[21] Implanon was introduced in the United States in 2006 and is no longer available, but many women still have this device in place. Nexplanon has been available in the United States since November 2011. It contains the same amount of etonogestrel and has the same flexibility and dimensions as Implanon. It contains 15 mg of barium sulfate to allow detectability by conventional radiographic imaging. Nexplanon also was developed with a novel applicator to facilitate 1-handed insertion.[22] Studies have shown that Nexplanon is bioequivalent to Implanon and has a comparable safety profile.[23] Like Implanon, the most frequently reported adverse side effects cited by women using Nexplanon are changes to menstrual bleeding patterns (28.2%), headache (18.6%), acne (13%), and weight gain (11.6%).[24]

Intrauterine Devices

Mirena has been available in the United States since December 2000. It is a polyethylene, 32- × 32-mm T-shaped frame with a drug reservoir containing 52 mg levonorgestrel. The initial release rate is 20 mcg/day, and the rate decreases to 10 mcg/day by the end of 5 years. This continuous release of levonorgestrel suppresses the endometrium, thickens cervical mucus, and inhibits sperm mobility and function inside the uterus. When the IUD is removed, endometrial morphology and cervical mucus return to normal. The most common adverse reactions are uterine/vaginal bleeding alterations (51.9%), amenorrhea (23.9%), intermenstrual bleeding and spotting (23.4%), abdominal/pelvic pain (12.8%), and ovarian cysts (12%).[25]

Skyla has been available in the United States since February 2013. It is a polyethylene, 30- × 28-mm T-shaped frame with a drug reservoir containing 13.5 mg levonorgestrel. The release rate of levonorgestrel into the uterine cavity is 14 mcg/day initially and decreases gradually over 3 years to 5 mcg/day. It is the smallest of the 3 IUDs on the US market and is indicated for use in nulliparous woman by the FDA. In an unpublished clinical trial described in the package insert, of 1432 women 18 to 35 years old who used Skyla for up to 3 years, the cumulative 3-year pregnancy rate was 0.9%. The most common side effects reported are bleeding pattern alterations, abdominal/pelvic pain, and ovarian cysts. Women can have amenorrhea with Skyla use but less commonly than with Mirena.[26]

ParaGard is a polyethylene, 32- × 36-mm T-shaped frame that has 176 mg of copper wire coiled around the vertical stem with a 68.7-mg copper sleeve on each side of the horizontal arm. It contains barium sulfate to make it radiopaque. It has been available to women in the United States since 1984 and can be used for contraception for at least 10 years. The most common side effects reported by women using ParaGard are heavier, longer periods, and spotting between menses.[27] The copper IUD is an extremely effective form of emergency contraception if it is placed within 5 days of unprotected intercourse. In this IUD, the primary contraceptive mechanism is inhibition of sperm function by the copper ions, which prevents fertilization. If fertilization has already occurred, the copper ions can prevent implantation in the endometrium.[28]

ADOLESCENT AWARENESS/ATTITUDES

Lack of knowledge is one of the main barriers to adolescent uptake of LARC. In a recent study examining young adults' knowledge of contraception, the variable most strongly associated with LARC use was high IUD knowledge.[29] Additional studies show that adolescents have little awareness of contraceptive methods other than oral contraceptives and Depo-Provera. Their knowledge of LARC methods is even more limited, especially pertaining to eligibility and side effects.[30] In a qualitative study about attitudes toward LARC among young women seeking abortion, information about LARC usually was obtained from family and friends and mostly pertained to negative experiences.[30,31]

When adolescents are educated about LARC, they have favorable attitudes regarding these methods. They feel that the long-acting and easy-to-forget nature of LARC is well suited to a young woman's lifestyle and desire to prevent an unintended pregnancy. However, many incorrectly believe their young age renders them ineligible for LARC and think the typical user is an older, married woman.[32] Whitaker et al[33] showed that a brief 3-minute oral education intervention regarding IUD insertion, benefits, and risks increased adolescent knowledge about LARC and resulted in more favorable attitudes toward IUDs. This study further demonstrated that adolescents can greatly benefit from discussion and education on LARC, and clinicians cannot predict based on demographics or reproductive history who will be interested in these contraceptives.[33] Accordingly, information about LARC methods should be included in all reproductive health discussions to give the adolescent the most comprehensive education regarding her contraceptive choices.

CLINICIAN AWARENESS/ATTITUDES

The ability of clinicians to recommend and insert LARCs is essential to increasing uptake. A 2012 American College of Obstetricians and Gynecologists (ACOG) Committee Opinion states LARC are "safe and appropriate contraceptive methods for most women and adolescents," including nulliparous females. They recommend counseling about LARC methods at all health care visits with sexually active adolescents, including preventive health, abortion, and prenatal and postpartum visits.[8] Likewise, the CDC Medical Eligibility Criteria (MEC) do not restrict the use of LARC in women younger than 20 years or for nulliparity and advises that the advantages of the IUD in this age group outweigh proven or theoretical risks.[9] Despite these recommendations, many clinicians do not include LARCs in their contraceptive counseling for a variety of reasons. Knowledge, skills, clinical environment, and physician attitudes all influence the likelihood of whether or not a physician will counsel or insert a LARC in adolescents.[32,34]

Lack of clinician knowledge and training are obstacles in offering LARC to adolescents. In national surveys, most pediatricians recommend abstinence as a favored method of contraception and identified lack of training in reproductive health care, especially regarding LARC, as a major barrier in providing care to adolescents.[35,36] A recent survey of general pediatricians and pediatric residents in the Chicago area showed that although most did offer at least 1 form of contraception to their patients, there were numerous misconceptions regarding contraception, especially pertaining to IUDs.[37] Further surveys of office-based and Title X clinicians in the United States have found that one-third have misconceptions about the safety of IUDs for nulliparous females, and most report infrequent provision of IUDs to these patients.[38] Despite recommendations from the CDC and ACOG, clinicians feel that characteristics associated with being a teen are concerns for LARC provision, including nulliparity and multiple sex partners.[32] Even when knowledge barriers are reduced, clinician attitudes affect the provision of LARC to adolescents. A survey of public high school-based health centers in New York City found that, despite high levels of knowledge about IUDs and their safety, only half of clinicians would be likely to recommend an IUD to a nulliparous patient or to those younger than 20 years.[39]

Another study demonstrated that although clinicians in both urban and rural areas have limited knowledge about LARC, clinicians in urban areas are more likely to use intrauterine contraception and hormonal implants compared with those in rural family planning clinics. The long-acting effects of LARC and the medically underserved nature of rural areas make LARC an ideal birth control method for adolescents living in these areas. However, because of rural health disparities, including a lack of clinicians, deficiencies in provider training, inadequate access to medical care, and differences in socioeconomic status, rural adolescents may face additional challenges to obtaining LARC.[40]

Appropriate training is essential in arming clinicians with the tools necessary to increase adolescent LARC use. Exposure to procedural women's health training is the strongest predictor of LARC provision, especially IUDs.[41] Physicians who insert IUDs during residency significantly increase their likelihood of inserting IUDs once they are in practice.[42] Residents who have not received LARC education and training may still have an interest in further training. A study at the University of Nebraska Medical Center demonstrated that pediatric residents do not consistently offer LARC to their adolescent patients, but a large portion are interested in learning more and gaining further training in placement of devices.[43]

LARC education and training should be integrated into residency and fellowship education so that clinicians are more comfortable with these contraceptive methods before they leave the training environment. In a recently published article, Zuckerman et al[44] highlight the importance of competency in discussing and administering all forms of contraception as an essential requirement for Adolescent Medicine fellowship training and best practice for Adolescent Medicine specialists. Zuckerman et al broaden the list of physicians who should be trained in LARC insertion to include not only Adolescent Medicine specialists and primary care pediatricians but pediatric emergency physicians as well. In an effort to ensure adequate pregnancy prevention by avoiding missed follow-ups, they discuss the importance of inserting LARC in the pediatric emergency department first, then referring to a family planning clinic for follow-up contraceptive care; they are currently piloting this effort at Boston Medical Center.[44] By arming clinicians with comprehensive contraception provision education during their training, important discussions with adolescents can be had at all preventive care and reproductive health visits, ultimately increasing LARC use.

COST

Perceived cost of LARC is a barrier for both adolescents and clinicians. Compared with shorter-acting contraceptives, the overall cost of LARC is lower because of its long duration of action. A retrospective cost-effectiveness study analyzed the actual cost of provision of both Implanon and oral contraceptives. In this study, Lipetz et al[45] showed that not only was Implanon more cost-effective, but after 12 months of use it was half the cost of oral contraceptives.[45] The CHOICE project is a prospective, observational study in St. Louis, Missouri, designed to promote the use of LARC, remove financial barriers to effective contraception, and evaluate use, satisfaction, and continuation of LARC and non-LARC methods. For adolescents, recent experiences of the CHOICE Project demonstrate that when contraceptives are provided at no cost along with comprehensive counseling that includes LARC methods, young women often choose LARC. In the CHOICE Project, 62% of adolescents aged 14 to 20 years chose a LARC.[19]

Clinicians also fear other indirect challenges related to the cost of LARC, including clinical time, funds, and staff needs. They cite that a history of low reimbursement from both public and private insurers for LARC caused them to absorb the extra costs and was a major challenge in providing these contraceptives.[32] In addition, clinicians also are concerned about not having enough time to perform effective contraceptive counseling in their busy clinic schedules. Using trained nonmedical professionals to do contraceptive counseling can be a solution to this problem. The CHOICE Project demonstrated that structured contraceptive counseling can be effectively provided by nonmedical professionals who are trained appropriately, saving time for clinicians and allowing them to perform other services.[46]

Reducing actual and perceived financial barriers to LARC has significant societal implications. In 2008, teen pregnancy and childbirth accounted for approximately $11 billion per year in costs to US taxpayers as a result of additional expenses in health care, foster care, incarcerations among children of teen parents, and lost tax revenue because of lower educational attainment and income of teen mothers.[47] Imperfect contraceptive adherence leads to many unplanned pregnancies. According to a recently published study by Trussell et al,[48] annual medical costs of unplanned pregnancies in the United States are estimated to be $4.6 billion, half of which are attributed to imperfect contraceptive adherence. If 10% of women aged 20 to 29 years switched from oral contraception to LARC, total costs would be reduced by $288 million per year.[48] Increased uptake of LARC can generate the health care savings cost by reducing contraceptive non-adherence and therefore unplanned pregnancy. When adolescents were provided with contraception at no cost, the CHOICE Project noted that there were significantly lower rates of teenage birth in the CHOICE cohort when compared nationally.[49]

Improvements in the coverage of LARC will be seen with new insurance policies under the Affordable Care Act.[50] Under the Affordable Care Act, women's preventive health care must be covered by new health plans with no cost sharing. The Health Resources and Services Administration health plan coverage guidelines, developed by the Institute of Medicine, will help ensure that women receive preventive services without having to pay a copayment, coinsurance, or a deductible. These guidelines include contraceptive methods and counseling under preventive services and state that all FDA-approved contraceptive methods, sterilization procedures, and patient education and counseling for all women of reproductive capacity are included.[51] These requirements apply to new private health plans starting August 2012. Existing plans are exempt from the requirement; however, the Department of Health and Human Services projects that most plans will lose their grandfathered status within a few years.[52] Requiring coverage of contraceptive services has generated much debate and objection from various religious groups. Currently, a religiously affiliated employer that objects to contraception coverage is not required to pay for contraceptive coverage for employees. However, the insurance company that it contracts with will have to provide coverage at no additional cost to the employee.[52]

POSTPARTUM/POSTABORTION INITIATION

Although the teen birthrate has been declining over the past 2 decades, more than 367,000 teens gave birth in 2010. Approximately 20% of these were repeat births.[53] Rapid repeat pregnancy is defined as a pregnancy within 2 years of previous pregnancy and occurs in roughly 35% of previously pregnant adolescents.[54] Teenagers who have appropriately spaced births, compared to those with rapid repeat pregnancies, have lower rates of adverse birth outcomes, including prematurity and stillbirth.[55] Improving access to LARC immediately after pregnancy may have a significant effect on preventing repeat unintended pregnancies.[56,57] In the postpartum period, 2 conditions for contraception are that the method should not cause after-effects in the development and growth of the baby and that the method should not interfere with breastfeeding. Updated recommendations regarding postpartum contraception also state that postpartum women should not use combined hormonal contraceptives during the first 21 days after delivery because of the increased risk of venous thromboembolism during this period.[58]

The CDC MEC recommend that it is safe to use contraceptive implants as well as both levonorgestrel-releasing IUDs and copper IUDs during the postpartum period.[59] Similarly, the ACOG 2012 Committee Opinion states that "Insertion of an IUD or implant immediately postpartum ensures reliable contraception for the adolescent when they are highly motivated to prevent pregnancy."[8] Despite these recommendations, adolescent use of LARC in the postpartum period is limited. Data from the Pregnancy Risk Assessment Monitoring System (PRAMS) demonstrate that 91% of sexually active teen mothers reported using postpartum contraception after the most recent birth, but only 1 in 5 reported using a LARC method.[53]

A primary risk factor for adolescent rapid repeat pregnancy is early resumption of sexual intercourse.[60] Waiting to discuss contraception until the traditional 6-week postpartum visit does not allow clinicians to always meet the goal of initiating contraception before the resumption of sexual activity and places this population at risk for rapid repeat pregnancy. In a prospective cohort study of adolescents who received Implanon 6 weeks after delivery, almost half had already engaged in sexual activity, and 2 were pregnant at the traditional postpartum visit.[61] A study by Tocce et al[62] evaluated the initiation of the etonogestrel implant within 14 days of delivery versus waiting until the 6-week postpartum visit for IUD insertion. Before implant insertion, all patients reported abstinence. Before IUD insertion, more than half reported intercourse, with condom use being their only birth control method.[62] Initiating LARC immediately postpartum not only increases the likelihood of adolescents having effective contraception before resuming sexual activity but also can increase contraception continuation rates, therefore decreasing repeat pregnancies.[63] Adolescents who received an etonogestrel implant immediately postpartum had higher continuation rates and lower repeat pregnancy rates compared to those who received any method of contraception more than 4 weeks after delivery.[63] To maximally affect rapid repeat pregnancies in women desiring contraception, contraceptive implants should be available at the time of delivery, and IUDs should be available immediately after delivery or at the earliest follow-up visit. Those who do not desire an immediate contraceptive should be offered a bridge method and should have earlier follow-up than the traditional postpartum visit.[54]

Similarly, teens who have had a therapeutic abortion are at high risk for repeat abortion.[64] Therefore, it is important not only to initiate LARC postpartum but immediately postabortion as well. Promoting access to LARCs for immediate use postabortion has the potential to reduce rates of repeat abortions. One prospective study demonstrated that fewer women who chose an IUD for postabortion use returned for a subsequent repeat abortion within 24 months.[65] Data from the CHOICE Project also indicate that women who were offered immediate postabortion contraception are more likely to choose the IUD and implant than women without a recent history of abortion.[66]

Contraceptive care provided postpartum and postabortion is not always possible because it can be complicated by cost restrictions and policy. For example, Title X funding for family planning services may not be used in programs with abortion services (42 USC §300 a-6). These polices are intended to discourage public funding of abortions but can effectively hinder contraceptive care. This is problematic because many women do not return for their postabortion follow-up visit and have shown that they would prefer to have the option of immediate insertion.[67] A Survey of National Abortion Federation member facilities found that although most offered LARC methods in their facilities, immediate postabortion placement of IUDs and implants occurred in less than half of the clinics. It was noted that state policies had a significant effect on coverage for contraception and the likelihood of LARC use. Immediate postabortion LARC provision was higher in states with private insurance contraceptive coverage mandates and Medicaid Family Planning Expansion programs.[68] One state has expanded Medicaid to pay clinicians for LARCs inserted immediately postpartum. Effective March 1, 2012, the South Carolina Department of Health and Human Services updated its policy to include reimbursement for LARC provided in a hospital setting postpartum.[69]

CONCLUSION

LARCs have been shown to be the most effective of all contraceptive methods. Moreover, they are safe and associated with superior satisfaction and continuation. Despite this, the use of LARC by adolescents remains low. To ensure that national public health goals are achieved and teen pregnancy is indeed a "Winnable Battle," it is imperative to address the largest obstacles to LARC provision. Increasing adolescent awareness of LARC, improving clinician education and training, reducing cost barriers, and providing LARC immediately postpartum/postabortion are necessary to achieve this goal and to help break the existing cycles of social, economic, and educational disadvantage that teen pregnancy causes.

References

1. Curtin S, Abma J, Ventura S, Henshaw S. Pregnancy rates for U.S. women continue to drop. *NCHS Data Brief.* Hyattsville, MD: National Center for Health Statistics; 2013;136:1-8. Available at: www.cdc.gov/nchs/data/databriefs/db136.pdf. Accessed January 14, 2014.
2. Singh S, Darroch J. Adolescent pregnancy and childbearing: levels and trends in developed countries. *Fam Plann Perspect.* 2000;32(1):14-23
3. US Department of Health and Human Services. Healthy People 2020: Overview. Available at: www.healthypeople.gov/2020/topicsobjectives2020/overview.aspx?topicId=13. Accessed January 25, 2014
4. National Research Council. *Initial National Priorities for Comparative Effectiveness Research.* Washington, DC: The National Academies Press; 2009
5. Frieden T. *2010 National Center for Health Statistics Keynote Address.* Hyattsville, MD: Department of Health and Human Services; 2010:1-4. Available at: www.cdc.gov/nchs/video/2010 nchs_frieden/frieden_keynote.pdf. Accessed January 25, 2014
6. Centers for Disease Control and Prevention, US Department of Health and Human Services. CDC winnable battles, teen pregnancy. August 2012. Available at: www.cdc.gov/winnablebattles/teenpregnancy/ppt/teenpregnancy_winnablebattles.pptx. Accessed January 25, 2014
7. Jennings V, Sinai I. Contraceptive failure in the United States. *Contraception.* 2012;85:331-332; author reply 332
8. Committee on Adolescent Health Care Long-Acting Reversible Contraception Working Group, The American College of Obstetricians and Gynecologists. Committee Opinion No. 539: adolescents and long-acting reversible contraception: implants and intrauterine devices. *Obstet Gynecol.* 2012;120:983-988
9. US Department of Health and Human Services, Centers for Disease Control and Prevention. US Medical Eligibility Criteria for Contraceptive Use, 2010. *MMWR Morb Mortal Wkly Rep.* 2010:59:1-88
10. Abma J, Martinez G, Copen C. Teenagers in the United States: sexual activity, contraceptive use, and childbearing, national survey of family growth 2006-2008. *Vital Health Stat 23.* 2010;(30):1-47
11. Raine TR, Foster-Rosales A, Upadhyay UD, et al. One-year contraceptive continuation and pregnancy in adolescent girls and women initiating hormonal contraceptives. *Obstet Gynecol.* 2011;117:363-371

12. Peipert JF, Zhao Q, Allsworth JE, et al. Continuation and satisfaction of reversible contraception. *Obstet Gynecol.* 2011;117:1105-1113
13. Rosenstock JR, Peipert JF, Madden T, Zhao Q, Secura GM. Continuation of reversible contraception in teenagers and young women. *Obstet Gynecol.* 2012;120:1298-1305
14. Winner B, Peipert JF, Zhao Q, et al. Effectiveness of long-acting reversible contraception. *N Engl J Med.* 2012;366:1998-2007
15. Finer LB, Jerman J, Kavanaugh ML. Changes in use of long-acting contraceptive methods in the United States, 2007-2009. *Fertil Steril.* 2012;98:893-897
16. Whitaker AK, Sisco KM, Tomlinson AN, Dude AM, Martins SL. Use of the intrauterine device among adolescent and young adult women in the United States from 2002 to 2010. *J Adolesc Health.* 2013:53:401-406
17. Berenson AB, Tan A, Hirth JM, Wilkinson GS. Complications and continuation of intrauterine device use among commercially insured teenagers. *Obstet Gynecol.* 2013;121:951-958
18. Russo JA, Miller E, Gold MA. Myths and misconceptions about long-acting reversible contraception (LARC). *J Adolesc Health.* 2013;52:S14-S21
19. Mestad R, Secura G, Allsworth JE, Madden T, Zhao Q, Peipert JF. Acceptance of long-acting reversible contraceptive methods by adolescent participants in the Contraceptive CHOICE Project. *Contraception.* 2011;84:493-498
20. Trussell J. Choosing a contraceptive: efficacy, safety, and personal consideration In: Hatcher R, Trussell J, Nelson A, Cates W, Kowal D, Policar M, eds. *Contraceptive Technology: Twentieth Revised Edition.* New York: Ardent Media; 2011:3;24
21. Wenzl R, van Beek A, Schnabel P, Huber J. Pharmacokinetics of etonogestrel released from the contraceptive implant Implanon®. *Contraception.* 1998;58:283-288
22. Mansour D. Nexplanon: what Implanon did next. *J Fam Plan Reprod Health Care.* 2010;36:187-189
23. Schnabel P, Merki-Feld G, Malvy A, Duijkers I, Mommers E, van den Heuvel. Bioequivalence and X-ray visibility of a radiopaque etonogestrel implant versus a non-radiopaque implant. *Clin Drug Investig.* 2012;32:413-422
24. Mommers E, Blum G, Gent TG, Peters KP, Sørdal TS, Marintcheva-Petrova M. Nexplanon, a radiopaque etonogestrel implant in combination with a next-generation applicator: 3-year results of a noncomparative multicenter trial. *Obstet Gynecol.* 2012;207:388.e1-388.e6
25. Mirena package insert. Wayne, NJ: Bayer Healthcare Pharmaceuticals; 2013
26. Skyla package insert. Wayne, NJ: Bayer Healthcare Pharmaceuticals; 2013
27. ParaGard package insert. Sellersville, PA: Teva Women's Health; 2011
28. Gemzell-Danielsson K, Berger C, Lalitkumar PGL. Emergency contraception: mechanisms of action. *Contraception.* 2013;87:300-308
29. Dempsey AR, Billingsley CC, Savage AH, Korte JE. Predictors of long-acting reversible contraception use among unmarried young adults. *Am J Obstet Gynecol.* 2012;206:526.e1-526.e5
30. Sokkary N, Mansouri R, Yoost J, et al. A multicenter survey of contraceptive knowledge among adolescents in North America. *J Pediatr Adolesc Gynecol.* 2013:26:274-276.
31. Rose SB, Cooper AJ, Baker NK, Lawton B. Attitudes toward long-acting reversible contraception among young women seeking abortion. *J Womens Health (Larchmt).* 2011;20:1729-1735
32. Kavanaugh ML, Frohwirth L, Jerman J, Popkin R, Ethier K. Long-acting reversible contraception for adolescents and young adults: patient and provider perspectives. *J Pediatr Adolesc Gynecol.* 2013;26:86-95
33. Whitaker AK, Johnson LM, Harwood B, et al. Adolescent and young adult women's knowledge of and attitudes toward the intrauterine device. *Contraception.* 2008;78:211-217
34. Rubin SE, Davis K, McKee MD. New York City physicians' views of providing long-acting reversible contraception to adolescents. *Ann Fam Med.* 2013;11:130-136
35. Pediatricians identify barriers to caring for adolescent patients. *AAP News.* 2000;16:39
36. Wilson SF, Strohsnitter W, Baecher-Lind L. Practices and perceptions among pediatricians regarding adolescent contraception with emphasis on intrauterine contraception. *J Pediatr Adolesc Gynecol.* 2013;26:281-284
37. Swanson KJ, Gossett DR, Fournier M. Pediatricians' beliefs and prescribing patterns of adolescent contraception: a provider survey. *J Pediatr Adolesc Gynecol.* 2013;26:340-345

38. Tyler CP, Whiteman MK, Zapata LB, et al. Health care provider attitudes and practices related to intrauterine devices for nulliparous women. *Obstet Gynecol.* 2012;119:762-771
39. Kohn JE, Hacker JG, Rousselle MA, Gold M. Knowledge and likelihood to recommend intrauterine devices for adolescents among school-based health center providers. *J Adolesc Health.* 2012;51:319-324
40. Vaaler ML, Kalanges LK, Fonseca VP, Castrucci BC. Urban–rural differences in attitudes and practices toward long-acting reversible contraceptives among family planning providers in Texas. *Womens Health Issues.* 2012;22:e157-e162
41. Greenberg KB, Makino KK, Coles MS. Factors associated with provision of long-acting reversible contraception among adolescent health care providers. *J Adolesc Health.* 2013;52:372-374
42. Rubin SE, Fletcher J, Stein T, Segall-Gutierrez P, Gold M. Determinants of intrauterine contraception provision among US family physicians: a national survey of knowledge, attitudes and practice. *Contraception.* 2011;83:472-478
43. French VA, Amoura NJ, LaCroix AE, Lyian, XM. *Long acting reversible contraception in adolescents: a survey of pediatric residents.* Manuscript in preparation
44. Zuckerman B, Nathan S, Mate K. Preventing unintended pregnancy: a pediatric opportunity. *Pediatrics.* 2014:133:181-183
45. Lipetz C, Phillips CJ, Fleming CF. The cost-effectiveness of a long-acting reversible contraceptive (Implanon) relative to oral contraception in a community setting. *Contraception.* 2009;79:304-309
46. Madden T, Mullersman JL, Omvig KJ, Secura GM, Peipert JF. Structured contraceptive counseling provided by the Contraceptive CHOICE Project. *Contraception.* 2013;88:243-249
47. Centers for Disease Control and Prevention, About Teen Pregnancy. Available at: www.cdc.gov/TeenPregnancy/AboutTeenPreg.htm. Accessed June 23, 2014
48. Trussell J, Henry N, Hassan F, Prezioso A, Law A, Filonenko A. Burden of unintended pregnancy in the United States: potential savings with increased use of long-acting reversible contraception. *Contraception.* 2013;87:154-161
49. Peipert JF, Madden T, Allsworth JE, Secura GM. Preventing unintended pregnancies by providing no-cost contraception. *Obstet Gynecol.* 2012;120:1291-1297
50. The Patient Protection and Affordable Care Act. March 23, 2010:111-148. Available at: www.gpo.gov/fdsys/pkg/PLAW-111publ148/pdf/PLAW-111publ148.pdf. Accessed July 21, 2014
51. Health Resources and Services Administration, US Department of Health and Human Services. Women's preventive services guidelines. Available at: www.hrsa.gov/womensguidelines/. Accessed June 23, 2014
52. Guttmacher Institute. Federal contraceptive coverage requirement emerges as major political issue despite accommodation for religiously affiliated employers. *Guttmacher Policy Review.* Winter 2012;15(1). Available at: www.guttmacher.org/pubs/gpr/15/1/gpr150120.html. Accessed January 15, 2014
53. Centers for Disease Control and Prevention. Vital signs: repeat births among teens—United States, 2007–2010. *MMWR Morb Mortal Wkly Rep.* 2013;62:249-255
54. Baldwin MK, Edelman AB. The effect of long-acting reversible contraception on rapid repeat pregnancy in adolescents: a review. *J Adolesc Health.* 2013;52:S47-S53
55. Smith GC, Pell JP. Teenage pregnancy and risk of adverse perinatal outcomes associated with first and second births: population based retrospective cohort study. *BMJ.* 2001;323:476
56. Blumenthal PD, Shah NM, Jain K, et al. Revitalizing long-acting reversible contraceptives in settings with high unmet need: a multi-country experience matching demand creation and service delivery. *Contraception.* 2013;87:170-175
57. Blumenthal PD, Voedisch A, Gemzell-Danielsson K. Strategies to prevent unintended pregnancy: increasing use of long-acting reversible contraception. *Hum Reprod Update.* 2011;17:121-137
58. World Health Organization, Department of Reproductive Health and Research. Combined hormonal contraceptive use during the postpartum period. Geneva, Switzerland: World Health Organization; 2010
59. Update to CDC's U.S. Medical Eligibility Criteria for Contraceptive Use, 2010. Revised recommendations for the use of contraceptive methods during postpartum period. *MMWR Morb Mortal Wkly Rep.* 2011;60:878-883

60. Kelly LS, Sheeder J, Stevens-Simon C. Why lightning strikes twice: postpartum resumption of sexual activity during adolescence. *J Pediatr Adolesc Gynecol.* 2005;18:327-335
61. Lewis LN, Doherty DA, Hickey M, Skinner SR. Implanon as a contraceptive choice for teenage mothers: a comparison of contraceptive choices, acceptability and repeat pregnancy. *Contraception.* 2010;81:421-426
62. Tocce K, Sheeder J, Python J, Teal SB. Long acting reversible contraception in postpartum adolescents: early initiation of etonogestrel implant is superior to IUDs in the outpatient setting. *J Pediatr Adolesc Gynecol.* 2012;25:59-63
63. Tocce KM, Sheeder JL, Teal SB. Rapid repeat pregnancy in adolescents: do immediate postpartum contraceptive implants make a difference? *Obstet Gynecol.* 2012;206:481.e1-481.e7
64. Mentula MJ, Niinimäki M, Suhonen S, Hemminki E, Gissler M, Heikinheimo O. Young age and termination of pregnancy during the second trimester are risk factors for repeat second-trimester abortion. *Obstet Gynecol.* 2010;203:107.e1-107.e7
65. Rose SB, Lawton BA. Impact of long-acting reversible contraception on return for repeat abortion. *Am J Obstet Gynecol.* 2012;206:37.e1-37.e6
66. Madden T, Secura GM, Allsworth JE, Peipert JF. Comparison of contraceptive method chosen by women with and without a recent history of induced abortion. *Contraception.* 2011;84:571-577
67. Stanek AM, Bednarek PH, Nichols MD, Jensen JT, Edelman AB. Barriers associated with the failure to return for intrauterine device insertion following first-trimester abortion. *Contraception.* 2009;79:216-220
68. Thompson KM, Speidel JJ, Saporta V, Waxman NJ, Harper CC. Contraceptive policies affect post-abortion provision of long-acting reversible contraception. *Contraception.* 2011;83:41-47
69. South Carolina Department of Health and Human Services. Long acting birth control device provided in a hospital setting. *MEDICAID Bulletin.* January 19, 2012. Available at: www.scdhhs.gov. Accessed June 23, 2014

Adolesc Med 025 (2014) 360–376

Child and Adolescent Feeding and Eating Disorders and the DSM-5: A Brave New World

Rollyn M. Ornstein, MD[a];
Debra K. Katzman, MD, FRCPC[b*]

[a]*Associate Professor of Pediatrics, Division of Adolescent Medicine and Eating Disorders, Penn State Hershey Children's Hospital/College of Medicine, Hershey, Pennsylvania;*
[b]*Professor of Pediatrics, Senior Associate Scientist, Research Institute, The Hospital for Sick Children and University of Toronto, Toronto, Ontario, Canada*

INTRODUCTION

In the newly published *Diagnostic and Statistical Manual of Mental Disorders*, Fifth Edition (DSM-5), the DSM-IV Feeding Disorders of Infancy or Early Childhood has been combined with the section on eating disorders. The new section called Feeding and Eating Disorders addresses feeding and eating disorders across the lifespan and includes (1) anorexia nervosa (AN); (2) bulimia nervosa (BN); (3) binge eating disorder (BED); (4) avoidant/restrictive food intake disorder (ARFID); (5) pica; (6) rumination disorder; (7) other specified feeding and eating disorder (OSFED), and (8) unspecified feeding and eating disorder (UFED). This article will describe the most recent changes to this section in the DSM-5 with a focus on the relevance to children and adolescents. The most significant changes are outlined in Table 1.

BACKGROUND

Reasons for the Change in DSM-IV

The main purpose in developing the DSM-5 section on Feeding and Eating Disorders was to create an evidence-based manual that would be useful for clini-

*Corresponding author:
E-mail address: debra.katzman@sickkids.ca

 ISSN 1934-4287

cians to accurately and consistently diagnose eating disorders across the lifespan. Two major issues that are relevant to children and adolescents with these disorders guided these changes. First, feeding and eating disorders can develop any time during the lifetime. Most psychiatric disorders start early in life, prior to adulthood. Therefore, it was critical to take a lifespan approach. As such, the first step was to consolidate the DSM-IV section on Feeding and Eating Disorders of Infancy or Early Childhood (Feeding Disorder of Infancy or Early Childhood [FDIC], pica, and rumination disorder) and the section on Eating Disorders into what is now Feeding and Eating Disorders. Next, the Eating Disorders Work Group reported that there were limitations to, as well as a lack of evidence regarding the clinical utility of, the DSM-IV diagnosis of FDIC. The diagnosis was rarely used, and there was little information on the characteristics of children who had the disorder. The DSM-5 presents a revised

Table 1
Significant changes made to the DSM-5

DSM-IV criteria ⟶	DSM-5 criteria
Anorexia Nervosa • Suggested weight cutoffs • Amenorrhea > 3 months	Anorexia Nervosa (AN) • Amenorrhea and numeric weight cutoffs eliminated • Developmental considerations incorporated • Addition of persistent behavior that interferes with weight gain to criterion B
Bulimia Nervosa • Binging and inappropriate compensatory behaviors twice weekly for the past 3 months	Bulimia Nervosa (BN) • Binging and inappropriate compensatory behaviors for at least once weekly for the past 3 months
Eating Disorder Not Otherwise Specified included Binge Eating Disorder (BED) in appendix • Binging twice weekly for the past 6 months	• Official recognition of Binge Eating Disorder (BED) • Binging once weekly for the last 3 months
Eating Disorder Not Otherwise Specified	• Eating Disorder Not Otherwise Specified eliminated • Avoidant/Restrictive Food Intake Disorder (ARFID) (Table 2) • Other Specified Feeding and Eating Disorders - Atypical AN (not underweight) - Purging disorder - Sub-threshold BN (<1×/wk or <3 mos) - Sub-threshold BED (<1×/wk or <3 mos) - Night eating syndrome • Unspecified Feeding and Eating Disorders
Feeding Disorders of Infancy or Early Childhood	• Feeding Disorders of Infancy or Early Childhood eliminated • Avoidant/Restrictive Food Intake Disorder (ARFID) (Table 2) • Pica • Rumination

conceptualization of this diagnostic category, which has been named ARFID. Furthermore, most children and younger adolescents who presented with disordered eating were classified in the heterogeneous DSM-IV diagnostic category of Eating Disorder Not Otherwise Specified (EDNOS). More than half of children and adolescents received this diagnosis despite having significant clinical and functional impairments.[1-3] This likely led to delayed or missed diagnoses, resulting in lack of necessary treatment for those who were clearly ill. The ARFID diagnosis was also developed to identify children and adolescents who presented with clinically significant restrictive eating problems, including some that met the DSM-IV criteria for EDNOS. The addition of ARFID, and modifications to criteria for existing diagnoses, is hoped to result in a reduction in the frequency of the EDNOS diagnosis, a major goal of the DSM-5.

Severity modifiers (mild, moderate, severe, and extreme) accompany the diagnostic criteria for AN, BN and BED, and elaborate on the degree of malnutrition or frequency of behaviors to provide additional case-based information.[4]

ANOREXIA NERVOSA

The diagnostic criteria for AN in the DSM-IV included 4 criteria and underscored critically low weight and pursuit of thinness as the primary symptoms. Because children and adolescents often failed to meet all 4 criteria, many young people ended up with a DSM-IV diagnosis of EDNOS, despite the fact that they clinically resembled adolescents and adults with AN. There are 2 types of AN: (1) restrictive type (no recurrent episodes of binge eating or purging behavior, 3 months prior to diagnosis); and (2) binge eating/purging type (recurrent episodes of binge eating or purging behavior within 3 months of diagnosis). A proper diagnosis is imperative to assuring evidence-based treatment, reducing the associated high morbidity and mortality, and improving the long-term outcome.

Several revisions to the diagnostic criteria for AN (Table 1) outlined here reflect the acknowledgement of the developmental differences, both physical and psychological, in children and young adolescents compared to older adolescents and adults, again reinforcing the lifespan approach.

Criterion A: Low Weight

The weight criterion in DSM-IV included "refusal to maintain body weight at or above a minimally normal weight for age and height, eg, 85% of that expected."[5] The example of "85% of that expected" was suggested as a guideline; however, in many instances, it was interpreted as doctrine. For example, if a patient was 86% of expected body weight (EBW), he or she would not be diagnosed as having AN, despite significant weight loss and obvious morbidity. As such, this cutoff had the potential to lead to adverse outcomes in such patients who were not diagnosed with AN and therefore were unable to obtain suitable treatment in a timely manner.[6] In addition, the methodology for determining "85% of EBW" varies both clinically and across research studies, leading to discrepancies in the prevalence of individuals who meet this guideline.[7] Finally, there does not seem to be a weight threshold whereby the signs and symptoms of malnutrition become clinically apparent. One study using body mass index (BMI) percentiles reported that adolescents with "partial AN" between 85% and 90% of median body weight (MBW) had the same medical complications as those who were less than 85% MBW.[1]

Children with eating disorders often present during critical times of physical growth and development, and, as such, deviations from individual growth trajectories, as opposed to absolute percentiles, should be taken into account. Skeletal growth in height without associated weight gain is a sign of a potential problem. Therefore, this indicator should be considered in the definition of low weight in the diagnosis of AN. This is especially true for children with premenarcheal-onset AN because linear growth slows down after menarche.[8] Additionally, younger patients with eating disorders are more likely to experience life-threatening complications with rapid weight loss, even if they do not meet strict DSM-IV criteria for AN.[2]

The revised criterion A now removes numeric cutoffs and incorporates developmental considerations. Finally, the word "refusal" has been removed because it was too pejorative and implied willful behavior within the individual's control. The utility of BMI-for-age percentiles in children and adolescents is discussed in the DSM-5.

Criterion B: Fear of Gaining Weight or Becoming Fat

In the DSM-IV, this cognitive criterion relied on the presence of formal operational thought and complex abstract reasoning; the former develops around 11 to 13 years of age and the latter develops into late adolescence.[6] Many younger patients do not acknowledge a fear of weight gain and may deny this as an impetus for their behavior. The DSM-5 has attempted to rely more on behaviors rather than cognitions, for example, skipping meals and other active food avoidance and caloric restriction, to capture those patients who may deny fear of weight gain or being fat despite their actions. There is also the possibility of using multiple informants (such as parents or guardians) to gather evidence of eating disorder behaviors and symptoms.

The concept of non–fat-phobic AN, which takes into account cultural differences and often applies to non-western cultures (eg, Asia, Africa) with diverse reasons for food refusal, including somatic complaints (eg, gastrointestinal), religious motives, need for control/self-discipline, and punishment of family,[9] has also been addressed in the DSM-5. These less typical presentations are subsumed in the revised criterion B.[4]

Criterion C: Body Image Disturbance

This criterion necessitates an understanding of the concept of self-worth as well as the perception of risk and long-term consequences, both of which younger patients may not yet appreciate from a developmental perspective. For this criterion, as with Criterion B, behavioral indicators should suffice when the young patient does not endorse distortion of body image. The word "denial" of the seriousness of the problem has been removed because it was felt to be stigmatizing and indicative of a volitional process.[4]

Criterion D: Amenorrhea

There has been a long-standing debate about whether amenorrhea or the absence of 3 consecutive menstrual cycles in postmenarchal females should remain as a criterion for AN.[10] AN is the only disorder in which an objective physical indicator of physiologic dysfunction is used as a criterion for a psychiatric diagnosis. If present, amenorrhea is usually a consequence of weight loss, although amenorrhea has been shown to precede weight loss in 20% of adolescents with AN.[11]

If amenorrhea were to have clinical utility, it should differentiate patients with eating disorders in some way. Recent findings in adult populations suggest that there are no significant clinical differences between patients with AN, with or without amenorrhea.[12,13] In fact, most differences among those who do and do not meet the amenorrhea criterion reflect weight and nutritional status, rather than providing useful diagnostic information. The amenorrhea criterion presents particular challenges in the pediatric population because many children and adolescents with eating disorders are premenarcheal, male, or may be on hormonal contraception. In addition, patients are not always forthcoming about their menstrual status, especially if they believe the presence of amenorrhea will require weight gain.[14] Finally, some patients who experience rapid weight loss may not have 3 absent menstrual cycles at the time of presentation despite clearly fitting the clinical picture of AN.

Amenorrhea has been eliminated in the DSM-5 criteria for AN. However, it can be used as an associated physiologic disturbance to support the diagnosis as well as a possible indicator of illness severity.[4]

Epidemiology

Anorexia nervosa has been described for centuries and remains a relatively uncommon disorder with a lifetime prevalence of 0.3% to 0.6% in adolescent females and somewhat higher percentages in adult populations.[15-17] Although there has been a stable incidence rate over the past several decades, there has been an increase in the incidence among 15- to 19-year-old females.[17] Studies in both community and clinical samples have demonstrated modest increases in the diagnosis of AN using the proposed DSM-5 criteria.[18,19] Even with the revisions stated earlier, there is controversy about the adequacy of the modifications with respect to the diagnosis of AN in children and adolescents.[20] Recent studies have demonstrated maintenance of validity with meticulous application of the new criteria.[21]

BULIMIA NERVOSA

Bulimia nervosa is defined by frequent episodes of binge eating followed by inappropriate compensatory behaviors (eg, self-induced vomiting; misuse of laxatives, diuretics, or other medication; fasting; or excessive exercising) to prevent weight gain and self-evaluation that is influenced by body shape and weight.

An episode of binge eating is defined as rapid consumption of an excessively large amount of food in a discrete period of time (larger than what most individuals would eat in a similar period of time under similar circumstances). Binge eating is exemplified by loss of control (LOC). It is often done in private and is associated with feelings of shame and guilt.[4]

The DSM-IV described binge eating and compensatory behaviors as needing to occur at least twice a week for a 3-month period to meet criteria for BN. In addition, there needed to be an undue emphasis on weight and shape with respect to self-worth. The illness could not occur during episodes of AN. The DSM-IV also subclassified BN as purging or nonpurging type, with the latter including compensatory behaviors such as exercising and fasting.[5] A review examining the clinical utility of the binge-purge frequency threshold have found that there are few differences between patients with higher and lower frequencies of episodes, including those who only use symptoms once a week. Less is known about outcomes of patients who were considered full versus partial syndrome BN.[22] Adolescents who met DSM-IV criteria for BN were quite similar to those with subthreshold BN with respect to severity of eating disorder symptomatology, medical complications, and psychiatric comorbidity.[23,24] In one study, almost half of adolescents who had symptoms of BN did not meet full criteria, mostly because of lower frequency of binge and purge episodes.[23] Similarly, in another study, one-fifth of adolescents diagnosed with EDNOS missed meeting full criteria for BN based on frequency of binge and purge episodes, and were classified as subthreshold BN. These patients were notably younger than those with BN, which may indicate that this type of presentation may signify an earlier stage in the development of full-syndrome BN.[25] Both BN and subthreshold BN have been shown to be associated with depression, low self-esteem, and suicidality.[26] In addition, subthreshold cases of eating disorders have serious physiologic complications.[1]

The DSM-5 diagnostic category for BN has reduced the threshold of binge-purge episodes to once per week over a 3-month period. In addition, the DSM-5 has removed the purging and nonpurging subtypes because there is little difference between them with respect to course or treatment response.[27]

Developmental aspects of symptoms and cognitions need to be taken into consideration when diagnosing a younger adolescent with BN. Younger patients may not comprehend the concept of LOC and therefore require concrete examples to understand this idea. Behaviors that may indicate a binge or LOC eating in children (those younger than 12 years) include secretive eating, food seeking in response to negative affect, eating in the absence of hunger, and food hoarding.[6] Research suggests that these behaviors may be more important in defining LOC than the consumption of objectively large quantities of food when assessing binge eating in children.[28,29]

Studies in nonclinical samples of children and adolescents have shown that disordered eating and cognitions, including objective or subjective binge eating, were more prevalent in overweight youth.[30,31] Additionally, subthreshold levels of dangerous weight loss behaviors, including purging, predict future eating disorder symptoms, as well as higher BMI, 5 years later.[32] Therefore, it is prudent to screen all overweight children and adolescents for eating disorder symptoms, including binge eating and compensatory behaviors.[1,26] The DSM-5 criteria for BN will hopefully facilitate earlier detection and treatment in younger patients.

Epidemiology

Bulimia nervosa is often characterized by a chronic course with intermittent periods of remission and relapse. It also has been associated with an increased mortality risk secondary to suicide.[33] In a large nationally representative sample of US adolescents, a lifetime prevalence of 1.3% for females and 0.5% for males was found for BN. Although the overall incidence of BN may be decreasing, it has remained stable in 10- to 19-year-old females. BN traditionally has been described as having an age of onset during middle to late adolescence, but several studies indicate that the age of onset of BN has been decreasing.[17] This may be attributed to increasing rates of childhood obesity and earlier age of menarche.[34] Studies in both adolescent and adult samples have shown a modest increase in the number of cases of BN when applying the DSM-5 criteria.[35,36] A preliminary study using the proposed DSM-5 criteria in a clinical sample of adolescents between 10 and 14 years old and those between 15 to 17 years old demonstrated an increase in the prevalence of BN from 2% to 6% and 16% to 24%, respectively.[36] Another study using a clinical sample of adolescents with eating disorders demonstrated an increase in the prevalence of BN from 7% to 12%.[19]

BINGE EATING DISORDER

In the DSM-IV, BED was incorporated into an appendix of disorders requiring further study. It is formally included as a diagnostic category in the DSM-5. In addition to the characteristics described earlier, the binge eating episodes must be associated with at least 3 of the following: eating more quickly than normal, eating until uncomfortable, eating despite not being hungry, avoidance of eating with others because of embarrassment over the quantity of food consumed, and feeling guilty/upset about the binge episode. Unlike BN, there are no associated compensatory behaviors.[5] Other revisions include a decrease in the duration of symptoms from 6 months to 3 months and a decrease in the threshold frequency for binge episodes from twice to once per week.[4] Studies in adults have shown that there is no significant difference in the severity of partial and full BED,[37] and there is little clinical utility in requiring the higher frequency of binge episodes.[22]

Epidemiology

Little is known about binge eating and BED in children and adolescents. Studies in adults with BED indicate that binge eating usually begins during late adolescence. However, there are 2 identified patterns of binge eating onset: 1 before and 1 after the start of dieting behaviors. The former pattern is associated with an earlier age (11-13 years) of onset of binge eating.[28] The prevalence of binge eating in girls, but not in boys, seems to increase with pubertal stage and age.[38] Retrospective studies have shown that childhood obesity and verbal bullying with respect to shape, weight, and eating are more common in individuals with BED.[39] It is not clear whether binge eating or BED in childhood and adolescence continues into adulthood. Longitudinal studies using DSM-IV criteria have identified BED in children and adolescents at rates between 3% and 10%.[40,41] The DSM-5 diagnostic category for BED likely will reveal more cases of eating disorder pathology.

AVOIDANT/RESTRICTIVE FOOD INTAKE DISORDER

Avoidant/Restrictive Food Intake Disorder is a new diagnostic category in the DSM-5 (Table 2) and represents one of the most significant revisions to the Feeding and Eating Disorder section. It has replaced FDIC but is also intended to capture some individuals who previously were given a diagnosis of EDNOS or certain patients who were diagnosed with early onset eating disorders using the Great Ormond Street (GOS) eating disorder classification system.[3] Together, FDIC, EDNOS and the GOS eating disorder classification system informed the development of ARFID. We will review these diagnostic groups in an effort to fully understand the impetus behind the inclusion of ARFID in the DSM-5.

Feeding Disorder of Infancy or Early Childhood

Historically, Feeding Disorder of Infancy or Early Childhood (FDIC) was rarely used; therefore, there is insufficient evidence to describe the clinical characteristics of this population.[42] One of the main issues with the diagnostic criteria for

Table 2
Avoidant/restrictive food intake disorder: diagnostic criteria

A. An eating or feeding disturbance (eg, apparent lack of interest in eating or food; avoidance based on the sensory characteristics of food; concern about aversive consequences of eating) as manifested by persistent failure to meet appropriate nutritional and/or energy needs associated with one (or more) of the following:
   - Significant weight loss (or failure to achieve expected weight gain or faltering growth in children)
   - Significant nutritional deficiency
   - Dependence on enteral feeding or oral nutritional supplements
   - Marked interference with psychosocial functioning

B. The disturbance is not better explained by lack of available food or by an associated culturally sanctioned practice

C. The eating disturbance does not occur exclusively during the course of anorexia nervosa or bulimia nervosa, and there is no evidence of a disturbance in the way in which a person's body weight or shape is experienced

D. The eating disturbance is not attributable to a concurrent medical condition or is not better explained by another mental disorder. When the eating disturbance occurs in the context of another condition or disorder, the severity of the eating disturbance exceeds that routinely associated with the condition or disorder and warrants additional clinical attention.

Specify if:
In remission: After full criteria for avoidant/restrictive food intake disorder were previously met, the criteria have not been met for a sustained period of time.

Source: American Psychiatric Association. *Diagnostic and Statistical Manual of Mental Disorders.* 5th ed. Washington, DC: American Psychiatric Association; 2013. Used with permission.

FDIC was the requirement that patients be younger than 6 years. Many patients were older than 6 years at the time of evaluation and therefore were given the diagnosis EDNOS. Additionally, FDIC excluded children who were growing normally despite abnormal eating patterns or nutritionally deficient or limited diets, but with sufficient caloric intake, possibly as a result of use of nutritional supplements. These patients often presented with clinically significant impairment, both physically and functionally.

Eating Disorder Not Otherwise Specified

A certain subset of children and younger adolescents who presented with restrictive eating but without weight and shape concerns were classified as having EDNOS. Such individuals did not fit the DSM-IV feeding and eating disorder diagnoses, nor did they meet the diagnostic criteria for AN, yet they experienced significant levels of impairment in development or functioning as well as potentially severe medical complications.[43]

The Great Ormond Street Eating Disorder Classification System

The Great Ormond Street (GOS) eating disorder classification system includes food avoidant emotional disorder (FAED), selective eating, functional dysphagia, AN, and BN, and seemed to be more reliable at both characterizing and identifying pediatric eating disorder patients than the DSM-IV.[3]

Food Avoidant Emotional Disorder

Food Avoidant Emotional Disorder (FAED) was first described as a combination of insufficient food intake and emotional disturbance, without meeting criteria for AN.[44] The GOS checklist adapted and further elucidated this group.[3] Patients with FAED can easily be confused with having AN because they usually present at a low weight with significant food restriction; however, they do not have weight or shape concerns. Additionally, children with FAED display more general psychopathology than similarly aged patients diagnosed with AN.[45] Children with FAED are more likely to experience somatic complaints, sadness, worries, or obsessionality interfering with eating and appetite, as well as generalized anxiety unrelated to food. However, it is usually poor intake and weight loss that bring them to clinical attention.[42,43,46,47]

Selective Eating

Selective eating, also known as "picky eating," although common in much younger children, can persist beyond toddlerhood/early childhood in some children, leading to significant psychosocial, and possibly physical, consequences. These patients are generally not underweight because they can obtain the required calories from preferred foods. However, their diets often are deficient in micronutrients. Some selective eaters can have sensory issues related to taste, smell, color, or texture, leading to a restricted range of foods eaten. For example, a child may present as eating only white or bland-colored foods, only pureed foods, only certain brands of food, or only hot or cold foods. Some children cannot tolerate the smell of certain foods to the point that they are unable to eat with family or friends. Studies have shown that a preponderance of boys have this presentation, and that children and adolescents with this disorder have a high degree of associated anxiety.[48,49]

Functional Dysphagia

Functional dysphagia (*globus hystericus*) is a fear of swallowing or an inability to eat or swallow food, especially solid or lumpy foods. Young people with this disorder generally fear gagging, choking, or vomiting, which often occurs after an actual traumatic episode or a witnessed episode. Some children present with food refusal specifically out of fear of vomiting, contamination, poisoning, or defecation. Many cases of acute food avoidance resulting from specific fears present as clinically ill; these children and adolescents will lose a significant percentage of their body weight in a short period of time. Again, these young people can easily be mistaken for patients with AN, but they are not concerned with their body weight or shape.[42]

Avoidant/Restrictive Food Intake Disorder: Summary

ARFID has expanded FDIC and subsumed a subset of patients who otherwise would have fallen into EDNOS or been classified according to the GOS system.

Patients with ARFID may present with clinically significant restrictive eating leading to weight loss or lack of weight gain, nutritional deficiencies, reliance on tube feeding or oral nutritional supplements, and/or disturbances in psychosocial functioning. Importantly, the avoidance or restriction of food cannot be better justified by another medical condition or psychiatric disorder; however, these disorders can coexist with the eating disorder as long as the aberrant eating behaviors necessitate further clinical attention (see Table 2).[4]

Because ARFID is a new diagnostic category, there is no validated assessment tool or formalized evaluation to aid clinicians in the diagnosis. Example questions to guide the clinician in making a diagnosis of ARFID are outlined in Table 3.[50]

Epidemiology

Recent studies have shown that the prevalence of ARFID in newly diagnosed patients presenting to adolescent medicine eating disorder programs ranges from 5% to 14%. In these studies, patients with ARFID were significantly

Table 3
Assessment of avoidant/restrictive food intake disorder in DSM-5

1. What is current food intake? This is to ascertain whether this represents an adequate age-appropriate amount or range (ie, is the diet sufficient in terms of energy, and does it include major food groups and essential micronutrients?).
2. Is diet supplemented by oral nutritional supplements or by enteral feeding? This is to ascertain whether there is a dependence on these other means of feeding.
3. Is the avoidance or restriction persistent? This is to ascertain whether this is an established rather than transient problem.
4. What are the patient's weight and height? This allows calculation of body mass index or body mass index percentile; comparison of the individual's previous weight and height percentiles; and assessment of whether growth is faltering and if weight has been lost or is static when it should be increasing.
5. Does the patient present with clinical or laboratory signs and symptoms of nutritional deficiency or malnutrition (eg, lethargy secondary to iron deficiency anemia or delayed bone age as a consequence of chronic restricted intake)?
6. Is there evidence of any significant distress or impairment to the individual's social and emotional development or functioning associated with the eating disturbance? This is to include in the case of children disruptions to normal family function that negatively affect the child.
7. Is the avoidance or restriction associated with a lack of interest in food or eating, or a failure to recognize hunger?
8. Is the avoidance or restriction based on sensory aspects of food such as appearance (including color), taste, texture, smell, or temperature?
9. Does the avoidance or restriction follow an aversive experience associated with intense distress, such as a choking incident, an episode of vomiting or diarrhea, or complications from a medical procedure such as an esophagoscopy?

From Bryant-Waugh R, Kreipe RE. Avoidant/restrictive food intake disorder in *DSM-5*. *Psychiatr Ann.* 2012;42(11):402-405. Reprinted with permission from Slack, Inc.

younger than those with other eating disorders.[19,51,52] Additionally, ARFID was found in 23% of young patients in a partial hospitalization program for eating disorders.[53]

PICA AND RUMINATION DISORDER

In the DSM-5, pica and rumination disorder were removed from Disorders Usually First Diagnosed in Infancy, Childhood, or Adolescence and added to the Feeding and Eating Disorders section, which reinforces that these diagnoses can be made for individuals of any age.

Pica

The hallmark of pica is the ingestion of 1 or more nonnutritive, nonfood substances on a continual basis for at least 1 month. The term *nonfood* was included in the DSM-5 to exclude the intake of diet products (eg, soda) with little to no nutritional value. This diagnosis cannot be made before the age of 2 years. In addition, the behavior cannot be part of a culturally advocated or socially normative practice. Pica can be a feature of other mental disorders (eg, developmental disabilities, autism spectrum disorder, schizophrenia) but is only given as a separate diagnosis if the eating behavior is serious enough to merit further clinical attention.[4]

Rumination Disorder

Rumination is the repeated, effortless regurgitation of recently eaten food over at least a 1-month period, occurring multiple times per week and often daily. It is not associated with nausea and is not part of any medical illness (eg, gastroesophageal reflux disease). However, the diagnosis can be made in conjunction with a medical condition as long as the medical condition does not solely explain the repeated regurgitation. Although the condition has been thought to occur most commonly in infants and the developmentally disabled, it does occur in children, adolescents, and adults of normal intelligence.[54] It may be hard to define the boundary between regurgitation and self-induced vomiting; however, as mentioned earlier, the behavior is effortless and does not serve as a method of weight control. Classically, rumination disorder has been underrecognized, especially in slightly older patients, leading to costly and unnecessary medical evaluations as well as misdiagnoses.[54]

Rumination is volitional in nature, and individuals may cough, use tongue or abdominal muscle contractions or movements, or place fingers in their mouths to help bring food back up. Patients with rumination disorder often seem to derive pleasure from the activity, and it may serve a self-soothing or self-stimulating function, especially in those with mental disabilities.[46] In others, it seems to be associated with anxiety. Oftentimes, clinicians can actually witness individuals engaging in the behavior. The DSM-5 specifies that the food may be rechewed, reswallowed, or spit out to include different patterns of behavior. In addition, the need for rumination to follow a period of normal functioning has been removed because this was too general, vague, and difficult to determine. Although regurgitation may be seen in other feeding and eating disorders, a separate diagnosis is only merited in pica.[54]

OTHER SPECIFIED FEEDING AND EATING DISORDERS

In an effort to further reduce the preponderance of EDNOS-type diagnoses, this category was renamed as OSFED, with identifiable subgroups.

Atypical Anorexia Nervosa

Changes to the description of atypical AN include a loosening of the weight criterion to incorporate individuals who are at or above a normal weight for age and/or height. This might include an individual who has all the features of AN but has not yet lost a significant amount of weight, eg, an obese/overweight adolescent who has rapidly lost weight but is still within or above the normal weight range.

Bulimia Nervosa (of Low Frequency and/or Limited Duration)

The diagnosis includes all the criteria for BN, except that the binge eating and inappropriate compensatory behavior(s) occur at a lower frequency and/or for less than 3 months.

Binge Eating Disorder (of Low Frequency and/or Limited Duration)

The diagnosis includes all the criteria for BED, except that the binge eating and inappropriate compensatory behavior(s) occur at a lower frequency and/or for less than 3 months.

Purging Disorder

The description of purging disorder (PD) as an atypical eating disorder is not a new concept, and it was included as an unnamed example in the DSM-IV.[5] It was typified by the frequent use of inappropriate compensatory behaviors by individuals with normal body weight after consuming small or normal amounts of food. It has more recently been studied as a clinically significant variant.[55] Despite a growing body of research on PD, the decision was made to leave it as an OSFED, with the hope that the inclusion of a name will facilitate both clinical understanding and more standardized research endeavors.[56] In the DSM-5, PD is described as recurrent purging behaviors (eg, self-induced vomiting, laxative, diuretic, or enema misuse) in an effort to affect weight or shape, without objective binge episodes. Those patients who engage in purging but also meet the diagnostic criteria for AN would be given a diagnosis of AN.[4] Of note, fasting and excessive exercise are not included in this definition, to distinguish it as more abnormal. In addition, purging to address weight or shape concerns distinguishes PD from culturally endorsed cleansing practices and vomiting because of anxiety.[56]

Night Eating Syndrome

This is the first time that night eating syndrome (NES) has ever been mentioned in the DSM. There is a debate as to whether NES represents a syndrome or a set of symptoms.[57] The succinct definition of NES in DSM-5 includes evening hyperphagia (consuming a substantial portion of daily calories after the evening meal) or nocturnal eating (waking up during the night and eating before returning to sleep).[4]

UNSPECIFIED FEEDING AND EATING DISORDERS

Those feeding and eating disorders that are clinically significant but do not meet the diagnostic criteria for any of the conditions already discussed fall into this category.

CONCLUSION

The DSM-5 section on Feeding and Eating Disorders was created to improve clinical utility, recognize a larger number of patients who were not being diagnosed with an eating disorder, decrease the frequency of the EDNOS diagnosis,[18,19,21] and adapt a lifespan approach to these disorders. Although it is too early to tell, new data suggest that the DSM-5 criteria for feeding and eating disorders will improve clinical utility and diagnostic accuracy.[58] Recent studies have demonstrated that the DSM-5 feeding and eating disorder criteria have the potential to assign eating disordered individuals to homogeneous diagnostic categories.[59] Additional work is needed to document its validity and clinical utility. The delineation of more specific and descriptive criteria may lead to earlier diagnosis and intervention, stimulate research into prevalence and incidence, facilitate the development of effective, evidence-based interventions, and inform prognosis and outcomes in children and adolescents with these disorders.

References

1. Peebles R, Hardy KK, Wilson JL, Lock JD. Are diagnostic criteria for eating disorders markers of medical severity? *Pediatrics.* 2010;125(5):e1193-e201
2. Madden S, Morris A, Zurynski YA, Kohn M, Elliot EJ. Burden of eating disorders in 5-13-year-old children in Australia. *Med J Austr.* 2009;190(8):410-414
3. Nicholls D, Chater R, Lask B. Children into DSM don't go: a comparison of classification systems for eating disorders in childhood and early adolescence. *Int J Eat Disord.* 2000;28(3):317-324
4. American Psychiatric Association. *Diagnostic and Statistical Manual of Mental Disorders.* 5th ed. Washington, DC: American Psychiatric Association; 2013

5. American Psychiatric Association. *Diagnostic and Statistical Manual of Mental Disorders*. 4th ed. Washington, DC: American Psychiatric Association; 1994
6. Bravender T, Bryant-Waugh R, Herzog D, et al. Classification of eating disturbance in children and adolescents: proposed changes for the DSM-V. *Eur Eat Disord Rev*. 2010;18(2):79-89
7. Thomas JJ, Roberto CA, Brownell KD. Eighty-five per cent of what? Discrepancies in the weight cut-off for anorexia nervosa substantially affect the prevalence of underweight. *Psychol Med*. 2009;39(5):833-843
8. Rosen DS. Physiologic growth and development during adolescence. *Pediatr Rev*. 2004;25(6):194-200
9. Becker AE, Thomas JJ, Pike KM. Should non-fat-phobic anorexia nervosa be included in DSM-V? *Int J Eat Disord*. 2009;42(7):620-635
10. Garfinkel PE, Lin E, Goering P, et al. Should amenorrhoea be necessary for the diagnosis of anorexia nervosa? Evidence from a Canadian community sample. *Br J Psychiatry*. 1996;168(4):500-506
11. Golden NH, Jacobson MS, Schebendach J, Solanto MV, Hertz SM, Shenker IR. Resumption of menses in anorexia nervosa. *Arch Pediatr Adolesc Med*. 1997;151(1):16-21
12. Attia E, Roberto CA. Should amenorrhea be a diagnostic criterion for anorexia nervosa? *Int J Eat Disord*. 2009;42(7):581-589
13. Roberto CA, Steinglass J, Mayer LE, Attia E, Walsh BT. The clinical significance of amenorrhea as a diagnostic criterion for anorexia nervosa. *Int J Eat Disord*. 2008;41(6):559-563
14. Abraham SF, Pettigrew B, Boyd C, Russell J, Taylor A. Usefulness of amenorrhoea in the diagnoses of eating disorder patients. *J Psychosom Obst Gynaecol*. 2005;26(3):211-215
15. Swanson SA, Crow SJ, Le Grange D, Swendsen J, Merikangas KR. Prevalence and correlates of eating disorders in adolescents: results from the national comorbidity survey replication adolescent supplement. *Arch Gen Psychiatry*. 2011;68(7):714-723
16. Stice E, Marti CN, Shaw H, Jaconis M. An 8-year longitudinal study of the natural history of threshold, subthreshold, and partial eating disorders from a community sample of adolescents. *J Abnorm Psychol*. 2009;118(3):587-597
17. Smink FR, van Hoeken D, Hoek HW. Epidemiology of eating disorders: incidence, prevalence and mortality rates. *Curr Psychiatry Rep*. 2012;14(4):406-414
18. Machado PP, Goncalves S, Hoek HW. DSM-5 reduces the proportion of EDNOS cases: evidence from community samples. *Int J Eat Disord*. 2013;46(1):60-65
19. Ornstein RM, Rosen DS, Mammel KA, et al. Distribution of eating disorders in children and adolescents using the proposed DSM-5 criteria for feeding and eating disorders. *J Adolesc Health*. 2013;53(2):303-305
20. Knoll S, Bulik CM, Hebebrand J. Do the currently proposed DSM-5 criteria for anorexia nervosa adequately consider developmental aspects in children and adolescents? *Eur Child Adolesc Psychiatry*. 2011;20(2):95-101
21. Keel PK, Brown TA, Holm-Denoma J, Bodell LP. Comparison of DSM-IV versus proposed DSM-5 diagnostic criteria for eating disorders: reduction of eating disorder not otherwise specified and validity. *Int J Eat Disord*. 2011;44(6):553-560
22. Wilson GT, Sysko R. Frequency of binge eating episodes in bulimia nervosa and binge eating disorder: diagnostic considerations. *Int J Eat Disord*. 2009;42(7):603-610
23. Binford RB, le Grange D. Adolescents with bulimia nervosa and eating disorder not otherwise specified-purging only. *Int J Eat Disord*. 2005;38(2):157-161
24. le Grange D, Loeb KL, Van Orman S, Jellar CC. Bulimia nervosa in adolescents: a disorder in evolution? *Arch Pediatr Adolesc Med*. 2004;158(5):478-482
25. Eddy KT, Celio Doyle A, Hoste RR, Herzog DB, le Grange D. Eating disorder not otherwise specified in adolescents. *J Am Acad Child Adolesc Psychiatry*. 2008;47(2):156-164
26. Ackard DM, Fulkerson JA, Neumark-Sztainer D. Stability of eating disorder diagnostic classifications in adolescents: five-year longitudinal findings from a population-based study. *Eat Disord*. 2011;19(4):308-322

27. van Hoeken D, Veling W, Sinke S, Mitchell JE, Hoek HW. The validity and utility of subtyping bulimia nervosa. *Int J Eat Disord.* 2009;42(7):595-602
28. Marcus MD, Kalarchian MA. Binge eating in children and adolescents. *Int J Eat Disord.* 2003;34(Suppl):S47-S57
29. Tanofsky-Kraff M, Yanovski SZ, Schvey NA, Olsen CH, Gustafson J, Yanovski JA. A prospective study of loss of control eating for body weight gain in children at high risk for adult obesity. *Int J Eat Disord.* 2009;42(1):26-30
30. Neumark-Sztainer D, Hannan PJ. Weight-related behaviors among adolescent girls and boys: results from a national survey. *Arch Pediatr Adolesc Med.* 2000;154(6):569-577
31. Tanofsky-Kraff M, Yanovski SZ, Wilfley DE, Marmarosh C, Morgan CM, Yanovski JA. Eating-disordered behaviors, body fat, and psychopathology in overweight and normal-weight children. *J Consult Clin Psychol.* 2004;72(1):53-61
32. Neumark-Sztainer D, Wall M, Guo J, Story M, Haines J, Eisenberg M. Obesity, disordered eating, and eating disorders in a longitudinal study of adolescents: how do dieters fare 5 years later? *J Am Diet Assoc.* 2006;106(4):559-568
33. Crow SJ, Peterson CB, Swanson SA, et al. Increased mortality in bulimia nervosa and other eating disorders. *Am J Psychiatry.* 2009;166(12):1342-1346
34. Day J, Schmidt U, Collier D, et al. Risk factors, correlates, and markers in early-onset bulimia nervosa and EDNOS. *Int J Eat Disord.* 2011;44(4):287-294
35. Sysko R, Roberto CA, Barnes RD, Grilo CM, Attia E, Walsh BT. Test-retest reliability of the proposed DSM-5 eating disorder diagnostic criteria. *Psychiatry Res.* 2012;196(2-3):302-308
36. Birgegard A, Norring C, Clinton D. DSM-IV versus DSM-5: implementation of proposed DSM-5 criteria in a large naturalistic database. *Int J Eat Disord.* 2012;45(3):353-361
37. Crow SJ, Stewart Agras W, Halmi K, Mitchell JE, Kraemer HC. Full syndromal versus subthreshold anorexia nervosa, bulimia nervosa, and binge eating disorder: a multicenter study. *Int J Eat Disord.* 2002;32(3):309-318
38. Field AE, Camargo CA Jr, Taylor CB, et al. Overweight, weight concerns, and bulimic behaviors among girls and boys. *J Am Acad Child Adolesc Psychiatry.* 1999;38(6):754-760
39. Fairburn CG, Doll HA, Welch SL, Hay PJ, Davies BA, O'Connor ME. Risk factors for binge eating disorder: a community-based, case-control study. *Arch Gen Psychiatry.* 1998;55(5):425-432
40. Johnson JG, Cohen P, Kotler L, Kasen S, Brook JS. Psychiatric disorders associated with risk for the development of eating disorders during adolescence and early adulthood. *J Consult Clin Psychol.* 2002;70(5):1119-1128
41. Morgan CM, Yanovski SZ, Nguyen TT, et al. Loss of control over eating, adiposity, and psychopathology in overweight children. *Int J Eat Disord.* 2002;31(4):430-441
42. Bryant-Waugh R, Markham L, Kreipe RE, Walsh BT. Feeding and eating disorders in childhood. *Int J Eat Disord.* 2010;43(2):98-111
43. Nicholls DE, Lynn R, Viner RM. Childhood eating disorders: British national surveillance study. *Br J Psychiatry.* 2011;198(4):295-301
44. Higgs JF, Goodyer IM, Birch J. Anorexia nervosa and food avoidance emotional disorder. *Arch Dis Child.* 1989;64(3):346-351
45. Cooper PJ, Watkins B, Bryant-Waugh R, Lask B. The nosological status of early onset anorexia nervosa. *Psychol Med.* 2002;32(5):873-880
46. Nicholls D, Bryant-Waugh R. Eating disorders of infancy and childhood: definition, symptomatology, epidemiology, and comorbidity. *Child Adolesc Psychiatr Clin N Am.* 2009;18(1):17-30
47. Pinhas L, Morris A, Crosby RD, Katzman DK. Incidence and age-specific presentation of restrictive eating disorders in children: a Canadian Paediatric Surveillance Program study. *Arch Pediatr Adolesc Med.* 2011;165(10):895-899
48. Timimi S, Douglas J, Tsiftsopoulou K. Selective eaters: a retrospective case note study. *Child Care Health Dev.* 1997;23(3):265-278
49. Nicholls D, Christie D, Randall L, Lask B. Selective eating: symptom, disorder or normal variant. *Clin Child Psychol Psychiatry.* 2001;6(2):257-270

50. Bryant-Waugh R, Kreipe RE. Avoidant/restrictive food intake disorder. *Psychiatr Ann.* 2012;42(11):402-405
51. Norris ML, Robinson A, Obeid N, Harrison M, Spettigue W, Henderson K. Exploring avoidant/restrictive food intake disorder in eating disordered patients: a descriptive study. *Int J Eat Disord.* 2014;47(5):495-499
52. Fisher MM, Rosen DS, Ornstein RM, et al. Characteristics of avoidant/restrictive food intake disorder in children and adolescents: a "new disorder" in DSM-5. *J Adolesc Health.* 2014;55(1):49-52
53. Nicely TA, Lane-Loney S, Masciulli E, Hollenbeak CS, Ornstein RM. Prevalence and characteristics of avoidant/restrictive food intake disorder in a cohort of young patients in day treatment for eating disorders. *J Eat Dis.* In press.
54. Chial HJ, Camilleri M, Williams DE, Litzinger K, Perrault J. Rumination syndrome in children and adolescents: diagnosis, treatment, and prognosis. *Pediatrics.* 2003;111(1):158-162
55. Striegel-Moore RH, Franko DL, Thompson D, Barton B, Schreiber GB, Daniels SR. An empirical study of the typology of bulimia nervosa and its spectrum variants. *Psychol Med.* 2005;35(11):1563-1572
56. Keel PK, Striegel-Moore RH. The validity and clinical utility of purging disorder. *Int J Eat Disord.* 2009;42(8):706-719
57. Striegel-Moore RH, Franko DL, Garcia J. The validity and clinical utility of night eating syndrome. *Int J Eat Disord.* 2009;42(8):720-738
58. Allen KL, Byrne SM, Oddy WH, Crosby RD. DSM-IV-TR and DSM-5 eating disorders in adolescents: prevalence, stability, and psychosocial correlates in a population-based sample of male and female adolescents. *J Abnorm Psychol.* 2013;122(3):720-732
59. Stice E, Marti CN, Rohde P. Prevalence, incidence, impairment, and course of the proposed DSM-5 eating disorder diagnoses in an 8-year prospective community study of young women. *J Abnorm Psychol.* 2013;122(2):445-457

Adolesc Med 025 (2014) 377–397

Transgender and Gender Nonconforming Youth

Michelle Forcier, MD, MPH[a*]; Johanna Olson, MD[b]

[a]Associate Professor of Clinical Pediatrics, Alpert School of Medicine, Brown University, Providence, Rhode Island; [b]Assistant Professor of Clinical Pediatrics, USC Keck School of Medicine, Los Angeles, California

PART 1: PARADIGM SHIFTS IN GENDER CARE

Gender Paradigm in Modern Culture

Gender, or who we are with respect to our maleness or femaleness, integrates our natal biologic features (chromosomes, hormones, anatomy), internal gender identity, and externalized gender roles and expression. Although gender is often confused with sexuality (innate romantic attraction, sexual orientation, and specific expressed behaviors), it is important for physicians to recognize these are different elements of psychosexual development, each presenting children, youth, and families with unique challenges (Figure 1).[1] All children and adolescents incorporate gender and sexuality in their physical and psychosocial growth and development, to create over time a mature adult sense of self and role in society.[2,3] For some children, gender is static and binary; for others, gender is more fluid and moves along a spectrum or range of typical cultural expectations.[4,5] All children will experiment with gender roles, activities, and expressions. However, for some children, gender nonconformity is often consistent, persistent, and insistent.

Gender nonconforming children may present to physicians at various ages, but certain trends seem to occur in clinical sites around the United States. Physicians who provide services for prepubertal, gender nonconforming children report more natal males asserting female gender identities presenting than natal females asserting male gender identities. In the peripubertal age range, there

---

*Corresponding author:
E-mail address: mforcier1205@gmail.com

 ISSN 1934-4287

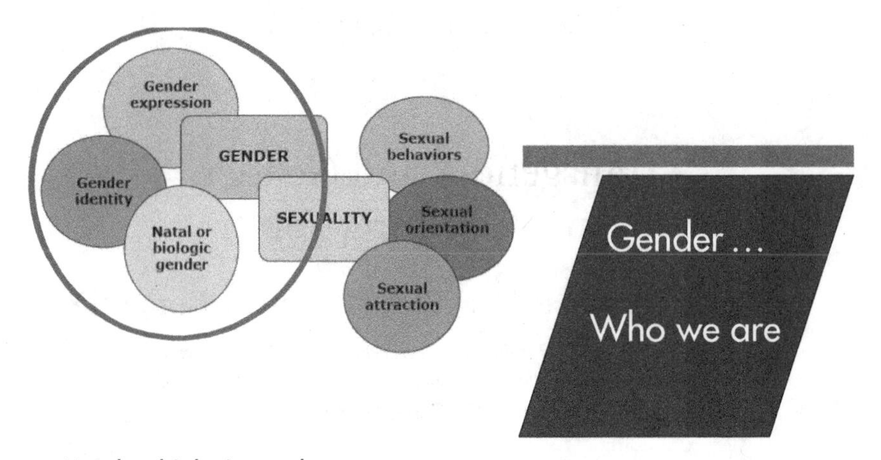

Natal or biologic gender: Brain, hormones, body parts assigning male or female gender, usually at birth

Gender identity: Person's basic sense of being male or female, especially as experienced in self-awareness and behavior

Gender expression: Ways in which person acts, presents self & communicates gender within a given culture

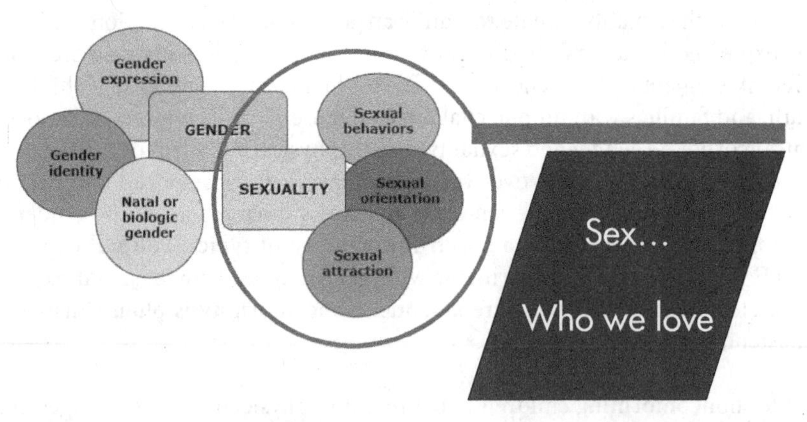

LGBTQQI: Lesbian, Gay, Bisexual, Transgender, Queer, Questioning, Intersex
YMSM: Young Men who have Sex with Men
YWSW: Young Women who have Sex with Women
Bisexual, pansexual, asexual, queer

Fig 1. Paradigm of gender and sexuality.

seems to be an increase in the number of natal females presenting to physicians with male gender identities. Patients also may present in adulthood, with or without prior gender nonconformity in their history. Whether or not more open recognition of gender and sexual minorities in modern western society is promoting the increase in numbers of clinically presenting gender nonconforming individuals, estimates regarding prevalence or incidence are unclear.[6-9]

Should We Use the Disease-Based Models of the Past?

A new diagnostic category, Gender Dysphoria, separate from Sexual Dysfunctions and Paraphilic Disorders, has been defined and included in the American Psychiatric Association's *Diagnostic and Statistical Manual of Mental Disorders*, Fifth Edition (DSM-5) with the "aim to avoid stigma and ensure clinical care for individuals who see and feel themselves to be a different gender than their assigned gender... It is important to note that gender nonconformity is not in itself a mental disorder...."[10] The gender identity disorder (GID) diagnosis has been dropped and is no longer appropriate. Rather, the critical element in making a diagnosis of gender dysphoria is the presence of clinically significant distress and impairment for at least 6 months related to experienced incongruence between assigned gender and gender identity. In youth, a diagnosis of gender dysphoria requires that the desire to be the other gender must be present and verbalized. Additionally, "the DSM-5 diagnosis adds a post-transition specifier for people who are living full-time as the desired gender (with or without legal sanction of the gender change). This ensures treatment access for individuals who continue to undergo hormone therapy, related surgery, or psychotherapy or counseling to support their gender transition."[10] New models of care have adapted useful psychological features while avoiding assigning pathology and stigmatization to what we understand as a more fluid and diverse range of gender identity and expression.

The *International Classification of Diseases, Tenth Revision* (ICD-10) is an anatomy-based billing tool that does not easily fit the care paradigms for gender nonconforming individuals. It contains multiple coding options that rely on outdated or inaccurate diagnostic frameworks.[11] We recommend avoiding coding options such as "gender identity disorder" (F64.1 adolescents/adults and F64.2 children), paraphilia unspecified (F65.9, formerly sexual gender identity disorder 320.9) because they do not accurately reflect the patient experience and may be used to deny insurance coverage for necessary treatments and services. ICD-10 coding that may be more appropriate for medical evaluation and care of gender diverse children may include endocrine disorder, unspecified (E34.9, formerly 259.9 endocrine disorder or disease of puberty, unspecified); other specific endocrine disorders (E34.8, formerly 259.8 endocrine disorder related to puberty); or other specified problems related to psychosocial circumstances (Z65.8, formerly V62.89 adolescent puberty related problems).

Developmental Approaches to Gender Diversity

Emerging views of gender eschew stigmatizing paradigms that rely on pathology, disease, and diagnostic approaches; rather, they embrace a cognitive and developmental perspective.[12-14] Using developmental models, a person's gender and sexuality may emerge and evolve as an individual grows, changes, and matures across the lifespan. Newer paradigms seek to avoid the historic dichotomization of gender into male and female and instead allow for a more fluid and flexible view of gender.[15] With a focus on developing identity, exploration of cultural roles, and successful integration into a healthy adulthood, the developmental perspective may promote proactive screening and anticipatory guidance at various junctures in child development. Emerging developmental perspectives suggest there may be value in more open discussions about gender play and expression in the early childhood years. Careful screening at key points in a child's development may offer opportunities to identify parental concerns, experiences of bullying and social stigma, and earlier more effective means of intervention. Developmentally appropriate conversations that screen for, or directly ask all youth to articulate, their gender experience open the door for youth to explicitly explore these and other potentially sensitive topics, enhancing trust, rapport, and communication that are essential to compassionate adolescent health care.

When parents of prepubertal children have questions regarding gender nonconformity, understanding gender in the context of overall child development may help physicians counsel parents and create a family environment supportive of all gender needs and expressions. Most children can verbally describe their own and other individuals' gender between ages 18 and 24 months. Children as young as 2 years start to demonstrate preference for toys, games, and types of play (physical vs cooperative) associated with gender stereotypes.[13,16,17] By the age of 4 years, children use gendered words ("he/him" and "she/her") and increasingly associate with same gender peers.[18] In the school-age years, children typically view gender and gender roles as static, bound by rules and established social conventions, with most play focused on stereotypical activities with same gender peers.[19-23] During the school-age years, many children begin to recognize personal characteristics that make them unique, including activities that suit specific gendered inclinations and interests, but often choose to balance or even subvert these as they strive for acceptance by peers.

Both medical professionals and parents should be confident that many children experiment with gender expression and social roles. For many children, gender experimentation can be time limited and does not reflect gender dysphoria or a desire to be another gender. For some prepubertal children, innate preferences and experience of self do not fit cultural expectations of masculinity or femininity. Gender nonconforming children may best be understood as those children or adolescents who, over time, present with a *consistent, persistent,* and *insistent* need to express outside the expectations of their assigned birth gender role or a feeling that their birth gender does not reflect their true gender.

Some children are quite clear about a cross-gender identity early in childhood. As soon as they have verbal skills, they may begin to express distress over name, anatomy, and presentation (hair, clothing), or they may specifically state they are or want to be the other gender.[24] A number of prepubertal children may not verbalize gender dysphoria or do not yet have the capacity to conceptualize or verbalize how internal gender identity is at odds with their natal gender. These children may initially present with behavioral, mood, and social problems before they mature and develop the concepts and language needed to address complex gender variations. Almost half of gender nonconforming youth have preexisting psychiatric diagnoses, including mood disorders (12%-35%), anxiety (16%-24%), suicide ideation and self harm (9%-22%), and suicide attempts (9%).[25-27]

For many gender nonconforming prepubertal youth, we cannot reliably predict or confirm a clear trajectory for adult gender and sexuality outcomes. Although this may be disconcerting for parents, medical professionals may focus on ways to support parents in supporting their child so that the child feels accepted and loved for who s/he authentically is.[28] It is critical for all children to feel safe, accepted, and loved as an essential aspect of a growing sense of and healthy self-esteem. In the ideal setting, parents adapt quickly, manage their own emotional reactions, and create a safe home setting that allows them to be emotionally present and appropriate for their child. Some parents need more time. After initial denial, dismay, or anger, many parents and caregivers eventually move toward acceptance, and often appreciation, for their gender nonconforming child.

Physicians may help parents balance support for their child's innate sense of self with tools to safely navigate social complexities and success in school and other peer networks. A more recent option for care includes social transitioning, the process of externally presenting in one's authentic gender by changing clothing, hairstyles, preferred name and pronouns, or a combination of these features. Social transitioning may be appropriate for prepubertal children with strong (consistent, persistent, and insistent) cross-gender identification who continue to assert a gender that differs from the one they were assigned at birth.[28-30] The process of social transition is entirely reversible, although not without potential complications and social consequences. Although there are no long-term outcome studies on social transitioning, the bulk of anecdotal experience seems to indicate that the positive benefits of being allowed to develop in one's identified gender seem to outweigh potential issues in the future for these strongly asserted cross-gender youth. With a focus on listening to the patient and allowing children to express their authentic self, children may transition to their asserted gender identity and continue this into puberty, or they may return to their birth gender if that is where their gender identity evolves over time.

Adolescent Gender Nonconformity

Although some gender nonconforming youth continue from prepuberty into puberty, steadfast in their transgender identity and expression, some youth only begin to identify as transgender during the onset of puberty.[28] Puberty, with its hormonal and physical changes, development of secondary sexual characteristics, and focus on peer and social acceptance, can be an incredibly difficult time for the gender nonconforming youth. If emerging gonadal hormones and anatomy are at odds with an adolescent's internal gender identity, then the adolescent experiencing discordance between gender identity and body gender may experience more dissonance in other areas of physical and mental health. The literature has begun to explore association and causality between poorer health outcomes and health disparities among gender nonconforming individuals of all ages.[31,32] All adolescents experiencing anxiety, depression, substance use, and homelessness should be directly asked about their gender identity and sexual behaviors because these negative psychosocial and mental health outcomes are associated with gender and sexual minority teens.[33,34] Self harm and suicidality are prevalent among gender nonconforming teens, reported as high as 40%.[35]

Unlike their prepubertal counterparts, the long-term trajectory for gender nonconforming peri- and postpubertal adolescents is much more predictable.[36] Limited data currently available strongly demonstrate that pubertal presentation of gender nonconformity, gender dysphoria, and a desire to be the other gender is quite predictive of a long-lasting transgender or gender nonconforming identity and expression.[36] In follow-up studies of gender dysphoric adolescents who underwent suppression of endogenous puberty, all youth have been reported to continue on to phenotypic gender transition with cross-sex hormones and/or gender confirmation surgeries.[26,27,37-41] Although parents are understandably concerned about life-changing decisions during adolescence, it is important to communicate to parents that it is rare for transgender postpubertal adolescents to regret gender transition, and return to their full natal gender.

PART 2: ADVANCES IN MEDICAL CARE FOR GENDER NONCONFORMING YOUTH

Earlier Screening for Gender Development

Using developmental models that embrace gender as a universal human attribute and allow for evolution and diversity across the lifespan, we may remedy the current inconsistent and inadequate systemized training in gender and sexual minority health and increase routine anticipatory guidance regarding gender and sexuality.[42,43] No studies addressing screening and anticipatory guidance for gender nonconformity have yet been reported in the literature. We can use the limited literature for sexual minority youth to extrapolate, understanding that we do an even less adequate job when it comes to gender. Many pediatric physicians feel uncomfortable or do not explore with adolescents their sexual attractions and behaviors despite evidence that adolescents not only welcome, but expect, physicians to ask about their burgeoning gender and sexual identities and feel that it is an important aspect of health care.[44,45] As many as 1 in 4 adolescents do not discuss sexual orientation during medical visits; again, gender is not even addressed in current studies.[42,46] The systematic lack of screening and of counseling and services creates overt and covert messaging to youth that gender nonconformity and sexual diversity are taboo and contributes further to existing negative stigma and isolation.[47,48] Lack of support, as well as more direct negative professional and social messages about gender and sexual diversity, increases minority stress and may contribute to poorer health outcomes over time.[49-52]

Conversely, positive and accepting reactions or actions seem to have long-term implications on the health and well-being of gender and sexual minorities.[53-55] Exploring gender and sexuality as a normative component during anticipatory guidance visits has value in (1) promoting opportunities for improved communication and support about identity development and social goal setting among parent(s) and all children; (2) creating a safe environment to discuss gender and sexual health needs in relation to family norms and social expectations; (3) creating a universal process that includes children who are less articulate or less free to express; (4) facilitating early identification and support of all gender and sexual minority youth; (5) establishing early mental health and parenting support for families; and (6) modeling support and acceptance to engage and promote a more tolerant society that embraces diversity. Early identification allows for earlier psychosocial support for the family and promotes the development of a coherent plan to explore complex feelings and innate needs within safe settings.[56]

Early Intervention: Timely Use of Puberty Blockers

Transgender youth undergoing an undesired endogenous puberty often experience distress, and this "wrong puberty" has a strong negative affect on emotional, academic, and family functioning.[6,35] Earlier identification and support of gender nonconforming youth may allow for more timely administration of gonadotropin-releasing hormone (GnRH) analogues (or puberty blockers) to halt puberty and give a youth and family time to sort out gender needs. Use of GnRH analogues at early Tanner stage 2 eliminates the development of undesired, permanent secondary sex characteristics, giving youth, families, and physicians time to explore gender identity. Blocking early puberty at Tanner stage 2 deters (1) unwanted physiologic and hormonal changes (menses in transgender males; erectile function for some but not all transgender females); (2) unwanted permanent physical changes associated with adult secondary sex characteristics (development of breasts and hips, fat deposition in transgender males; male pattern face and body hair; voice changes; heavier larger musculoskeletal structure in transgender females); (3) future costly gender confirming surgeries; and (4) continued or progressively worsening dissonance and body dysphoria as teens progress through pubertal changes that do not match developing gender identity.

Multiple medical and mental health professional organizations recommend the use of puberty blockers for gender nonconforming youth just starting puberty, with addition of cross-sex hormones later in adolescence.[57-60] GnRH agonists such as leuprolide, triptorelin, and histrelin bind pituitary GnRH receptors, interrupting normal postpubertal pulsatile stimulation. Blockers downregulate secretion of gonadotropins (luteinizing hormone [LH] and follicle-stimulating hormone [FSH]) reverting to prepubertal low testosterone and estradiol levels. Because GnRH analogues cost between $3000 to $18,000 per year and insurance coverage for these medications is inconsistent and absent in many cases, some youth do not have this option for early intervention. Improvements in coding and medical diagnosis may improve insurance coverage, but for uninsured or underinsured families and youth experiencing homelessness, these expensive medications are too often financially out of reach. Some physicians may utilize medroxyprogesterone 150 mg intramuscularly every 6 to 12 weeks as an alternative method to block the hypothalamic gonadal axis and stop menses. Medroxyprogesterone is a less effective mechanism for suppressing puberty (Table 1).[58]

Table 1
Recommended hormone therapy for puberty blocking and menstrual suppression

Gonadotropin-releasing hormone analogues	Dosing	Tips
Leuprolide depot Lupron (Also Viadur, Eligard)	• Intramuscular (IM) injection monthly or every 3 months • Low end of dosing 7.5 mg to high end 22.5 mg • Commonly start at 11.25 mg every 12 weeks	Contains gluten
Histrelin (Supprelin, Vantas)	• 50-mg implant requiring outpatient insertion into upper arm • Can last up to 2 years	Gluten-free
Goserelin (Zoladex) **Triptorelin (Triptorelin)**	• 3.6-, 10.8-mg implant • IM 3.75 mg every 4 weeks, 11.25 mg every 12 weeks, 22.5 mg every 24 weeks	Injection is in the buttocks
Menstrual blockers	All provide additional birth control benefits if patient is sexually active	Male patient may not want more "female" hormones
Medroxyprogesterone acetate (Depo-Provera)	• 150 mg IM injection every 12 weeks	Less expensive but less effective than GnRH analogues to block puberty
Extended cycling of estrogen-progestin hormones	• Daily "birth control" pills with menses every 3 to 12 months • Can suppress hypothalamic-pituitary-ovarian axis • Offers less frequent menses or year round extended cycling	
Levonorgestrel intrauterine device	• Lasts 5 to 7 yrs • Offers excellent contraception • 50% report amenorrhea in 1 year; 80% in 2 yrs • Requires pelvic exam and insertion	Males may not like uterine procedure or device

GnRH agonists have been used in children experiencing central precocious puberty for many years, and they appear to be safe and well tolerated in the transgender community. Side effects of this medicine are rare and include pain and vasovagal episodes with injection. Current data suggest that short-term use of GnRH agonists offers more benefits than known negative long-term effects on brain development, metabolism, and bone health in gender nonconforming youth.[60] Physicians may consider baseline bone density evaluation when patients have multiple risk factors for osteoporosis in later adult years. More commonly, some adolescents presenting in later adolescence (Tanner stage 4 or 5) may experience menopausal-type symptoms as hormones shift from adult levels of estrogen or testosterone to prepubertal levels. Hot flashes, irritability, concentration issues, and depression may occur with this hormone shift.[59] The potential for mood changes in any youth with significant preexisting mental health disorders should be monitored closely by patients, parents, therapists, and medical professionals. Clinical experience reports most adolescents experience positive feelings of satisfaction in halting "the wrong puberty" and relief in blocking further development of natal secondary gender characteristics. Although blockers may help stop progression of an incongruent puberty, GnRH analogues do not improve or eradicate gender dysphoria, unlike cross-gender hormone therapy and gender confirmation surgeries (GCS). It is essential to understand that available data report most gender dysphoric adolescents who are receiving GnRH agonists not only wish to continue blockers but also eventually seek phenotypic gender transition with cross-gender hormones in order to continue to align their bodies with their internal gender identities.[38-40,60]

Outcomes for gender nonconforming youth who have used puberty blockers do not seem to indicate significant medical morbidity or mortality, unlike the significant morbidity and mortality experienced by transgender individuals who are not offered medical intervention. Continued physical development in a puberty that differs from one's asserted gender identity leads to a host of permanent physical changes, only some of which can be altered with future surgical correction. Continued or worsening dissonance between brain identity and body development has been historically linked to poorer physical and mental health outcomes in transgender individuals, including anxiety, depression, suicidality, homelessness, substance use, acquisition of human immunodeficiency virus (HIV), and economic disparities.[31,61-66] Again, poorer health outcomes are precipitated by minority stress, internalized transphobia, social isolation, and effects of social stigma.[67] The harm of not acting or of withholding treatment, in addition to the reversibility of GnRH agonists, argues for more widespread and earlier use in adolescents with significant questions and concerns regarding their gender identity (Figure 2).

Older GnRH agonists are intramuscular long-acting agents administered every 1 or 3 months. Newer agents utilize subcutaneous implantable devices that slow release the GnRH agonist histrelin over 1 to 2 years. Medication effectiveness is monitored at 3- to 6-month intervals in order to assure continued suppression of endogenous hormones and pubertal development. These visits also allow physicians to continue

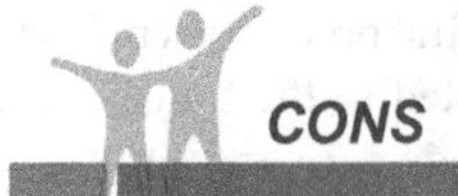

CONS	PROS
• Controversial, outcomes data rare • Possible temporary adverse effect on bone density □ Reversible once hormones initiated □ BMD normal in teens with precocious puberty treatment □ Height reduction (MTF) if started early □ Not necessarily a bad thing □ Negligible impact on height for FTMs • Lack of secondary sex characteristics compared to peers • Expensive! Insurance sometimes covers	• Delays decision to undergo cross hormone therapy until child is older • Prevents undesired irreversible pubertal changes • Decreases distress, with mental health/self esteem benefits • Prevents need for costly and invasive surgery as adult • Cosmetic congruency as adult leading to passing & greater social & financial opportunities

Puberty Blocking

Delemarre-van de Waal, EuropJEndo 2006

MTF= asserted female, natal male
FTM= asserted male, natal female

Fig 2. Pros and cons of puberty blocking.

supporting the patient and family as they explore their transition process. Endogenous LH and gender hormones (testosterone or estradiol) may be monitored along with height, weight and, other growth parameters, with GnRH dosage or timing adjusted to maintain prepubertal levels and effective block of ongoing puberty changes.[58] Although no real data exist at present, absence of gender hormones may delay growth plate closure and may allow early adolescents to continue to grow in height along the youth's genetic growth potential even as secondary gender physical characteristics are suppressed. Continued cognitive, emotional, and social development congruent with their peers also should be followed. Youth who are undergoing pubertal suppression should be engaged as individually needed in mental health services in order to support any mental health concerns, as well as potentially help prepare youth for the challenges associated with gender transition in adolescence.

PART 3: CROSS-GENDER HORMONES AND TRANSITION CARE IN ADOLESCENCE AND YOUNG ADULTHOOD

Consent Model of Medical Care for Cross-Gender Hormones

Phenotypic gender transition is not just about hormones (although that is what most youth are focused on) but is more about supporting youth in a continued pathway for healthy transition. Dose and timing guidelines for the administration of cross-gender hormones are available in the 2009 Endocrine Guidelines and other sources.[58] Timing and dosing considerations include age and gender of youth, adolescent and parent(s) consent, concurrent use of GnRH analogues, and degree of desired masculinization or feminization. Guidelines suggest age 16 years for initiation of cross-gender hormones based on arbitrary legal age of consent in earlier international studies.[58] With emerging data and outcomes gained by these earlier studies, many guidelines and practices have dropped the "gatekeeper" approach in favor of a consent-based model more tailored to individual patient needs.[28,57] For some youth who have a clear and unchanging transgender identification, it may be more appropriate to consider starting cross-gender hormones closer to average age of puberty, estimated as between 12 and 13 years for transgender females and between 13 and 14 years for transgender males. Again, timing for any aspect of transition care depends on patient readiness, support, and ability to move forward in a safe and healthy trajectory.

Rare contraindications to starting cross-gender hormones in children and teens include inability to provide informed consent, ongoing pregnancy, hormone-sensitive tumor, or allergy to medication components. Consent-based models recommend detailed medical history and psychosocial assessment of the patient's gender identity and transition goals; offering but not necessarily requiring referral to mental health resources for assistance with transition planning or other psychiatric comorbidities; and timing of gender hormones based on patient characteristics, including stage of puberty, readiness for transition, support for transition, and other psychosocial factors. As with many other pediatric medications, use of cross-gender hormones for the purpose of treating transgender youth is off-label, but physicians can reassure parents that significant clinical experience demonstrates their effectiveness and safety in treating gender dysphoria.[58]

Fertility is a major concern for many parents who are considering consenting to their adolescent's use of cross-gender hormones. Youth who use GnRH agonists early in Tanner stage 2 and move on to cross-gender hormones will not develop oocytes or sperm viable for future genetic reproduction. Therefore, this regimen essentially eliminates the option for future genetic childbearing or offspring. Parenthood is still an option but would require assisted reproduction, surrogacy, or adoption. If genetic offspring are important to the patient and family, it may be wise to delay use of cross-gender hormones. Referrals to reproductive and fertility specialists are an option for sperm banking and oocyte storage but continue to be very expensive and not generally covered by health insurance. Although sperm and embryo banking offer successful assisted reproductive options, oocyte and ovarian banking is still more experimental, requires a complex hormonal and retrieval process, and has less successful outcomes. In our current health care environment, genetic fertility preservation options are expensive and, in our experience, not available or prioritized by most adolescents. Regardless, a clear and detailed consent process regarding the likelihood of infertility must occur, involving the patient and parents, when involved. Given their long-standing internal struggle with gender, many gender nonconforming youth have thought through fertility issues with unexpected sophistication and insight, often reporting that personhood and identity come before and ultimately outweigh genetic reproduction. Fertility issues are often a greater challenge for parents who may have difficulty recognizing their child's emerging sexual development and mourn the loss of future genetic grandchildren. Youth who use cross-gender hormones later in puberty must understand that cross-gender hormones may not provide reliable contraception. Lack of adult penile and scrotal tissue development in youth who are suppressed early in Tanner stage 2 may present challenges for surgeons during gender confirmation procedures in transgender women and may require new surgical approaches to vulvovaginoplasties.

Cross-Gender Hormones

Existing guidelines recognize that a variety of medical, psychiatric, and mental health professionals are capable of and competent in assessing gender nonconformity, so although many patients might benefit from extensive treatment and support from a mental health specialist, required or mandated therapy is not necessary for all patients to begin or plan transition care.[57] For adolescents, mental health professionals may provide resources for parents and families to most appropriately support their teen, but they also offer opportunities to explore complex emotions and experiences; ensure success of gender transition in the context of their particular family, school, neighborhood, and other cultural milieus; develop ongoing interpersonal resiliency and self esteem; work on social and communication skills useful to transitioning to their identified gender; evaluate and treat coexisting mental health concerns that may impede successful transition and impair positive self-regard; educate and model acceptance of diversity and fluidity; and assist in transition preparation and planning.[68,69] Existing mental health conditions should not preclude youth from initiating cross-gender hormones but should be addressed with appropriate mental health therapy and medication if necessary.

Exogenous 17 β-estradiol is used for feminization and creates secondary gender characteristics desired by many transgender identified females. For teens who have undergone early puberty blocking at Tanner stage 2, feminization includes breast development, female fat distribution, softening of skin, prevention of male pattern face and body hair, and continued higher voice pitch. Estrogen will not undo previous secondary sexual characteristics already present in those teens in Tanner stage 3 and above (eg, change voice pitch, remove already present male pattern hair, change male skeletal structure). Estrogen is available in a variety of formulations. We avoid oral synthetic or conjugated estrogens (ethinyl estradiol or Premarin) because they are difficult to monitor and have higher risk of venous thromboembolic events (VTEs).[70,71] Sublingual use of oral 17 β-estradiol theoretically avoids first-pass effects, minimizing hepatic induction of procoagulant factors and proteins, and offers potential advantages, including negligible risk for deep vein thrombosis or pulmonary thromboembolism, compared to oral counterparts.[72,73] Use of estradiol valerate as an intramuscular injection is an alternative. Intramuscular injections can be taught and self-administered every 2 weeks. Each method has its pros and cons but both are equally efficacious.

Individuals who identify as masculine need exogenous testosterone if they wish to develop male secondary sexual characteristics. Testosterone with puberty blockers may prevent menarche or induce amenorrhea after 1 to 3 months of use. Testosterone also deepens voice pitch, creates male pattern fat distribution and muscle bulk, creates male pattern facial and body hair, and enlarges the clitoris to resemble a small neophallus. Injected oil-based testosterone esters (cypionate and enanthate) are most commonly used, are safe, and offer good effect. Testosterone is available in a variety of formulations. Subcutaneous injections are rapidly becoming preferred over intramuscular injections because the smaller needle and subcutaneous injection are less painful, easier, better tolerated, and equally efficacious.[74] Topical testosterone often is less desirable in youth because gels are inconsistently absorbed by patients and may be unintentionally absorbed by close contacts or sexual partners.

When GnRH agonists are used, both estradiol and testosterone may be effective at lower doses. Dosing of gender hormones is titrated to achieve desired gender effects and average adult gender hormone levels while minimizing adverse effects. Titration that is too low and too slow can be frustrating and problematic. Too low or slow titrating may not suppress the ovaries or testes, allowing continued secondary gender development, menses, or erections. Doses that are too high may increase risk of possible side effects or rare adverse events related to cross-gender hormones including mood changes, liver enzyme (aspartate aminotransferase [AST]) elevation, and lipid profile changes. Effects of testosterone to monitor include polycythemia, acne, male pattern baldness, and male pattern cardiovascular risks. Effects of estradiol include stimulation of pituitary tissue (prolactinoma), increased risk of VTEs, and erectile dysfunction.

Aftercare and Follow-Up for Transitioning or Transitioned Youth

Follow-up is especially important during the first 1 to 2 years after initiation of hormone therapy, when expected effects of cross-gender hormone therapy primarily occur. Regular follow-up to monitor physical changes should include an assessment of development, growth parameters, side effects and adverse effects, hormone levels, and metabolic changes (Table 2). Regular visits also provide an opportunity to monitor psychosocial development and support healthy decision-making during a time of rapid change and emerging social roles and expression. When a teen is on a stable dose of hormones without adverse side effects, visit frequency may decrease according to need.

Table 2
Aftercare and follow-up of transgender youth over time

Gender hormones (specific follow-up)	Primary care follow-up (health maintenance)
Medications adjusted to • Desired physical response • Prevention of side effects • Prevention of adverse events • Average hormone range for asserted gender Vitals • Weight (appetite changes, risk for eating disorders) • Blood pressure (BP) (spironolactone)	Review potential for medication interactions HEADDSSS interview, screening, counseling, including • Mental health screening for depression, anxiety, self harm, risk for suicide higher in transgender populations than in the general population • Substance use • Violence (abuse, interpersonal, bullying) • Sexually transmitted infection (STI) prevention
Laboratory tests • Testosterone • Liver function (AST) • Lipid panel • Complete blood count (CBC) (hemoglobin [Hb], testosterone) • Prolactin (estradiol) • Potassium (spironolactone)	Age appropriate health screening • Hypertension, hyperlipidemia, diabetes Screen for STIs in sexually active patients • Urine, rectal, or oral gonorrhea • Chlamydia depending on specific sexual behaviors • Syphilis • Human immunodeficiency virus (HIV) • Hepatitis
Physical examination Many gender nonconforming individuals are body dysphoric. Physical examinations should be conducted with great sensitivity and respect. • FTM (asserted male, natal female) chest • MTF (asserted female, natal male) testes/penis	Provide age and diagnostically appropriate, sensitive, safe examinations for those with extreme body dysphoria • Pap cervical cancer screening • Breast/chest carcinoma screening • Pelvic examination for STI diagnosis • Skin examination for self harm
Reproductive health considerations: • MTF at high risk for STIs, HIV • Consider pre- or post-HIV prophylaxis as needed • Cross-gender hormones *not* considered birth control, address contraceptive needs • Testosterone has teratogenic properties	Pregnancy prevention, family planning counseling

The use of a developmental model that allows for fluidity and movement along a spectrum can help physicians avoid assumptions as they begin to create a personal care plan. Asking each patient detailed questions regarding specific gender goals assures youth that their physician is listening and tailoring care to their identified needs and goals. Not all gender nonconforming youth wish to be at the diametric end of the gender binary. Some identified males do not identify with a very muscular or hairy body habitus and may require lower dose of testosterone than other patients. Some transgender females enjoy using their penis or need their penis to function for sexual activity. Some youth who identify as gender queer or androgenous may want no hormones or lower levels of hormones to maintain a more androgynous effect. Over the long term, gender hormones have benefit for continued development along with bone, cognitive, and emotional health, but which hormone and at what level are less certain.

Although caring for gender nonconforming children and adolescents requires thorough assessment for gender identity and gender expression, changes over time and experience related to gender identity, gender goals, and transition planning do not necessarily indicate that the initial transition plan was in error or was harmful to the youth. Children are able to express and contribute to decision-making about their gender identity and expression; and teens often are mature enough to understand and adequately consent to potentially irreversible decisions about gender, sexuality, and fertility. Physicians who have carefully listened to an adolescent expressing gender dysphoria and have adapted a safe social and healthy medical transition plan are providing care according to present known needs and risks, as opposed to withholding treatment for a low likelihood of future changes. It should be reassuring that with careful assessment, clear communication and expectations, and active engagement in an overall healthy transition plan, it is extremely unlikely that postpubertal youth will change their mind; an overwhelming majority of youth will continue taking blockers, will continue on to taking cross-gender hormones, and, when financially viable, often will consider options for gender confirmation surgeries. Waiting too long or doing nothing may be antithetical to the medical Hippocratic oath when it comes to gender nonconforming children.

Transition Is About More than Hormones

Although youth often focus on "When can I start hormones?," physicians and parents should help youth have a broader and more inclusive transition plan. Medical professionals can support gender nonconforming youth and their parents or caregivers by discussing with whom and how to disclose to family, friends, and social peers; preparing and educating the school system, including both staff and students; planning for how to respond and manage bullying and other socially stigmatizing interactions; and providing any medical documentation necessary for changes in name, gender, passports, and other official documents. Some families decide it is best for the young person to be nondisclosed by transitioning to the asserted gender in a new school, community, and other social settings. This may entail the school and some adults knowing that the child is gender nonconforming but the general population assuming the asserted gender is the child's assigned gender at birth. Other children and families come out openly and publically with good support and success. As with early social transition, safety is the single most critical aspect of any transition plan. Safety and a positive experience are essential priorities, even as we encourage parents to allow children to express and be themselves. Caregivers may ask for a "safe letter" or may ask physicians to interact with schools and other social agencies so that other professionals understand that their child is gender nonconforming and receiving appropriate medical and mental health care (Table 3). There is no

Table 3
Medical legal safe letter for gender confirmation

- Safe letter from professional persons, knowledgeable and supportive of your child or teen, that reaffirms the child's emerging gender identity
  - Physician or therapist name, medical or professional ID, state license number
  - Date started care, and if continued care
  - Description that the patient has M/F natal gender but has been evaluated and is in appropriate medical and mental health care for gender nonconforming or transgender asserted identity as F/M
  - Recommendations about continued activities in asserted gender
  - List of any necessary medications, devices, or surgeries as appropriate
  - Recommendations for continued support and appropriateness of transition plan
- Parents may additionally include
  - Reports, evaluations, or other input from other professionals who have provided care or therapy for the child or teen
  - Professional recommendations that the child or teen be supported in the asserted gender
    - Use of appropriate bathroom or locker room
    - Placement in gender-appropriate school lines, play group, sports teams
    - Expression of asserted gender with hair, clothes, shoes, makeup, and other accessories

one right way to disclose or transition. Transitioning is a very personal, family, community, and situation-specific decision that should focus on safety, support, and acceptance.[28,75-78]

Transgender adolescents and young adults who are from socially rigid environments face bullying, social isolation, and ostracization; discrimination in work and housing; physical and sexual assault; and death by hate crime.[79] Data suggest that transgender women, transgender persons of color, and HIV-affected people of color experience a greater risk of violence and homicide than other lesbian, gay, bisexual, transgender, queer and questioning (LGBTQQ) and HIV-affected persons.[80] Although significant concerns about potential violence and abuse and risk of other social and economic difficulties are real, fear and risk should not outweigh a youth's asserted need and desire to transition to his or her authentic gender identity.

Future Directions and Conclusion

Family acceptance, even when controlling for confounding characteristics, continues its protective effects with ongoing young adult positive health outcomes, such as improved self-esteem, social support, and general health, and is protective against negative outcomes, such as suicide, depression, and substance abuse.[81] Simons et al[82] saw more limited protective effects against acquisition of sexually transmitted infections (STIs) and generally lower support and health markers for transgender patients. Adults have retrospectively identified a variety of needs for successful parenting, including access to information and education, social awareness, peer support, and access to educated medical professionals.[83]

With time and increasing experience, we have learned more about the trajectory and outcomes of gender nonconforming youth and transgender adults. Many physicians now feel more confident offering an informed consent or shared decision-making model, rooted in the understanding that it is the youth themselves who determine the direction and pace of their transitions and establish a gender identity, expression, and role that is right for them. Earlier support, social transition, and individualized application of GnRH analogues and cross-gender hormones may create a very different outcomes profile for a new generation of transgender youth as they go through a single congruent puberty and are more comfortable and confident in passing into their asserted gender. It is our hope that we are entering a new era of care for gender nonconforming youth. As more and more individuals feel safe and free to express gender nonconformity in our present culture, medical professionals need to offer universal anticipatory screening, support, and interventions that promote potentially lifesaving therapies for this previously at-risk population of youth and adults. Modeling and promoting care that is accepting and welcoming of all gender identities and expression establish new benchmarks that other adults and professionals can aim to achieve as they work with children and families. In this patient-by-patient, clinic-by-clinic, and community-by-community way, we can begin to create a larger and long-term cultural shift toward appreciation of differences and diversity.

References

1. Money J. The concept of gender identity disorder in childhood and adolescence after 39 years. *J Sex Marital Ther*. 1994;20:163-177
2. Kohlberg LA. A cognitive-developmental analysis of children's sex role concepts and attitudes. In: Maccoby EE, eds. *The Development of Sex Differences*. Stanford, CA: Stanford University Press; 1966:82-173
3. Stollter RJ. *Sex and Gender*. New York: Science House; 1968
4. Bockting WO. Psychotherapy and the real-life experience: from gender dichotomy to gender identity. *Sexologies*. 2008;17:211-224
5. Diamond LM, Butterworth M. Questioning gender and sexual identity: dynamic links over time. *Sex Roles*. 2008;59:365-376
6. De Vries AL, Cohen-Kettenis PT. Clinical management of gender dysphoria in children and adolescents: the Dutch approach. *J Homosex*. 2012;59:301-320
7. Wood H, Sasaki S, Bradley SJ, et al. Patterns of referral to a gender identity service for children and adolescents (1976-2011): age, sex ratio, and sexual orientation. *J Sex Marital Ther*. 2013;39:1-6
8. Zucker KJ, Bradley SJ, Owen-Anderson A, Kibblewhite SJ, Cantor JM. Is gender identity disorder in adolescents coming out of the closet? *J Sex Marital Ther*. 2008;34:287-290
9. Pleak RR. Gender-variant children and transgender adolescents. *Child Adolesc Psychiatr Clin N Am*. 2011;20:xv-xx
10. Gender dysphoria. Available at: www.dsm5.org/Documents/Gender Dysphoria Fact Sheet.pdf. Accessed December 9, 2013
11. World Health Organization. *The ICD 10 Classification of Mental and Behavioral Disorders: Clinical Descriptions and Diagnostic Guidelines*. Geneva, Switzerland: World Health Organization; 1992
12. Fausto-Sterling A. *Sexing the Body: Gender Politics and the Construction of Sexuality*. New York: Basic Books; 2000
13. Ruble DN, Martin CL. Gender development. In: Eisenberg N. ed. *Handbook of Child Psychology: Volume 3. Personality and Social Development*. 5th ed. New York: Wiley; 1998:933-1016

14. Ruble DN, Martin, CL, Berenbaum SA. Gender development, In: Eisenberg E, Damon W, Lerner RM, eds. *Handbook of Child Psychology: Volume 3, Social, Emotional, and Personality Development.* 6th ed. Hoboken, NJ: John Wiley & Sons; 2006:858-932
15. Wiseman M, Davidson S. Problems with binary gender discourse: using context to promote flexibility and connection in gender identity. *Clin Child Psychol Psychiatry.* 2012;17:528-537
16. Serbin LA, Poulin-Dubois D, Colburne KA, Sen MG, Eichstedt JA. Gender stereotyping in infancy: visual preferences for and knowledge of gender-stereotyped toys in the second year. *Int J Behav Dev.* 2001;25:7-15
17. Zosuls KM, Ruble DN, Tamis-Lemonda CS, Shrout PE, Bornstein MH, Greulich FK. The acquisition of gender labels in infancy: implications for gender-typed play. *Dev Psychol.* 2009;45:688-701
18. Lobel TE, Bar-David E, Gruber R, Lau S, Bar-Tal Y. Gender scheme and social judgments: a developmental study of children from Hong Kong. *Sex Roles.* 2000;43:19-42
19. Martin CL, Ruble D. Children's search for gender cues. *Curr Dir Psychol Sci.* 2004;13:67-70
20. Egan SK, Perry DG. Gender identity: a multidimensional analysis with implications for psychosocial adjustment. *Dev Psychol.* 200;37:451-463
21. Carver P. Gender identity and adjustment in middle childhood. *Sex Roles.* 2003;49:95-109
22. Maccoby EE. *The Two Sexes: Growing Up Apart, Coming Together.* 5th printing. Boston: First Harvard University Press Belknap; 2003
23. Perrin EC. *Sexual Orientation in Child and Adolescent Health Care.* New York: Kluwer Academic/Plenum Publishers; 2002
24. Cohen-Kettenis PT. Gender identity disorders. In: Gillberg C ed. *A Clinician's Handbook of Child and Adolescent Psychiatry.* Cambridge: Cambridge University Press; 2005:695-725
25. de Vries AL, Doreleijers TA, Steensma TD, Cohen-Kettenis PT. Psychiatric comorbidity in gender dysphoric adolescents. *J Child Psychol Psychiatr.* 2011;52:1195-1202
26. Spack NP, Edwards-Leeper L, Feldman HA, et al. Children and adolescents with gender identity disorder referred to a pediatric medical center. *Pediatrics.* 2012;129:418-425
27. Khatchadourian K, Amed S, Metzger DL. Clinical management of youth with gender dysphoria in Vancouver. *J Pediatr.* 2014;164(4):906-911
28. Olson J, Forbes C, Belzer M. Management of the transgender adolescent. *Arch Pediatr Adolesc Med.* 2011;165:171-176
29. Ehrensaft D. From gender identity disorder to gender identity creativity: true gender self child therapy. *J Homosex.* 2012;59(3):337-356
30. Sherer I, Rosenthal SM, Ehrensaft D, Baum J. Child and Adolescent Gender Center: a multidisciplinary collaboration to improve the lives of gender nonconforming children and teens. *Pediatr Rev.* 2012;33(6):273-275
31. Institute of Medicine. Committee on Lesbian, Gay, Bisexual, and Transgender Health Issues and Research Gaps and Opportunities. *The Health of Lesbian, Gay, Bisexual, and Transgender People: Building a Foundation for Better Understanding.* Washington, DC: National Academies Press; 2011
32. Health risks and needs of lesbian, gay, bisexual, transgender, and questioning adolescents position statement. *J Pediatr Health Care.* 2011;25:A9-A10
33. Robinson JP, Espelage DL. Peer victimization and sexual risk differences between lesbian, gay, bisexual, transgender, or questioning and nontransgender heterosexual youths in grades 7-12. *Am J Public Health.* 2013;103:1810-1819
34. Rice E, Barman-Adhikari A, Rhoades H, et al. Homelessness experiences, sexual orientation, and sexual risk taking among high school students in Los Angeles. *J Adolesc Health.* 2013;52:773-778
35. Grossman AH, D'Augelli AR. Transgender youth and life-threatening behaviors. *Suicide Life Threat Behav.* 2007;37:527-537
36. Kreukels BP, Cohen-Kettenis PT. Puberty suppression in gender identity disorder: the Amsterdam experience. *Nat Rev Endocrinol.* 2011;7:466-472
37. Wallien MS, Cohen-Kettenis PT. Psychosexual outcome of gender-dysphoric children. *J Am Acad Child Adolesc Psychiatry.* 2008;47:1413-1423
38. Cohen-Kettenis PT, van Goozen SH. Sex reassignment of adolescent transsexuals: a follow-up study. *J Am Acad Child Adolesc Psychiatry.* 1997;36:263-271

39. Smith YL, van Goozen SH, Cohen-Kettenis PT. Adolescents with gender identity disorder who were accepted or rejected for sex reassignment surgery: a prospective follow-up study. *J Am Acad Child Adolesc Psychiatry.* 2001;40:472-481
40. Murad MH, Elamin MB, Garcia MZ, et al. Hormonal therapy and sex reassignment: a systematic review and meta-analysis of quality of life and psychosocial outcomes. *Clin Endocrinol.* 2010; 72:214-231
41. de Vries ALC, Steensma TD, Doreleijers TAH, Cohen-Kettenis PT. Puberty suppression in adolescents with gender identity disorder: a prospective follow-up study. *J Sex Med.* 2011;8:2276-2283
42. Obedin-Maliver J, Goldsmith ES, Stewart L, et al. Lesbian, Gay, bisexual, and transgender-related content in undergraduate medical education. *JAMA.* 2011;306:971-977
43. Henry-Reid L, O'Connor KG, Klein JD, et al. Current pediatrician practices in identifying high-risk behaviors of adolescents. *Pediatrics.* 2010;125:e741-e747
44. East J, Rayes F. Pediatricians' approach to the health care of lesbian, gay, and bisexual youth. *J Adolesc Health.* 1998;23:191-193
45. Meckler GD, Elliott MN, Kanouse DE, Beals KP, Schuster MA. Nondisclosure of sexual orientation to a physician among a sample of gay, lesbian, and bisexual youth. *Arch Pediatr Adolesc Med.* 2006;160:1248-1254
46. Allen LB, Glicken AD, Beach RK, Naylor KE. Adolescent health care experience of gay, lesbian and bisexual young adults. *J Adolesc Health.* 1998;23:212-220
47. Makadon HJ. Ending LGBT invisibility in health care: the first step in ensuring equitable care. *Cleve Clin J Med.* 2011;78:220-224
48. Sison AC, Greydanus DE. Deconstructing adolescent same-sex attraction and sexual behavior in the twenty-first century: perspectives for the clinician prim care. *Clin Office Pract.* 2007;34:293-304
49. Meyer IH. Prejudice, social stress, and mental health in lesbian, gay, and bisexual populations: conceptual issues and research evidence. *Psychol Bull.* 2003;129:674-697
50. Meyer IH. Minority stress and mental health in gay men. *J Health Soc Behav.* 1995;36(1):38-56
51. Brooks VR. *Minority Stress and Lesbian Women.* Lexington, MA: Lexington Books; 1981
52. Poteat T, German D, Kerrigan D. Managing uncertainty: a grounded theory of stigma in transgender health care encounters. *Soc Sci Med.* 2013;84:22-29
53. Needham BL, Austin EL. Sexual orientation, parental support and health during the transition to young adulthood. *J Youth Adolesc.* 2010;39:1189-1198
54. Bouris A, Guilamo-Ramos V, Pickard A, et al. A systematic review of parental influences on the health and well-being of lesbian, gay, and bisexual youth: time for a new public health research and practice agenda. *J Prim Prev.* 2010;31:273-309
55. Ryan C, Huebner D, Diaz RM, Sanchez J. Family rejection as a predictor of negative health outcomes in white and Latino lesbian, gay, and bisexual young adults. *Pediatrics.* 2009;123:346-352
56. Malpas J. Between pink and blue: a multi-dimensional family approach to gender nonconforming children and their families. *Fam Process.* 2011;50:453-470
57. World Professional Association for Transgender Health. Standards of Care for the Health of Transsexual, Transgender, and Gender Nonconforming People Version 7. Available at: admin.associationsonline.com/uploaded_files/140/files/Standards%20of%20Care,%20V7%20Full%20Book.pdf. Accessed June 10, 2014
58. Hembree WC, Cohen-Kettenis P, Delemarre-van de Waal HA, et al. Endocrine treatment of transsexual persons: an Endocrine Society clinical practice guideline. *J Clin Endocrinol Metab.* 2009;94:3132-3154
59. Kiesel LA, Rody A, Greb RR, Szilágyi A. Clinical use of GnRH analogues. *Clin Endocrinol.* 2002;56(6):677-687
60. Delemarre-van de Waal HA, Cohen-Kettenis PT. Clinical management of gender identity disorder in adolescents: a protocol on psychological and paediatric endocrinology aspects. *Eur J Endocrinol.* 2006;155(Suppl 1):S131-S137
61. Coulter RW, Kenst KS, Bowen DJ, Scout. Research funded by the National Institutes of Health on the Health of Lesbian, Gay, Bisexual, and Transgender Populations. *Am J Public Health.* 2014;104:e105-e112

62. McKay B. Lesbian, gay, bisexual, and transgender health issues, disparities, and information resources. *Med Ref Serv Q.* 2011;30(4):393-401
63. Russell ST, Ryan C, Toomey RB, Diaz RM, Sanchez J. Lesbian, gay, bisexual, and transgender adolescent school victimization: implications for young adult health and adjustment. *J Sch Health.* 2011;81:223-230
64. Kreiss JL, Patterson DL. Psychosocial issues in primary care of lesbian, gay, bisexual, and transgender youth. *J Pediatr Health Care.* 1997;11:266-274
65. Coker TR, Austin SB, Schuster MA. Health and healthcare for lesbian, gay, bisexual, and transgender youth: reducing disparities through research, education, and practice. *J Adolesc Health.* 2009;45:213-215
66. Fredriksen-Goldsen KI, Cook-Daniels L, Kim HJ, et al. Physical and mental health of transgender older adults: an at-risk and underserved population. *Gerontologist.* Available at: caringandaging.org/wordpress/wp-content/uploads/2013/04/Physical-and-mental-health-of-transgender-older-adults-An-at-risk-and-underserved-population.pdf. Accessed June 27, 2014
67. Poteat T, German D, Kerrigan D. Managing uncertainty: a grounded theory of stigma in transgender health care encounters. *Soc Sci Med.* 2013;84:22-29
68. Bockting W. Counseling and mental health care for transgender adults and loved ones. *Int J Transgend.* 2006;9(3/4):35-82
69. Anton B. Proceedings of the American Psychological Association for the legislative year 2008: minutes of the annual meeting of the Council of Representatives, February 22-24, 2008, Washington, DC, and August 13 and 17, 2008, Boston, MA, and minutes of the February, June, August, and December 2008 meetings of the Board of Directors. *Am Psychol.* 2008;64:372-453
70. Toorians AW, Thomassen MC, Zweegman S, et al. Venous thrombosis and changes of hemostatic variables during cross-sex hormone treatment in transsexual people. *J Clin Endocrinol Metab.* 2003;88:5723-5729
71. Smith NL, Blondon M, Wiggins KL, et al. Lower risk of cardiovascular events in postmenopausal women taking oral estradiol compared with oral conjugated equine estrogens. *JAMA Intern Med.* Available at: http://archinte.jamanetwork.com/. Accessed January 2, 2014
72. L'hermite M, Simoncini T, Fuller S, Genazzani AR. Could transdermal estradiol + progesterone be a safer postmenopausal HRT? A review. *Maturitas.* 2008;60:185-201
73. Wren BG, Day RO, McLachlan AJ, Williams KM. Pharmacokinetics of estradiol, progesterone, testosterone and dehydroepiandrosterone after transbuccal administration to postmenopausal women. *Climacteric.* 2003;6:104-111
74. Kovac JR, Rajanahally S, Smith RP, Coward RM, Lamb DJ, Lipshultz LI. Patient satisfaction with testosterone replacement therapies: the reasons behind the choices. Patient satisfaction with testosterone replacement therapies: the reasons behind the choices. Available at: onlinelibrary.wiley.com.revproxy.brown.edu/doi/10.1111/jsm.12369/abstract. Accessed January 2, 2014
75. Society for Adolescent Health and Medicine. Recommendations for promoting the health and well-being of lesbian, gay, bisexual, and transgender adolescents: a position paper of the Society for Adolescent Health and Medicine. *J Adolesc Health.* 2013;52(4):506-510
76. American Academy of Pediatrics Committee on Adolescence. Office-based care for lesbian, gay, bisexual, transgender, and questioning youth. *Pediatrics.* 2013;132(1):198-203
77. The American Academy of Child and Adolescent Psychiatry. Sexual orientation, gender identity and civil rights. 2009 Policy Statement. Available at: www.aacap.org/AACAP/Policy_Statements/2009/Sexual_Orientation_Gender_Identity_and_Civil_Rights.aspx. Accessed December 27, 2013
78. Corrigan PW, Kosyluk KA, Rüsch N. Reducing self-stigma by coming out proud. *Am J Public Health.* 2013;103:794-800
79. Greytak EA, Kosciw JG, Diaz EM. Harsh realities: the experiences of transgender youth in our nation's schools. Available at: www.umass.edu/stonewall/uploads/listWidget/25125/trans%20youth%20in%20schools.pdf. Accessed June 10, 2014
80. Report from the National Coalition of Anti-Violence Programs (NCAVP). 2013 ed. Lesbian, gay bisexual, transgender, queer and HIV-affected hate violence in 2012. Available at: www.avp.org/storage/documents/ncavp_2012_hvreport_final.pdf. Accessed January 2, 2014

81. Ryan C, Russell ST, Huebner D, Diaz R, Sanchez J. Family acceptance in adolescence and the health of LGBT young adults. *J Child Adolesc Psychiatr Nurs.* 2010;23:205-213
82. Simons L, Schrager SM, Clark LF, Belzer M, Olson J. Parental support and mental health among transgender adolescents. *J Adolesc Health.* 2013;53:791-793
83. Riley EA, Clemson L, Sitharthan G, Diamond M. Surviving a gender-variant childhood: the views of transgender adults on the needs of gender-variant children and their parents. *J Sex Marital Ther.* 2013;39:241-263

Adolesc Med 025 (2014) 398–408

Pediatric Bipolar Disorder and Mood Dysregulation: Diagnostic Controversies

Benjamin N. Shain, MD, PhD[a*]

[a]*Vice Chair, Department of Psychiatry, Head, Division of Child and Adolescent Psychiatry, NorthShore University HealthSystem, Deerfield, Illinois*

INTRODUCTION

Once thought to be rare in adolescents and nearly nonexistent in younger children, bipolar disorder has been diagnosed increasingly over the past 15 years[1,2] and accounted for 26% of primary discharge diagnoses among psychiatrically hospitalized adolescents in the United States.[3] The various types of bipolar disorder have an estimated prevalence of 4% of children and adolescents in the general population.[4]

Children and adolescents with bipolar disorder may have a variety of impairments, including severe depression, high risk of suicide, psychosis, impulsive and dangerous behaviors, social and cognitive deficits, and frequent comorbidity with other psychiatric disorders, including substance use disorders, attention-deficit/hyperactivity disorder (ADHD), anxiety disorders, oppositional defiant disorder, and conduct disorder.[1] Patients often blame others for their difficulties and have little recognition of their own roles in their troubles. Bipolar disorder is particularly challenging to diagnose because of changing symptoms, difficulty in accurate recollection of history, need to consider a range of bipolar diagnoses, overlap of symptoms with other conditions, and high prevalence of comorbid conditions. Management may be difficult because of medication limitations, including troublesome adverse medication effects, lack of full response, prescription of multiple medications, and incomplete prevention of relapse.[1] Poor adherence to prescribed dosing is common.[5]

Bipolar disorder has long been described as encompassing a spectrum of disorders, with variation in severity, duration and frequency of episodes, degree of

*Corresponding author:
E-mail address: aias@ix.netcom.com

 ISSN 1934-4287

impairment, and types of symptoms.[1,6,7] Classification of child and adolescent bipolar disorder has been particularly challenging because of the explosive increase in use of the diagnosis and the large number of patients with atypical symptoms, particularly with regard to duration and type of mania or maniclike episodes.

The salient feature of all bipolar diagnoses is the presence, at some point in time, of mania, hypomania, or manic features.[8] Mania is a distinct period of abnormally and persistently elevated, expansive, or irritable mood and abnormally and persistently increased goal-directed activity or energy, lasting at least 1 week and accompanied by at least 3 (at least 4 if mood only irritable) associated symptoms: inflated self-esteem, less need for sleep, more talkative, flight of ideas or racing thoughts, distractibility, increased directed or nondirected activity, and excessive involvement in activities that have a high potential for painful consequences. The mood disturbance is severe enough to include marked impairment in social or occupational functioning, necessitates hospitalization, or is associated with psychotic symptoms. Hypomania has the same criteria except for severity and duration (severity is change in functioning but not marked impairment, and duration is at least 4 rather than 7 days) (see Shain et al for a recent comprehensive review of diagnosis and management of adolescent bipolar disorder and the collaborative role of the pediatrician[7]). The rest of this article focuses on diagnostic controversies in pediatric bipolar and related disorders. The term *pediatric* is used interchangeably with *child* and *adolescent*.

HISTORY OF BIPOLAR DIAGNOSES IN CHILDREN AND ADOLESCENTS

Common but Atypical

A school of thought advanced in the late 1990s was that pediatric mania is common (16% in 1 study of psychiatrically referred preadolescents) but atypical by adult standards because it generally includes irritability rather than euphoria, is chronic rather than episodic, and often is comorbid with ADHD.[9,10] The irritability in children is characterized by "affective storms"; severe and prolonged temper outbursts that may include yelling, crying, threatening, throwing, and other aggression toward people or property; and persistent anger or quickness to anger between outbursts. Manic adolescents show more tendency to euphoria than do children, but irritability still is predominant. Chronic, nonepisodic mania is seen in both children and adolescents, with the tendency toward rapid-cycling, mixed states. *Mixed* refers to rapid alternation between mania and depression or dysphoric mania, a state characterized by an unpleasant, usually angry, mood and other symptoms of mania. *Rapid cycling* is defined as more than 4 mood episodes in 12 months that meet criteria for mania, hypomania, or major depressive episode.[8] Faster cycles are referred to in the literature as "ultra-rapid" (episodes lasting a few days to a few weeks) and "ultradian" (mood variation within a 24-hour period).[11]

The construct in the late 1990s was that mania, especially in children, is strongly comorbid with ADHD, with studies showing 60% to 90% of pediatric bipolar patients also having an ADHD diagnosis. There is considerable symptom overlap with mania because symptoms of ADHD include excessive talking, high activity level, and impulsivity, and ADHD is associated with negative emotionality and reduced behavioral inhibition. Evidence supporting overlap between ADHD and mania included diagnostic assessment with the overlapping criteria removed,[12] family aggregation studies, and response of children diagnosed with mania to treatment with mood-stabilizing medication.

This view of chronic, irritable mania highly comorbid with ADHD has been associated with considerable controversy.[13] Clinical descriptions of mania have been stable for years and consist of a *distinct* period of elevated or irritable mood along with well-established associated features. Continuous mania has never been a diagnostic feature of bipolar disorder. The view was also questioned with skepticism regarding the validity of the family history studies and the reported high rate of pediatric bipolar disorder compared to the lower lifetime prevalence in adults.

SEVERE MOOD DYSREGULATION

The pediatric bipolar diagnostic controversy has focused on whether the disorder in children and adolescents is different from the disorder in adults with regard to manic symptoms, particularly duration (the need for at least 7 days for mania and 4 days for hypomania vs the frequent occurrence of daily or hourly mood changes in children and adolescents); distinctiveness (the need for clear and sharp differences from the previous mood state vs less distinction between states in child and adolescents); and type (at least some euphoria is typical in adults vs the common, exclusively irritable state seen in children and adolescents). An excellent review of the literature comparing youths who meet *Diagnostic and Statistical Manual of Mental Disorders* (DSM) criteria for bipolar disorder with those who are atypical with regard to duration, distinctiveness, or type of mania is provided by Leibenluft.[14]

Leibenluft et al suggested research diagnostic criteria for 3 clinical phenotypes of pediatric bipolar disorder: narrow, intermediate, and broad.[15] Although these are not part of the DSM, they have been helpful in characterizing the atypical presentation of bipolar and other mood symptoms in children and adolescents. Narrow phenotype bipolar disorder includes at least 1 episode of mania or hypomania that meets full DSM (DSM-IV-TR[16] is used) mania or hypomania criteria and requires the presence of elation and/or grandiosity. Elation and grandiosity were argued by Geller et al[12] to be core bipolar features. The episode must meet full duration criteria (at least 7 days for mania and 4 days for hypomania), be a clear switch from another mood state (depressed, mixed state, euthymic), be different from the child's or adolescent's baseline mood, and simultaneously include the associated symptoms of mania/hypomania.

Intermediate phenotype bipolar disorder also includes at least 1 episode of mania or hypomania that meets full DSM mania/hypomania criteria except for duration (episodes shorter than 4 days but lasting at least 1 day) *or* the mania/hypomania is exclusively irritable rather than euphoric. Mood cycling remains a required feature.

Broad phenotype bipolar is characterized by chronic irritability that is present for at least 1 year and on most days does not include mood cycling. This diagnosis overlaps other disorders because irritability is a common diagnostic criterion, present in at least 6 different DSM diagnoses, including mania, oppositional defiant disorder, generalized anxiety disorder, dysthymic disorder, posttraumatic stress disorder, and major depressive episode. The broad phenotype is characterized by high reactivity to negative emotional stimuli. Hyperarousal is present, which is defined by the presence of at least 3 of the following: insomnia, agitation, distractibility, racing thoughts or flight of ideas, pressured speech, and intrusiveness. The broad phenotype has been referred to as the research diagnosis of severe mood dysregulation (SMD).

A number of differences have been found between youth with SMD and those with full criteria for bipolar disorder. SMD is common, with a lifetime prevalence of 3.3% among children and adolescents 9 to 19 years of age in a community sample, compared to only 0.1% for youth meeting full criteria for bipolar disorder.[17] Most affected children and adolescents with SMD had comorbid psychiatric disorders, most frequently disruptive behavior disorders (ADHD, conduct disorder, and oppositional defiant disorder). Children and adolescents with SMD were 7 times more likely to develop depression as young adults compared with those without SMD. In a longitudinal study, episodic and chronic irritability were associated with different groups of psychiatric diagnoses at a later date. Youth with a mean age of 13.8 years at time 1 were followed up at time 2 (mean age 16.2 years) and time 3 (mean age 22.1 years).[18] Episodic irritability at time 1 was associated with simple phobia at time 2. Chronic irritability at time 1 was associated with ADHD at time 2 and major depression at time 3. In a subsequent, 20-year follow-up study, irritability at first assessment was associated with the following diagnoses at 20-year follow up: depressive disorders (14.5%), obsessive-compulsive disorder (4%), agoraphobia (4.3%), generalized anxiety disorder (2.9%), and bipolar disorder (1.6%).[19] Regression analysis adjusting for baseline disorders showed that irritability only predicted depression and generalized anxiety and not bipolar disorder. With respect to the associated disruptive behavior disorders, data from 2 British surveys, which included 3-year follow-ups, demonstrated different disorders associated with the different dimensions of youth oppositionality. The irritable dimension was associated with later depression and anxiety, the headstrong dimension with ADHD and conduct disorder at follow-up, and the hurtful dimension only with conduct disorder.[20]

In another study, there was also a significant difference in the diagnoses of parental bipolar disorders, comparing parents of offspring with narrow phenotype bipolar disorder versus those with SMD: 33.3% of parents of children with narrow phenotype bipolar disorder were found to have bipolar disorder compared to only 2.7% of parents of children with SMD.[21] No other diagnoses were found to be significantly different between the 2 sets of parents.

Measures of pathophysiology also differed between children and adolescents with SMD and those with narrow phenotype bipolar disorder. Whereas children and adolescents in both groups showed greater arousal while doing a task designed to elicit frustration,[22] EEG measures during the frustration task showed differences between the groups. This finding suggests that narrow phenotype patients have more difficulty modulating their attention in the context of higher emotional demands, similar to results associated with depression and anhedonia, whereas those with SMD had EEG patterns suggesting attentional problems unrelated to emotion, similar to results with ADHD. Differences were also seen in cognitive flexibility, the ability to adapt to changing environmental conditions, with greater impairment in the narrow phenotype group.[23] Cognitive flexibility with regard to rewards is thought to be relevant, because both depression (symptoms include diminished interest and pleasure in activities and feelings of worthlessness) and mania (symptoms include increased pursuit of pleasurable activities, increased goal-directed activity, and increased self-esteem or grandiosity) may result in impaired reward processing. Facial-emotion labeling, a measure of social impairment, showed similar deficits between narrow phenotype and SMD groups, with both groups showing more social impairment than controls and youth with anxiety, major depression, ADHD, or conduct disorder.[24] However, the type of psychosocial impairments differed, with deficient social reciprocity skills correlating with facial-emotion labeling deficits in the narrow phenotype group and dysfunctional family relationships correlating with facial-emotion labeling deficits in the SMD group.[25]

The research concepts of the 3 pediatric bipolar phenotypes and SMD have not been adopted for clinical use but are a prelude to the creation of a new diagnosis, "disruptive mood dysregulation disorder," in DSM-5.

DSM-5

Disruptive Mood Dysregulation Disorder

Concerns that youth with anger outbursts and chronic irritability have been increasingly misdiagnosed as having bipolar disorder[14] led to the creation of disruptive mood dysregulation disorder (DMDD),[26] a new diagnosis in the *Diagnostic and Statistical Manual of Mental Disorders*, Fifth Edition (DSM-5).[8] Criteria for

DMDD (Table 1) are severe and persistent temper outbursts occurring 3 or more times per week for at least 12 months and accompanied by irritable or angry mood between outbursts, with a minimum age of diagnosis of 6 years and a maximum age of onset of 10 years. Patients who meet criteria for both DMDD and oppositional defiant disorder are given the diagnosis of DMDD. Criteria for DMDD are somewhat different from those for the research diagnosis of SMD. The SMD requirement for hyperarousal (at least 3 of following: insomnia, agitation, distractibility, racing thoughts or flight of ideas, pressured speech, and intrusiveness) is not included in the DMDD criteria, thereby reducing the diagnostic criteria overlap with ADHD. In addition, the age, duration, and persistence criteria are somewhat different between DMDD and SMD. DMDD is placed in the DSM-5 section for depressive disorders rather than that for bipolar and related disorders, emphasizing the greater relatedness to depression than to mania.

Table 1
Disruptive mood dysregulation disorder

A. Severe recurrent temper outbursts manifested verbally (eg, verbal rages) and/or behaviorally (eg, physical aggression toward people or property) that are grossly out of proportion in intensity or duration to the situation or provocation.
B. The temper outbursts are inconsistent with developmental level.
C. The temper outbursts occur, on average, 3 or more times per week.
D. The mood between temper outbursts is persistently irritable or angry most of the day, nearly every day, and is observable by others (eg, parents, teachers, peers).
E. Criteria A-D have been present for 12 or more months. Throughout that time, the individual has not had a period lasting 3 or more consecutive months without all of the symptoms in Criteria A-D.
F. Criteria A and D are present in at least 2 of 3 settings (ie, at home, at school, with peers) and are severe in at least 1 of these.
G. The diagnosis should not be made for the first time before age 6 years or after age 18 years.
H. By history or observation, the age at onset of Criteria A-E is before 10 years.
I. There has never been a distinct period lasting more than 1 day during which the full symptom criteria, except in duration for a manic or hypomanic episode, have been met.

Note: Developmentally appropriate mood elevation, such as occurs in the context of a highly positive event or its anticipation, should not be considered as a symptom of mania or hypomania.

J. The behaviors do not occur exclusively during an episode of major depressive disorder and are not better explained by another mental disorder (eg, autism spectrum disorder, posttraumatic stress disorder, separation anxiety, disorder, persistent depressive disorder [dysthymia]).

Note: This diagnosis cannot coexist with oppositional defiant disorder, intermittent explosive disorder, or bipolar disorder, though it can coexist with others, including major depressive disorder, attention-deficit/hyperactivity disorder, conduct disorder, and substance use disorders. Individuals whose symptoms meet criteria for both disruptive mood dysregulation and oppositional defiant disorder should only be given the diagnosis of disruptive mood dysregulation disorder. If an individual has ever experienced a manic or hypomanic episode, the diagnosis of disruptive mood dysregulation should not be assigned.

K. The symptoms are not attributable to the physiological effects of a substance or to another medical or neurological condition.

From American Psychiatric Association. *Diagnostic and Statistical Manual of Mental Disorders*. 5th ed. Arlington, VA: American Psychiatric Association: 2013. Used with permission.

Concerns about the DMDD diagnosis began before the release of DSM-5. Axelson et al analyzed data obtained from 706 children aged 6 to 12 years who participated in the Longitudinal Assessment of Manic Symptoms study.[27] The analysis waived the DMDD requirement for lack of coexistence with oppositional defiant disorder to better examine the overlap. At intake, 26% of the sample met criteria for DMDD. Children with DMDD had higher rates of oppositional defiant disorder and conduct disorder but not mood, anxiety, or attention-deficit/hyperactivity disorders. Conversely, most of the children with oppositional defiant disorder and conduct disorder met criteria for DMDD. Additionally, no differences in symptom severity were found between children diagnosed with DMDD versus those who were not. Over the 2-year follow up, 40% of the sample met DMDD criteria at least once, with half of these meeting criteria at only 1 of the assessments. DMDD was not associated with parental psychiatric history. The authors concluded that the diagnosis of DMDD may have limited utility based on lack of diagnostic stability, lack of differences of both type of symptoms and symptom severity from oppositional defiant disorder and conduct disorder, and lack of association with parental disorders.

Copeland et al analyzed data obtained from 3 community samples, 1 made up of preschool children (ages 2-5 years) and the other 2 made up of older children and adolescents.[28] The analysis waived requirements for minimum age and lack of coexistence with oppositional defiant disorder. Nearly half of the children and adolescents in the older samples had severe temper outbursts, but after criteria for frequency, irritable mood, duration, and age were applied, the prevalence of DMDD dropped to about 1%. The preschool sample showed a similar pattern but had higher percentages of other diagnoses, including 81% who had severe temper outbursts but only 3.3% who met full DMDD criteria (except for age). Concern was expressed that making the diagnosis of DMDD is highly dependent on applying criteria for frequency, persistence, and duration but that this type of information often is difficult for patients and caregivers to recall accurately.[26] Comorbidity was frequent with all common psychiatric disorders, and the concordance was exceptionally high with oppositional defiant disorder. Nearly all participants diagnosed with either DMDD or oppositional defiant disorder also had the other disorder, causing the authors to question the classification of DMDD as only a mood disorder. In addition, unexpectedly, Copeland et al found only partial overlap between DMDD and SMD, with only 39% of youth with SMD meeting criteria for DMDD. This brings into question the validity of applying results from studies of SMD to children with DMDD. The diagnosis of DMDD does not seem to solve the pediatric bipolar classification problem, although further research is indicated.

"Other Specified" and "Unspecified" Bipolar and Related Disorder

The other major change of importance to the diagnosis of pediatric bipolar disorder in DSM-5 is deletion of the diagnosis of "bipolar disorder not otherwise specified," which clinicians used to diagnose most children and adolescents with bipolar disorder. DSM-5 introduces 2 new diagnoses: "other specified bipolar and related disorder," and "unspecified bipolar and related disorder."

Other specified bipolar and related disorder requires a presentation that includes "symptoms characteristic of bipolar" (left undefined) that causes significant distress or impairment but does not meet full criteria for any disorder in the bipolar and related disorders diagnostic class. This diagnosis is used in situations where the clinician chooses to communicate the specific reason why the presentation does not meet full criteria for another bipolar disorder, potentially leading to documentation of important diagnostic information for clinical or research purposes. Unspecified bipolar and related disorder has the same criteria as other specified bipolar and related disorder except that the clinician chooses *not* to communicate the specific reason for lack of full criteria, as in situations where insufficient information is available.

Some inferences can be made as to the meaning of "symptoms characteristic of bipolar" that "do not meet the full criteria for any of the disorders in the bipolar and related disorders diagnostic class." The salient feature of bipolar is one or more episodes of mania or hypomania. Full criteria for a bipolar diagnosis can be lacking in 1 of 2 ways: (1) full criteria for hypomania are met (past or present), but there was never a major depressive episode and duration criteria for cyclothymia (1 year for children and adolescents, 2 years for adults) are not met; or (2) full criteria for mania or hypomania at any time are lacking, other than by the exclusionary criteria of causation of symptoms by a substance or other medical condition. It is important to note that a presentation meeting full criteria for mania at any time is always another diagnosis (bipolar I disorder or 1 of the psychotic disorders).

Failing to meet full criteria for mania or hypomania is the reason of primary importance for the difficulty in diagnosing bipolar disorder in children and adolescents. As discussed earlier, mania and hypomania require a distinct period (4 days or more for hypomania and 7 days or more for mania) of abnormally and persistently elevated, expansive, or irritable mood and increased activity or energy, both during the same time period as 3 or more (4 or more if mood is only irritable) associated symptoms (inflated self-esteem or grandiosity, less need for sleep, more or pressured speech, flight of ideas or racing thoughts, distractibility, increased activity or energy, and activities with potential for painful consequences). Typically children and adolescents do not meet full criteria for bipolar because they do not meet the criteria for duration of the mania/hypomania episode. It also may be challenging to elicit the required associated symptoms for the same historical period of time.

The lack of duration criteria may be further subdivided into presentations of distinct episodes lasting 1 to 3 days versus those that last less than 1 day. Mood changes related to external reasons, such as euphoria associated with a new romance or feeling better around friends, do not count. Research criteria, such as the intermediate phenotype described earlier, generally have adopted at least a 1-day minimum for mood state duration. This was done in part for practical reasons because making the diagnosis relies on eliciting the 3 or 4 associated symptoms during the same period of time. When the mood state lasts less than 1 day, diagnosis becomes more challenging and unreliable. DSM-5 does not note any such difference between 1 to 3 days and less than 1 day. An important unanswered question is how short an episode may be and still be an episode. A work-around answer is that an episode may be any length as long as it is distinct, observable by others, reflects a change in functioning, and is clearly accompanied by at least the minimum 3 or 4 associated symptoms. Obtaining this history may be challenging. See Shain et al for interviewing suggestions and use of "red flag" symptoms (summarized in Table 2) that may raise suspicion for a bipolar or mood dysregulation diagnosis.[7] "Red flag" symptoms are *not* diagnostic by themselves; rather, the presence of 1 or more such symptoms suggests the possibility of a diagnosis of bipolar or mood dysregulation disorder.

SUMMARY

Pediatric bipolar disorder, once thought rare, has gone through stages of conceptualization. DSM criteria were reinterpreted such that children and adolescents, particularly those with ADHD, were commonly diagnosed with bipolar disorder and thought to be atypical by adult standards. Research criteria separated pediatric

Table 2
Examples of interview questions

"Red flag" symptom	Question examples
Rage outbursts	"Do you lose your temper?" If so, ask about frequency, duration, triggers, and what happens.
Episodes of requiring little sleep	"Do you ever have nights when you have lots of energy, do not need to sleep much, and do lots of things?" If so, "Are you tired the next day?"
Spontaneous mood shifts	"Do you find yourself suddenly angry or extremely happy for no apparent reason?" If so, ask about frequency and duration of the moods.
Running away, sneaking out at night, spending money, hypersexuality	"Have you even run away or snuck out of the house at night?" "Do you have time when you spend a lot of money or when you feel that you cannot control your sexual urges?"
Grandiosity	"Do you have times when you feel that nothing can happen to you?" "Do you have times when you greatly overestimate your talents or abilities?"
Agitation or mania with antidepressant	"Have you ever taken medication for depression?" If so, "Did you have any side effects?" "Did you ever become very edgy or much more happy or angry than is typical for you?"

From Shain BN; Committee on Adolescence. Collaborative role of the pediatrician in the diagnosis and management of bipolar disorder in adolescents. *Pediatrics.* 2012;130:e1725.

bipolar patients into 3 phenotypes, including a research diagnosis of "severe mood dysregulation." DSM-5 largely maintained previous criteria for bipolar disorder at all ages and created a new diagnosis called "disruptive mood dysregulation disorder," categorized as a depressive disorder, for persistently angry or irritable patients with symptoms of childhood onset. However, the controversy regarding the diagnosis of pediatric bipolar disorder continues. Progress has been made in the classification of children and adolescents with mood symptoms who are predominantly irritable or angry, but lack of clarity remains regarding classification of children and adolescents with "symptoms characteristic of bipolar disorder" who do not meet criteria for bipolar I disorder, bipolar II disorder, or cyclothymia.

References

1. American Academy of Child and Adolescent Psychiatry. Practice parameters for the assessment and treatment of children and adolescents with bipolar disorder. *J Am Acad Child Adolesc Psychiatry*. 2007;46(1):107-122
2. Carlson G. Early onset bipolar disorder: clinical and research considerations. *J Clin Child Adolesc Psychol*. 2005;34:331-342
3. Bladder JC, Carlson GA. Increased rates of bipolar disorder diagnoses among U.S. child, adolescent, and adult inpatients, 1996-2004. *Biol Psychiatry*. 2007;62(2):107-114
4. Kowatch RA, Fristad MA, Findling RL, Post RM, eds. *Clinical Manual for Management of Bipolar Disorder in Children and Adolescents*. Washington, DC: American Psychiatric Association; 2009
5. Drotar D, Greenley RN, Demeter CA, et al. Adherence to pharmacological treatment for juvenile bipolar disorder. *J Am Acad Child Adolesc Psychiatry*. 2007;46(7):831-839
6. Akiskal H, Pinto O. The evolving bipolar spectrum. *Psychiatr Clin North Am*. 1999;22(3):517-534
7. Shain BN; Committee on Adolescence. Collaborative role of the pediatrician in the diagnosis and management of bipolar disorder in adolescents. *Pediatrics*. 2012;130:e1725-e1742
8. American Psychiatric Association. *Diagnostic and Statistical Manual of Mental Disorders*. 5th ed. Arlington, VA: American Psychiatric Association; 2013
9. Biederman J. Resolved: mania is mistaken for ADHD in prepubertal children, affirmative. *J Am Acad Child Adolesc Psychiatry*. 1998;37(10):1091-1093
10. Biederman J, Mick E, Faraone SV, Spencer T, Wilens TE, Wozniak J. Pediatric mania: a developmental subtype of bipolar disorder. *Biol Psychiatry*. 2000;48:458-466
11. Kramlinger K, Post R. Ultra-rapid and ultradian cycling in bipolar affective illness. *Br J Psychiatry*. 1996;168:314-323
12. Geller B, Williams M, Zimmerman B, Frazier J, Beringer L, Warner KL. Prepubertal and early adolescent bipolarity differentiate from ADHD by manic symptoms, grandiose delusions, ultra-rapid or ultradian cycling. *J Affect Disord*. 1998;51:81-91
13. Klein RG, Pine DS, Klein DF. Resolved: mania is mistaken for ADHD in prepubertal children, negative. *J Am Acad Child Adolesc Psychiatry*. 1998;37(10):1093-1096
14. Leibenluft E. Severe mood dysregulation, irritability, and the diagnostic boundaries of bipolar disorder in youths. *Am J Psychiatry*. 2011;168:129-152
15. Leibenluft E, Charney DS, Towbin KE, Bhangoo RK, Pine DS. Defining clinical phenotypes of juvenile mania. *Am J Psychiatry*. 2003;160:430-437
16. American Psychiatric Association. *Diagnostic and Statistical Manual of Mental Disorders*. 4th ed, text revision. Washington, DC: American Psychiatric Association; 2000
17. Brotman MA, Schmajuk M, Rich BA, et al. Prevalence, clinical correlates, and longitudinal course of severe mood dysregulation in children. *Biol Psychiatry*. 2006;60:991-997
18. Leibenluft E, Cohen P, Gorrindo T, Brook JS, Pine DS. Chronic versus episodic irritability in youth: a community-based, longitudinal study of clinical and diagnostic associations. *J Child Adolesc Psychopharmacol*. 2006;16(4):456-466

19. Stringaris A, Cohen P, Pine DS, Leibenluft E. Adult outcomes of youth irritability: a 20-year prospective community-based study. *Am J Psychiatry*. 2009;166:1048-1054
20. Stringaris A, Goodman R. Longitudinal outcome of youth oppositionality: irritable, headstrong, and hurtful behaviors have distinctive predictions. *J Am Acad Child Adolesc Psychiatry*. 2009;48(4):404-412
21. Brotman MA, Kassem L, Reising MM, et al. Parental diagnoses in youth with narrow phenotype bipolar disorder or severe mood dysregulation. *Am J Psychiatry*. 2007;164:1238-1241
22. Rich BA, Schmajuk M, Perez-Edgar KE, Fox NA, Pine NA, Leibenluft E. Different psychophysiological and behavioral responses elicited by frustration in pediatric bipolar disorder and severe mood dysregulation. *Am J Psychiatry*. 2007;164:309-317
23. Dickstein DP, Nelson EE, McClure EB, et al. Cognitive flexibility in phenotypes of pediatric bipolar disorder. *J Am Acad Child Adolesc Psychiatry*. 2007;46(3):341-365
24. Guyer AE, McClure EB, Adler AD, et al. Specificity of facial expression labeling deficits in childhood psychopathology. *J Child Psychol Psychiatry*. 2007;48(9):863-871
25. Rich BA, Grimley ME, Schmajuk M, Blair KS, Blair RJR, Leibenluft E. Face emotion labeling deficits in children with bipolar disorder and severe mood dysregulation. *Dev Psychopathol*. 2008;20:529-546
26. Axelson D. Taking disruptive mood dysregulation disorder out for a test drive. *Am J Psychiatry*. 2013;170(2):136-139
27. Axelson D, Findling RL, Fristad MA, et al. Examining the proposed disruptive mood dysregulation disorder diagnosis in children in the longitudinal assessment of manic symptoms study. *J Clin Psychiatry*. 2012;73(10):1342-1350
28. Copeland WE, Angold A, Costello EJ, Egger H. Prevalence, comorbidity, and correlates of DSM-5 proposed disruptive mood dysregulation disorder. *Am J Psychiatry*. 2013;170(2):173-179

Adolesc Med 025 (2014) 409–424

Celiac Disease and Gluten-Related Disorders

Stefano Guandalini, MD[a*]; Hilary Jericho, MD[b]

[a]*Professor and Chief Section of Gastroenterology, Hepatology and Nutrition, Department of Pediatrics, University of Chicago Medicine, Chicago, Illinois. Founder and Medical Director, University of Chicago Celiac Disease Center;* [b]*Assistant Professor, Section of Gastroenterology, Hepatology and Nutrition, Department of Pediatrics, University of Chicago Medicine, Chicago, Illinois*

INTRODUCTION

In the past few years, remarkable progress has been made in our knowledge of gluten-related disorders. A better understanding of the pathophysiology of celiac disease and of the growing list of environmental factors that play a role in its development has led to new therapeutic horizons. At the same time, increased awareness has resulted in improved rates of diagnosis. The growing recognition of other disorders related to gluten (or wheat) ingestion has originated a widespread belief that a gluten-free diet (GFD) might be beneficial for many more individuals than celiac patients alone. This review will examine the state of the art of these conditions, with particular emphasis on the implications most relevant to adolescents.

WHEAT INGESTION CAUSES DIFFERENT DISORDERS

Wheat (and related cereals rye and barley) contains gluten. After about 6 decades of its description in modern times (as a result of the work of Dr Samuel Gee[1] in 1888) celiac disease (CD) was finally discovered to be triggered by ingestion of this plant storage protein. Subsequently, it became clear that wheat may also cause unrelated allergic symptoms, and in the past few years a new entity, currently called non-celiac gluten sensitivity (NCGS), has been described.[2] Thus, our current knowledge of the panorama of disorders caused by wheat (mostly by its gluten) includes 3 different entities: wheat allergy, CD, and NCGS (Figure 1).

*Corresponding author:
E-mail address: sguandalini@peds.bsd.uchicago.edu

 ISSN 1934-4287

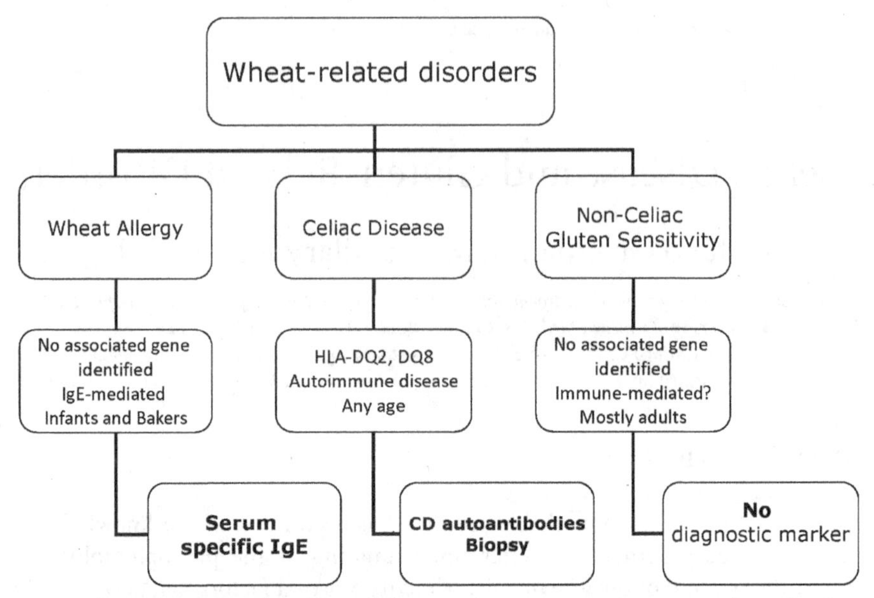

Fig 1. Wheat-related disorders. Three different entities are currently recognized as related to gluten (or wheat) ingestion: wheat allergy, celiac disease, and non-celiac gluten sensitivity. Although prevalence, main pathogenetic mechanisms, and diagnostic tools are available for wheat allergy and celiac disease, none are currently known for non-celiac gluten sensitivity, a term that may well be inclusive of various disorders (see text for discussion).

HOW DID WHEAT AND GLUTEN-RELATED DISORDERS COME TO BE?

For the first 240,000 years of his history, *Homo sapiens* lived without any wheat-related disorders. This was not the result of lack of awareness, poor diagnostic techniques, or the fact that humankind had different gene pools. It was the result of the fact that there simply *was* no wheat or gluten. But what happened just about 12,000 years ago changed our way of life forever: the Neolithic era agricultural revolution, which sprung from the incidental observation that seeds that had fallen from some wild plants later generated other similar plants. Thus, man learned that food-bearing plants could actually be cultivated. Soon the hunter-gatherer way of life was replaced by domestication of crops and animals, enabling people to live sedentary lives next to their sources of food. Permanent settlements arose, beginning in the area of the Middle East called the Fertile Crescent (a term coined by the University of Chicago archaeologist James H. Breasted), creating previously unforeseen forms of social, cultural, economic, and political institutions.

All was good: However, this also meant that we began eating foods that our ancestors were never exposed to, foods containing "strange" proteins that, although edible, could prove to be hard or impossible to fully digest. In addition, plenty of new antigenic molecules were presented to our gut. In other words, evolution had provided us with the ability to show immunologic tolerance to food antigens that have been the staple of our diet over many hundreds of thousands of years. The domestication of wild animals and the cultivation of cereals (in the fertile Crescent, especially wheat and barley) generated a plethora of completely new antigens in the diet to which our gut immune system was not accustomed. Proteins from cow, goat, and donkey milks, birds' eggs, and cereals such as wheat and barley all suddenly became new and major components of man's diet.

Not everybody adapted: Food allergies and intolerances appeared, and among them were wheat allergy and CD.

WHEAT ALLERGY

Wheat is a common food allergen, along with milk, soy, eggs, peanuts, fish, and shellfish. Recent epidemiologic data from North America show that the prevalence of food allergy in children has increased.

In the United States, the prevalence of reported food allergy increased 18% from 1997 through 2007 in children younger than 18 years ($P < .01$), and outpatient visits because of allergy tripled between 1993 and 2006 ($P < .01$). In 2009, almost 4% of US children younger than 18 years had reported food allergy,[3] with an economic effect recently estimated at about $25 billion per year.[4] Wheat elicits an allergy that is an immunoglobulin E (IgE)-mediated phenomenon, well known to occur especially in selected populations: infants and bakers (in whom inhaled wheat can trigger asthma, a professional hazard). More recently, a distinct clinical manifestation of wheat allergy has been identified, part of a group of rare, very severe acute disorders caused by allergy to various food proteins and triggered by physical exercise: wheat-induced, exercise-dependent anaphylaxis.[5]

In the case of children, allergen specific IgE (sIgE) antibodies to foods, including wheat, typically appear within the first 2 years of life. Most children eventually will tolerate the allergy-inducing foods, including wheat,[6] although wheat allergy may persist into adolescence in a significant minority of patients.[7]

In children, IgE-mediated reactions to wheat typically have a rapid onset, within minutes to 2 hours from the time of ingestion. Symptoms can involve many organ systems, including the skin, lungs, and gastrointestinal tract. Common presentation in up to 80% of children includes gastrointestinal manifestations such as nausea, abdominal pain, vomiting, and diarrhea, followed by skin involvement (20%-40%) such as erythema, pruritus, and urticaria. Respiratory symptoms such as cough, wheezing, and rhinorrhea are present in 4% to 25% of children.[8]

We lack a well-accepted set of criteria for the diagnosis of food allergies.[9] Diagnosis is further complicated by the observation that detection of food-specific

IgE implies sensitization but does not necessarily indicate clinical allergy. Therefore, diagnosis requires a careful medical history, laboratory studies, and, in many cases, an oral food challenge to confirm a diagnosis.[8] The National Institute of Allergy and Infectious Diseases (NIAID) guidelines specifically recommends *against* using intradermal testing and total serum IgE levels as methods of diagnosis. The NIAID does state that skin prick tests and sIgE testing may be of assistance in identifying foods that provoke an IgE-mediated food reaction but cannot be used alone to diagnose food allergies. These tests have very high sensitivity but poor specificity and must be interpreted along with clinical presentation and possible food challenge.[10,11] Oral food challenges can be used to diagnose food allergies, and the double-blind placebo-controlled food challenge remains the gold standard; however, it is expensive, time consuming, and rarely acceptable in clinical practice. Single-blind and open food challenges are diagnostic only if no symptoms are elicited, indicating no food allergy, or if objective symptoms correlate with medical history and are supported by laboratory testing, which would then indicate a food allergy.

Therefore, in patients, especially infants, very young children, and those who are exposed to flour on the job (eg, bakers, as mentioned earlier), the possibility of allergy to wheat must be considered and properly addressed.

CELIAC DISEASE

We now understand CD to be a complex autoimmune disease triggered by the ingestion of gluten (the major storage protein in wheat, barley, and rye) in genetically predisposed individuals. It causes elevated titers of celiac-specific autoantibodies and results in variable degrees of inflammation of small intestine and a wide range of gastrointestinal and extra-intestinal complaints.

The availability and widespread use of specific and sensitive serologic markers, such as serum tissue transglutaminase (tTG) IgA antibody levels, a powerful screening tool,[12] has resulted in remarkable advances in our understanding of the true prevalence of CD and of its increase. In fact, the prevalence of CD seems to have increased at a remarkable pace during the past few decades.[13-18] Several factors probably are combining to cause this rapid increase, including modalities of delivery,[19,20] early life infections,[21] exposure to antibiotics,[22] infant feeding practices,[23,24] and even socioeconomic status,[25,26] possibly linked to the effect of the "hygiene hypothesis," according to which a decreased prevalence of infections and exposure to environmental antigens skews the development of the immune system toward predisposition for allergic and autoimmune disorders. The current prevalence of CD is estimated to be 3 to 13 per 1000, with a higher prevalence among first-degree relatives of known CD patients.[27,28] However, only a limited portion of the expected celiac patients actually are recognized, with proportions varying among different countries. In the United States, even though CD overall prevalence should be around 1%, only about 15% of this population (including children and adults) has been diagnosed and therefore can be treated.[29] This phenomenon of underdiagnosis likely is a result of a combination of inadequate awareness and a high prevalence of asymptomatic patients, and seems to be quite widespread.

CD is a complex multifactorial disease that develops in genetically predisposed individuals as a result of the influence of environmental factors. The genetic asset necessary to develop CD is in part known. In fact, human leukocyte antigen (HLA) class II genotypes defined as DQ2 and DQ8 have been found to be crucially necessary predisposing factors. However, it also is clear that other genes are involved because most individuals who carry these haplotypes do not develop CD. Genome-wide association studies are actively underway to fully characterize the genetic constellation behind the predisposition to develop CD, and so far about 40 additional genes (all involved in immune reactions but providing only minor contributions) have been identified.[30] As for the environment, in addition to the only necessary factor of gluten, multiple environmental factors are now known to be key players. Among them are the infant's gut microbiota, the amount and timing of initial exposure to gluten, early infections, and feeding patterns.[27,31,32]

Gluten is a heterogeneous molecule. The gluten fractions that are toxic to celiac patients are a mixture of alcohol-soluble proteins called gliadins. Gliadins are rich in glutamine and proline residues, which even the healthy human intestine cannot fully digest.[33] As a result, intact gliadin peptides are left in the lumen, and some cross the intestinal barrier. These fragments then come into contact with the intracellular enzyme tTG, which deamidates them, changing their shape and increasing their negative charges, thereby generating peptides ideally suited for capture by the HLA-DQ2 or DQ8 molecules expressed on the surface of the lamina propria-associated antigen-presenting cells. These cells are mostly dendritic cells whose proinflammatory status is enhanced by IL-15 in the lamina propria. Once bound to DQ2 or DQ8, gliadin peptides are presented to $CD4^+$ T cells, which triggers the inflammatory reaction (see Abadie et al[34] for a full review of CD pathophysiology).

The end result of autoimmune-triggered inflammation of the small intestine is a variable degree of mucosal damage, typically more severe proximally than distally. Marsh[35] described in great detail the progression from simple infiltration of lymphocytes into the epithelium to extreme damage (ie, total villous atrophy), and his description is widely, although not universally, used in pathology reports from duodenal biopsies.

What are the consequences of active small intestinal inflammation? A wide variety of clinical presentations have been described, and, although gastrointestinal manifestations are obviously present and in many cases prominent, basically all systems and organs can be involved.

Table 1 lists the main clinical presentations of CD and their prevalent age distributions.

Diagnosing CD is a process that first requires a high degree of suspicion. Based on the heterogeneous list of signs and symptoms, CD can be considered a chameleon, and its identification is far from simple. Although gastrointestinal symptoms because of malabsorption (eg, diarrhea, abdominal pain) are common and require prompt evaluation for CD, by no means are they universally present. In fact, there is evidence that CD presentation in children and teenagers has changed over time, moving from a malabsorptive disorder causing gastrointestinal symptoms and malnutrition to a more subtle condition causing a variety of extra-intestinal manifestations.[36-40] It is this variety of presentations, and the fact that CD also may be entirely asymptomatic, that is responsible for the dismal rate of diagnoses around the globe.

Table 1
Main clinical presentations of celiac disease*

Sign or symptom	Age most commonly involved
Vomiting	Infancy
Diarrhea	All ages
Abdominal bloating	All ages
Abdominal pain	Child to adult
Constipation	Child to adolescent
Failure to thrive	Infancy and early childhood
Weight loss	Child to adult
Hypertransaminasemia and other liver issues	Adolescent to adult
Anorexia	Infancy and early childhood
Fatigue	Adolescent to adult
Delayed puberty	Adolescent
Short stature	Child to adolescent
Anemia	Adolescent to adult
Dermatitis herpetiformis	Adolescent to adult
Dental enamel defects	Child to adult
Aphthous ulcers	Child to adult
Arthritis	Adolescent to adult
Osteopenia	Adolescent to adult
Osteoporosis	Adult
Unexplained infertility (in women)	Adult
Headaches	Adolescent to adult
Numbness/neuropathy	Adults
Idiopathic seizures	Child to adult
Sad mood	Infancy to early childhood
Psychiatric disorders	Adolescent to adult

*In many textbooks and publications about celiac disease (CD), gastrointestinal presentations were (and are) grouped under the term "typical" CD, whereas all extra-intestinal manifestations are called "atypical." This originated from the fact that for many decades CD was thought to be restricted to symptoms and signs of malabsorption, and all extra-intestinal manifestations were considered rare or at least not belonging to the classic presentation.

CD is often associated with other conditions, namely, other autoimmune disorders (the best known example is type 1 diabetes) and some syndromes (the most common is Down syndrome). Furthermore, its prevalence is much higher in first-degree relatives of known celiac patients. Hence, these populations represent groups in which CD must be suspected, even in the absence of suggestive symptoms.

Once suspected, CD can be effectively screened by detecting serum levels of celiac-specific autoantibodies, such as tTG IgA or antiendomysium IgA (EMA).[41] Another class of antibodies valuable in screening (especially in very young children in whom tTG could be negative[42,43]) and following up in patients with CD are the antideamidated gliadin peptides (DGP), both –IgA and –IgG, which are generated in the small intestinal mucosa against gliadin peptides after they have been modified by tTG.[44]

Currently, it is universally recommended that tTG IgA and total serum IgA be the first line of screening because of the very high sensitivity of the tTG-IgA test.[28,41,45] Total serum IgA needs to be determined in order to ascertain that the individual is able to produce tTG IgA. Celiac patients are IgA deficient more often than the general population[46] and therefore may have a falsely negative tTG IgA. Under these circumstances, both tTG IgG[47-49] and DGP IgG[50] can be useful as markers of CD.

In 1990, the European Society of Pediatric Gastroenterology, Hepatology and Nutrition (ESPGHAN) published diagnostic criteria that have been universally applied for more than 20 years in both pediatric and adults patients.[51] Although they have reduced from 3 to only 1 the number of biopsy procedures needed for a firm diagnosis, they still called for the indispensable role of demonstrating the flattening of small intestinal mucosal villi in patients with a consistent history and laboratory findings. In 2012, an ad hoc task force of ESPGHAN published revised criteria and produced an evidence-based algorithm that allowed physicians to skip the duodenal biopsy under certain circumstances, namely, in children and teenagers showing a history and genetic asset compatible with CD, a highly elevated titer (more than 10 times the upper limit of normal) of tTG-IgA, and a positive titer of EMA.[52] Although this simplified approach seems valid because it possesses a positive predictive value close to 100%, it needs to be applied with great care. Children with gastrointestinal complaints diagnosed without endoscopy may have additional disorders that would go undiagnosed by skipping this procedure. In our retrospective experience, 12% of our celiac patients who would have qualified for skipping the biopsy showed *additional* diagnoses, including eosinophilic esophagitis, at endoscopy.[53]

Figure 2 shows an algorithm (based in part on the ESPGHAN guidelines[52]) that synthesizes the diagnostic steps recommended for a child or teenager suspected of having CD. The first step is identifying the subject to be tested. Tables 1 and 2

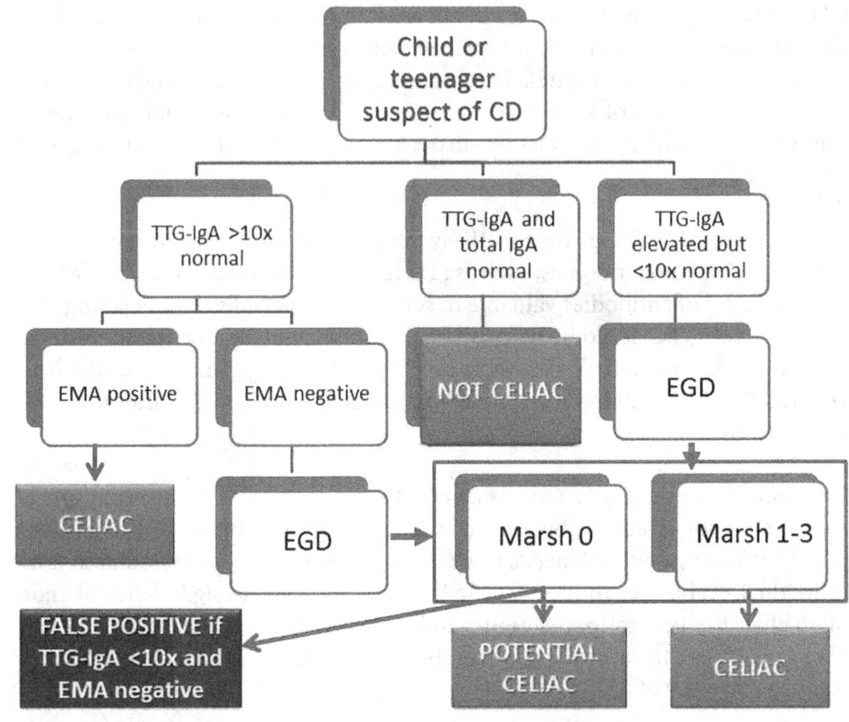

Fig 2. Suggested diagnostic algorithm. See text for a detailed description of the recommended diagnostic steps.

list the presentations that require screening. The adolescent patient with normal tTG IgA need not be considered celiac given the high sensitivity of the test.

If the subject has a positive tTG IgA, then the titer becomes important. Titers that are more than 10 times the upper limit of normal prompt the pediatric gastroenterologist to check the EMA, and if that result also is clearly positive, then

Table 2
Populations to be screened for celiac disease

- All conditions listed in Table 1 not explained by another diagnosis
- First-degree relatives of celiac patients
- Autoimmune conditions
  - Type 1 diabetes
  - Autoimmune thyroiditis
  - Autoimmune hepatitis
  - Addison disease
- Genetic disorders
  - Down syndrome
  - Turner syndrome
  - Williams syndrome
  - Immunoglobulin A (IgA) deficiency

the diagnosis of CD can be considered definitive. On the contrary, EGD would be necessary if the EMA proved negative or in all cases where the tTG IgA increase did not reach the threshold of more than 10 times normal. It is recommended that at least 4 biopsy samples be taken from the distal duodenum and 1 to 2 from the bulb; otherwise, the diagnostic yield might be jeopardized.[45,52,54] This is in striking contrast to alarming findings from adult gastroenterology practices, which report that adherence to recommendations calling for these biopsies is poor, particularly in busy practices with high volumes of patients where patients who undergo EGD to rule out CD still may not undergo biopsy procedures at all![55-58]

The pathology test results of the duodenal biopsies guide the final diagnosis. Pathology changes showing Marsh type 1 to 3 lesions confirm the diagnosis, whereas the call is more delicate for those with Marsh 0 lesions. The Marsh 0 patient can be defined as "potential" if tTG IgA is elevated more than 10 times or EMA are positive. However, if EMA are negative and tTG IgA is less than 10 times normal, then the possibility of a false-positive tTG IgA must be considered. Such patients, if they are asymptomatic, should remain on a gluten-containing diet and be carefully monitored. More complex is the decision about the need for a GFD for true "potential" celiac children and adolescents who are asymptomatic. The literature reports variable percentages (30%-60%) of evolution into full-blown CD when these patients are left on gluten, including the possibility of some patients eventually becoming serologically negative.[59-61] It seems that potential CD patients show low-grade inflammation that likely could be the result of active regulatory mechanisms preventing the progression toward mucosal damage.[62] In essence, although research is active in the area with the aim of being able to predict which patients would develop full-blown CD if left on gluten, the state of the art presently is such that we do not have this capacity, so the decision on whether or not to place potential celiac patients on a GFD must be taken with great care, on an individual basis, and be properly agreed on by the caregivers and the physician.

A strict, lifelong adherence to a GFD is still the only available treatment option for patients diagnosed with CD. The GFD typically results in a complete return to health, as recently shown in Sweden in a large epidemiologic investigation, which found that a GFD effectively reduces symptoms and health care utilization in adults with CD.[63] In addition, a survey in Finland showed that screen-detected children with CD can attain satisfactory dietary adherence and benefit from treatment similar to symptom-detected patients.[64] However, adherence to the diet has proved to be difficult at all ages, but particularly for teenagers, for whom the diet may be very challenging psychologically and socially. Occasions such as birthday parties, sleepovers, eating out, and even snack time at school can be difficult to navigate. A survey of college students with CD revealed that the students were motivated to adhere to the diet but experienced challenges related to dining services and social situations.[65] In spite of good response to the diet and evidence that a GFD generally offers adequate amounts of macro- and micronutrients in adolescents, studies have documented unsatisfactory rates of adherence in older children and adolescents.[66,67] The main reasons for poor adherence are the poor palatability of gluten-free foods, the need for avoidance of traveling and eating out at restaurants, and concerns regarding the difficulty in finding gluten-free foods.[68] The recent introduction by the FDA of a rule indicating 20 ppm (parts per million) as the maximum amount of gluten allowed in foods labeled as "gluten-free" (a rule going into effect as of August 2014) will certainly help celiac families in their constant search for safe foods.[69]

The quality of life (QoL) for teenagers with CD is affected not only by the disease but also by its treatment. A survey of celiac children and their parents showed that although QoL total scores were similar between celiac children and their healthy counterparts, the scores of children with CD were significantly lower in the "leisure" dimension.[70] Scores also were significantly lower in the social field for parents of children with CD.[70] A study of celiac patients showed that the effects of the disease on daily living and of the need for adherence to the GFD were rated much worse by young patients and by those with extraintestinal symptoms than by those with classic symptoms.[71] The same higher degree of unhappiness was expressed by patients who were asymptomatic and detected by screening in at-risk groups. Additionally, young and "extra-intestinal" patients on GFD reported more frequent dietary lapses and a negative attitude toward the disease.[71] Negative perceptions were associated with dissatisfaction with the quality of doctor-patient communication and younger age at diagnosis. Thus, it is evident that effective doctor-patient communication is essential to minimizing the disease burden, particularly in young and screen-detected asymptomatic patients.

Although at present the GFD remains the only treatment available for CD, evidence has emerged in recent years that its efficacy is not as complete as previously thought. Whereas full histologic remission seems to be achieved by about 75% of pediatric patients,[72] complete remission apparently is seen in only a small percentage of adult cases.[73,74] Given this finding and considering the difficulty with adherence and the reduced quality of life, it is not surprising that research into alternatives to the GFD for treatment of celiac patients is very active (reviewed by Freeman[75] and Mukherjee et al[76]). It is likely that some of the alternatives will come to fruition in the next year or 2, but with the caveat that a true cure, although certainly possible, might take much longer.[77]

NON-CELIAC GLUTEN SENSITIVITY

The third disorder of the group, NCGS, is not a newcomer as the general public seems to believe. The first indication that non-celiac individuals may show an adverse reaction to gluten dates back to 1978, when Ellis and Linaker[78] reported the case of a 43-year-old woman who had abdominal pain, bloating, and diarrhea that responded to gluten withdrawal but relapsed upon its reintroduction, in the absence of CD and with normal duodenal biopsies both on and off gluten. However, the report went largely unnoticed, and it was only in recent years that this entity was rediscovered and redefined with the exact same nomenclature given to it by Ellis and Linaker.[2,78] The diagnosis of NCGS now is enormously popular, such that today a large number of self-appointed experts have appeared in the media, many claiming a prevalence of up to 50% in the general population.

In reality, because NCGS is currently characterized by the lack of any objective diagnostic parameter (no biomarker is available), it is not possible to define its prevalence, and it is quite difficult even to define its connotations in precise terms. As a possible indication of true prevalence, surveys performed in the United States have shown that a mere 0.6% of the population follows a strict daily GFD without having been diagnosed with CD and therefore could be cautiously thought of as having NCGS.[29]

Keeping in mind the uncertainties about this poorly defined entity, it seems safe to state that there are patients in whom CD and wheat allergy have been excluded, who report adverse effects when eating gluten-containing foods and improvement when avoiding them. The most frequently reported symptoms are[79,80]

- Abdominal bloating and gassiness
- Abdominal discomfort or pain
- Diarrhea
- Tiredness
- "Foggy mind"
- Headache
- Joint pain

Although antibodies to native gliadin have been found to occur slightly more commonly in these patients than in healthy controls, no consistent laboratory abnormalities have been identified.[81-83] No biomarker has been found for these patients.

To complicate matters further, it now has become clear that patients with self-reported NCGS, when put on a diet low in fermentable oligosaccharides, disaccharides, monosaccharides, and polyols (FODMAP), experienced a sharp reduction of their irritable bowel syndrome (IBS)-like symptoms.[84] When these patients were re-exposed to gluten in the context of an ongoing low-FODMAP diet, they did not report any worsening of symptoms compared to an otherwise identical, placebo GFD.[84] Of note, foods typically used in a GFD are very low in FODMAP, whereas normal, gluten-containing foods tend to have a high FODMAP content (Table 3).[85] Therefore, it is possible, and indeed likely, that at least a substantial portion of the patients who are considered to have NCGS are simply experiencing IBS-like symptoms because of ingestion of FODMAP-rich foods,[86] hence leaving gluten innocent.[87]

Table 3
Common sources of FODMAP

Food component	Dietary form	Common sources
Fructose	Free monosaccharide constituent (fructose in excess of glucose)	Apple, pear, watermelon, honey, high fructose corn syrup, asparagus, artichoke
Lactose	Free disaccharide	Milk, yogurt, ice cream, soft cheese
Fructose	Fructo-oligosaccharide (FOS) and inulin	Wheat, rye, barley, garlic, leek, onion, asparagus, artichoke, peach, persimmon, watermelon, pistachio, inulin
Polyols	Sorbitol, mannitol, xylitolmaltitol, isomalt	Apple, pear, plum, apricot, nectarine, mushroom, cauliflower, reduced caloric sweetener
Calacto-oligosaccharides (GOS)	Raffinose, stachyose	Legumes, chickpeas, lentils

FODMAP = fermentable oligosaccharides, disaccharides, monosaccharides. and polyols.
From Biesiekierski JR, Muir JG, Gibson PR. Is gluten a cause of gastrointestinal symptoms in people without celiac disease? *Curr Allergy Asthma Rep*. 2013;13(6):631-638, with permission.

Furthermore, there is evidence that another family of wheat-associated, but not gluten-related, proteins found in wheat (α-amylase/trypsin inhibitor [ATI]) activates an innate immune mucosal response and is able to elicit the release of proinflammatory cytokines in cells from celiac and non-celiac patients. Therefore, ATI possibly has causative role in some patients who report adverse effects when ingesting wheat.[88]

CONCLUSION

Non-celiac gluten sensitivity is still an ill-defined entity, with vague, celiac-like symptoms and no current identified biomarker. It is possible that this umbrella term will be determined to encompass those with true gluten intolerance, possibly involving the innate immune system, as well as FODMAP-sensitive patients and even patients responsive to ATI. Thus, the well-documented favorable clinical response shown by some patients with IBS to the withdrawal of gluten may not be the result of gluten after all[89] and the definition of NCGS may well be a misnomer. This condition should indeed more objectively be referred to as "Self-reported adverse reactions upon ingestion of wheat-based foods" until we have explored better its etiology, pathophysiology, diagnostic markers, and natural history.

References

1. Gee SJ. On the Celiac Affection. *St. Bartholomew's Hospital Reports*. 1888;24:17-20
2. Ludvigsson JF, Leffler DA, Bai JC, et al. The Oslo definitions for coeliac disease and related terms. *Gut*. 2013;52(1):43-52

3. Branum AM, Lukacs SL. Food allergy among children in the United States. *Pediatrics.* 2009;124(6): 1549-1555
4. Gupta R, Holdford D, Bilaver L, Dyer A, Holl JL, Meltzer D. The economic impact of childhood food allergy in the United States. *JAMA Pediatr.* 2013;167(11):1026-1031
5. Levy J, Levy-Carrick N. Wheat Allergy. In: Fasano A, ed. *A Clinical Guide to Gluten-Related Disorders.* Philadelphia, PA: Lippincott Williams & Wilkins; 2013:54-70
6. Kotaniemi-Syrjanen A, Palosuo K, Jartti T, et al. The prognosis of wheat hypersensitivity in children. *Pediatr Allergy Immunol.* 2010;21(2 Pt 2):e421-428
7. Keet CA, Matsui EC, Dhillon G, Lenehan P, Paterakis M, Wood RA. The natural history of wheat allergy. *Ann Allergy Asthma Immunol.* 2009;102(5):410-415
8. Sicherer SH, Sampson HA. Food allergy. *J Allergy Clin Immunol.* 2010;125(2 Suppl 2):S116-125
9. Chafen JJ, Newberry SJ, Riedl MA, et al. Diagnosing and managing common food allergies: a systematic review. *JAMA.* 12 2010;303(18):1848-1856
10. Sampson HA, Ho DG. Relationship between food-specific IgE concentrations and the risk of positive food challenges in children and adolescents. *J Allergy Clin Immunol.* 1997;100:444-451
11. Sampson HA. Utility of food-specific IgE concentration in predicting symptomatic food allergy. *J Allergy Clin Immunol.* 2001;107:891-896
12. Reilly NR, Fasano A, Green PH. Presentation of celiac disease. *Gastrointest Endosc Clin N Am.* 2012;22(4):613-621
13. Dydensborg S, Toftedal P, Biaggi M, Lillevang ST, Hansen DG, Husby S. Increasing prevalence of coeliac disease in Denmark: a linkage study combining national registries. *Acta Paediatr.* 2012; 101(2):179-184
14. Vilppula A, Kaukinen K, Luostarinen L, et al. Increasing prevalence and high incidence of celiac disease in elderly people: a population-based study. *BMC Gastroenterol.* 2009;9:49
15. Lohi S, Mustalahti K, Kaukinen K, et al. Increasing prevalence of coeliac disease over time. *Aliment Pharmacol Ther.* 2007;26(9):1217-1225
16. Mustalahti K, Catassi C, Reunanen A, et al. The prevalence of celiac disease in Europe: results of a centralized, international mass screening project. *Ann Med.* 2010;42(8):587-595
17. Catassi C, Kryszak D, Bhatti B, et al. Natural history of celiac disease autoimmunity in a USA cohort followed since 1974. *Ann Med.* 2010;42(7):530-538
18. Ludvigsson JF, Rubio-Tapia A, van Dyke CT, et al. Increasing incidence of celiac disease in a north american population. *Am J Gastroenterol.* 2013;108(5):818-824
19. Decker E, Hornef M, Stockinger S. Cesarean delivery is associated with celiac disease but not inflammatory bowel disease in children. *Gut Microbes.* 2011;2(2):91-98
20. Marild K, Stephansson O, Montgomery S, Murray JA, Ludvigsson JF. Pregnancy outcome and risk of celiac disease in offspring: a nationwide case-control study. *Gastroenterology.* 2012;142(1):39-45 e33
21. Myleus A, Hernell O, Gothefors L, et al. Early infections are associated with increased risk for celiac disease: an incident case-referent study. *BMC Pediatr.* 2012;12:194
22. Marild K, Ye W, Lebwohl B, et al. Antibiotic exposure and the development of coeliac disease: a nationwide case-control study. *BMC Gastroenterol.* 2013;13:109
23. Ivarsson A, Myleus A, Norstrom F, et al. Prevalence of childhood celiac disease and changes in infant feeding. *Pediatrics.* 2013;131(3):e687-694
24. Myleus A, Ivarsson A, Webb C, et al. Celiac disease revealed in 3% of Swedish 12-year-olds born during an epidemic. *J Pediatr Gastroenterol Nutr.* 2009;49(2):170-176
25. Whyte L, Kotecha S, Watkins W, Jenkins H. Coeliac disease is more common in children with high socio-economic status. *Acta Paediatr.* 2014;103(3):289-294
26. Kondrashova A, Mustalahti K, Kaukinen K, et al. Lower economic status and inferior hygienic environment may protect against celiac disease. *Ann Med.* 2008;40(3):223-231
27. Lionetti E, Castellaneta S, Pulvirenti A, et al. Prevalence and natural history of potential celiac disease in at-family-risk infants prospectively investigated from birth. *J Pediatr.* 2012;161(5):908-914
28. Hill ID, Dirks MH, Liptak GS, et al. Guideline for the diagnosis and treatment of celiac disease in children: recommendations of the North American Society for Pediatric Gastroenterology, Hepatology and Nutrition. *J Pediatr Gastroenterol Nutr.* 2005;40(1):1-19

29. Rubio-Tapia A, Ludvigsson JF, Brantner TL, Murray JA, Everhart JE. The prevalence of celiac disease in the United States. *Am J Gastroenterol.* 2012;107(10):1538-1544; quiz 1537, 1545
30. Trynka G, Hunt KA, Bockett NA, et al. Dense genotyping identifies and localizes multiple common and rare variant association signals in celiac disease. *Nat Genet.* 2011;43(12):1193-1201
31. Ludvigsson JF, Fasano A. Timing of introduction of gluten and celiac disease risk. *Ann Nutr Metab.* 2012;60 Suppl 2:22-29
32. Sellitto M, Bai G, Serena G, et al. Proof of concept of microbiome-metabolome analysis and delayed gluten exposure on celiac disease autoimmunity in genetically at-risk infants. *PLoS One.* 2012;7(3):e33387
33. Hausch F, Shan L, Santiago NA, Gray GM, Khosla C. Intestinal digestive resistance of immunodominant gliadin peptides. *Am J Physiol Gastrointest Liver Physiol.* 2002;283(4):G996-G1003
34. Abadie V, Sollid LM, Barreiro LB, Jabri B. Integration of genetic and immunological insights into a model of celiac disease pathogenesis. *Annu Rev Immunol.* 2011;29:493-525
35. Marsh MN. Gluten, major histocompatibility complex, and the small intestine. A molecular and immunobiologic approach to the spectrum of gluten sensitivity ('celiac sprue'). *Gastroenterology.* 1992;102(1):330-354
36. Garampazzi A, Rapa A, Mura S, et al. Clinical pattern of celiac disease is still changing. *J Pediatr Gastroenterol Nutr.* 2007;45(5):611-614
37. Lebenthal E, Shteyer E, Branski D. The changing clinical presentation of celiac disease. In: Fasano A, Troncone R, Branski D, eds. *Frontiers in celiac disease.* Basel, Switzerland: S Karger AG; 2008: 18–22
38. Maki M, Kallonen K, Lahdeaho ML, Visakorpi JK. Changing pattern of childhood coeliac disease in Finland. *Acta Paediatr Scand.* 1988;77(3):408-412
39. Roma E, Panayiotou J, Karantana H, et al. Changing pattern in the clinical presentation of pediatric celiac disease: a 30-year study. *Digestion.* 2009;80(3):185-191
40. Lo W, Sano K, Lebwohl B, Diamond B, Green PH. Changing presentation of adult celiac disease. *Dig Dis Sci.* 2003;48(2):395-398
41. Giersiepen K, Lelgemann M, Stuhldreher N, et al. Accuracy of diagnostic antibody tests for coeliac disease in children: summary of an evidence report. *J Pediatr Gastroenterol Nutr.* 2012;54(2):229-241
42. Amarri S, Alvisi P, De Giorgio R, et al. Antibodies to Deamidated Gliadin Peptides: An Accurate Predictor of Coeliac Disease in Infancy. *J Clin Immunol.* 2013;33(5):1027-1030
43. Barbato M, Maiella G, Di Camillo C, et al. The anti-deamidated gliadin peptide antibodies unmask celiac disease in small children with chronic diarrhoea. *Dig Liver Dis.* 2011;43(6):465-469
44. Aleanzi M, Demonte AM, Esper C, Garcilazo S, Waggener M. Celiac disease: antibody recognition against native and selectively deamidated gliadin peptides. *Clin Chem.* 2001;47(11):2023-2028
45. Rubio-Tapia A, Hill ID, Kelly CP, Calderwood AH, Murray JA. ACG Clinical Guidelines: Diagnosis and Management of Celiac Disease. *Am J Gastroenterol.* 2013;108(5):656-676
46. Cataldo F, Marino V, Ventura A, Bottaro G, Corazza GR. Prevalence and clinical features of selective immunoglobulin A deficiency in coeliac disease: an Italian multicentre study. Italian Society of Paediatric Gastroenterology and Hepatology (SIGEP) and "Club del Tenue" Working Groups on Coeliac Disease. *Gut.* 1998;42(3):362-365
47. Dahlbom I, Olsson M, Forooz NK, et al. Immunoglobulin G (IgG) anti-tissue transglutaminase antibodies used as markers for IgA-deficient celiac disease patients. *Clin Diagn Lab Immunol.* 2005;12(2):254-258
48. Korponay-Szabo IR, Dahlbom I, Laurila K, et al. Elevation of IgG antibodies against tissue transglutaminase as a diagnostic tool for coeliac disease in selective IgA deficiency. *Gut.* 2003;52(11): 1567-1571
49. Villalta D, Alessio MG, Tampoia M, et al. Testing for IgG class antibodies in celiac disease patients with selective IgA deficiency. A comparison of the diagnostic accuracy of 9 IgG anti-tissue transglutaminase, 1 IgG anti-gliadin and 1 IgG anti-deaminated gliadin peptide antibody assays. *Clin Chim Acta.* 2007;382(1-2):95-99
50. Villalta D, Tonutti E, Prause C, et al. IgG antibodies against deamidated gliadin peptides for diagnosis of celiac disease in patients with IgA deficiency. *Clin Chem.* 2010;56(3):464-468

51. Walker-Smith JA, Guandalini S, Schmitz J, Shmerling DH, Visakorpi JK. Revised criteria for diagnosis of coeliac disease. Report of a Working Group of ESPGAN. *Arch Dis Child.* 1990;65:909-911
52. Husby S, Koletzko S, Korponay-Szabo IR, et al. European Society for Pediatric Gastroenterology, Hepatology, and Nutrition guidelines for the diagnosis of coeliac disease. *J Pediatr Gastroenterol Nutr.* 2012;54(1):136-160
53. Guandalini S, Newland C. Can we really skip the biopsy in diagnosing symptomatic children with celiac disease? *J Pediatr Gastroenterol Nutr.* 2013;57(4):e24
54. Bai JC, Fried M, Corazza GR, et al. World gastroenterology organisation global guidelines on celiac disease. *J Clin Gastroenterol.* 2013;47(2):121-126
55. Lebwohl B, Bhagat G, Markoff S, et al. Prior endoscopy in patients with newly diagnosed celiac disease: a missed opportunity? *Dig Dis Sci.* 2013;58(5):1293-1298
56. Lebwohl B, Genta RM, Kapel RC, et al. Procedure volume influences adherence to celiac disease guidelines. *Eur J Gastroenterol Hepatol.* 2013;25(11):1273-1278
57. Lebwohl B, Kapel RC, Neugut AI, Green PH, Genta RM. Adherence to biopsy guidelines increases celiac disease diagnosis. *Gastrointest Endosc.* 2011;74(1):103-109
58. Parakkal D, Du H, Semer R, Ehrenpreis ED, Guandalini S. Do gastroenterologists adhere to diagnostic and treatment guidelines for celiac disease? *J Clin Gastroenterol.* 2012;46(2):e12-20
59. Biagi F, Trotta L, Alfano C, et al. Prevalence and natural history of potential celiac disease in adult patients. *Scand J Gastroenterol.* 2013;48(5):537-542
60. Kurppa K, Ashorn M, Iltanen S, et al. Celiac disease without villous atrophy in children: a prospective study. *J Pediatr.* 2010;157(3):373-380, 380.e371
61. Tosco A, Salvati VM, Auricchio R, et al. Natural history of potential celiac disease in children. *Clin Gastroenterol Hepatol.* 2011;9(4):320-325; quiz e336
62. Borrelli M, Salvati VM, Maglio M, et al. Immunoregulatory pathways are active in the small intestinal mucosa of patients with potential celiac disease. *Am J Gastroenterol.* 2013;108(11):1775-1784
63. Norstrom F, Sandstrom O, Lindholm L, Ivarsson A. A gluten-free diet effectively reduces symptoms and health care consumption in a Swedish celiac disease population. *BMC Gastroenterol.* 2012;12:125
64. Kinos S, Kurppa K, Ukkola A, et al. Burden of illness in screen-detected children with celiac disease and their families. *J Pediatr Gastroenterol Nutr.* 2012;55(4):412-416
65. Panzer RM, Dennis M, Kelly CP, et al. Navigating the gluten-free diet in college. *J Pediatr Gastroenterol Nutr.* 2012;55(6):740-744
66. Kautto E, Ivarsson A, Norstrom F, et al. Nutrient intake in adolescent girls and boys diagnosed with coeliac disease at an early age is mostly comparable to their non-coeliac contemporaries. *J Hum Nutr Diet.* 2014;27(1);41-53
67. Theethira TG, Dennis M, Leffler DA. Nutritional consequences of celiac disease and the gluten-free diet. *Exp Rev Gastroenterol Hepatol.* 2014;8(2):123-129
68. Roma E, Roubani A, Kolia E, Panayiotou J, Zellos A, Syriopoulou VP. Dietary compliance and life style of children with coeliac disease. *J Hum Nutr Diet.* 2010;23(2):176-182
69. Food, Drug Administration HHS. Food labeling: gluten-free labeling of foods. Final rule. *Federal register.* 2013;78(150):47154-47179
70. de Lorenzo CM, Xikota JC, Wayhs MC, Nassar SM, de Souza Pires MM. Evaluation of the quality of life of children with celiac disease and their parents: a case-control study. *Qual Life Res.* 2012; 21(1):77-85
71. Ukkola A, Maki M, Kurppa K, et al. Patients' experiences and perceptions of living with coeliac disease - implications for optimizing care. *J Gastrointestin Liver Dis.* 2012;21(1):17-22
72. Bardella MT, Velio P, Cesana BM, et al. Coeliac disease: a histological follow-up study. *Histopathology.* 2007;50(4):465-471
73. Lebwohl B, Murray JA, Rubio-Tapia A, Green PH, Ludvigsson JF. Predictors of persistent villous atrophy in coeliac disease: a population-based study. *Aliment Pharmacol Ther.* 2014;39(5):488-495
74. Lanzini A, Lanzarotto F, Villanacci V, et al. Complete recovery of intestinal mucosa occurs very rarely in adult coeliac patients despite adherence to gluten-free diet. *Aliment Pharmacol Ther.* 2009;29(12):1299-1308

75. Freeman HJ. Non-dietary forms of treatment for adult celiac disease. *World J Gastrointest Pharmacol Ther.* 6 2013;4(4):108-112
76. Mukherjee R, Kelly CP, Schuppan D. Nondietary therapies for celiac disease. *Gastrointest Endosc Clin N Am.* 2012;22(4):811-831
77. McAllister CS, Kagnoff MF. The immunopathogenesis of celiac disease reveals possible therapies beyond the gluten-free diet. *Sem Immunopathol.* 2012;34(4):581-600
78. Ellis A, Linaker BD. Non-coeliac gluten sensitivity? *Lancet.* 1978;1(8078):1358-1359
79. Volta U, De Giorgio R. New understanding of gluten sensitivity. *Nat Rev Gastroenterol Hepatol.* 2012;9(5):295-299
80. Biesiekierski JR, Newnham ED, Irving PM, et al. Gluten causes gastrointestinal symptoms in subjects without celiac disease: a double-blind randomized placebo-controlled trial. *Am J Gastroenterol.* 2011;106(3):508-514; quiz 515
81. Catassi C, Bai JC, Bonaz B, et al. Non-Celiac Gluten sensitivity: the new frontier of gluten related disorders. *Nutrients.* 2013;5(10):3839-3853
82. Francavilla R, Cristofori F, Castellaneta S, et al. Clinical, serologic, and histologic features of gluten sensitivity in children. *J Pediatr.* 2014:164(3):463-467.e1
83. Volta U, Tovoli F, Cicola R, et al. Serological tests in gluten sensitivity (nonceliac gluten intolerance). *J Clin Gastroenterol* 2012;46(8):680-685
84. Biesiekierski JR, Peters SL, Newnham ED, et al. No effects of gluten in patients with self-reported non-celiac gluten sensitivity after dietary reduction of fermentable, poorly absorbed, short-chain carbohydrates. *Gastroenterology.* 2013;145(2):320-328.e323
85. Biesiekierski JR, Rosella O, Rose R, et al. Quantification of fructans, galacto-oligosacharides and other short-chain carbohydrates in processed grains and cereals. *J Hum Nutr Diet.* 2011;24(2): 154-176
86. Biesiekierski JR, Muir JG, Gibson PR. Is gluten a cause of gastrointestinal symptoms in people without celiac disease? *Curr Allergy Asthma Rep.* 2013;13(6):631-638
87. Vanga R, Leffler DA. Gluten sensitivity: not celiac and not certain. *Gastroenterology.* 2013;145(2): 276-279
88. Junker Y, Zeissig S, Kim SJ, et al. Wheat amylase trypsin inhibitors drive intestinal inflammation via activation of toll-like receptor 4. *J Exp Med.* 2012;209(13):2395-2408
89. Vazquez-Roque MI, Camilleri M, Smyrk T, et al. A controlled trial of gluten-free diet in patients with irritable bowel syndrome-diarrhea: effects on bowel frequency and intestinal function. *Gastroenterology.* 2013;144(5):903-911. e903.

Adolesc Med 025 (2014) 425–437

Implementation of Health Care Transition in Clinical Practice

Sarah J. Beal[a], PhD; Abigail Nye[a,b*], MD;
Jennifer M. Shoreman[a,b], MD; Darcey L. Thornton[a,b], MD;
Jason F. Woodward[a,b], MD, MS

[a]*Division of Adolescent and Transition Medicine, Cincinnati Children's Hospital Medical Center, Cincinnati, Ohio;* [b]*College of Medicine, University of Cincinnati, Cincinnati, Ohio*

Discussion of the transition to adult health care has increased in the past 5 years.[1] Health care transition is the planned movement from child-centered to adult-oriented medical systems. It involves preparing youth to assume autonomy for their health care, understand their health conditions, effectively manage their health needs, and navigate the medical system.[2,3] Guidelines endorsed by the American Academy of Pediatrics (AAP), American Academy of Family Physicians (AAFP), and American College of Physicians (ACP)[1] and by the National Center for Healthcare Transition Improvement (Got Transition[4]) recommend that health care transition be part of general practice for youth *with* and *without* special health care needs.

Importantly, shifts to adult health care occur at a vulnerable time for many young adults. Developmentally, adolescents and young adults are preparing to take on new social roles in areas of education, work, independent living, financial management, intimate relationships, and parenting.[5] These changes occur at a faster rate than at any other point in the lifespan. Adolescents and young adults need to have optimal physical and mental health to successfully navigate these shifting roles.[6,7] However, recent evidence indicates that health declines during the transition to

*Corresponding author:
E-mail address: Abigail.Nye@cchmc.org
Authors are listed in alphabetical order; all authors contributed equally to this manuscript. We thank Jan Clavey for her instrumental help in compiling and editing sections from the authors, as well as Dr Frank Biro for his feedback on an earlier draft. Sarah Beal's time was supported in part by funds from the Bureau of Health Professions (BHPr), Health Resources and Services Administration (HRSA), Department of Health and Human Services (DHHS), under Grant # T32 HP10027.

 ISSN 1934-4287

adulthood.[8] This decline includes increased rates of mortality, substance abuse, onset of mental health disorders, and unintended pregnancy in young adulthood compared to adolescence.[9] Addressing these disparities in health requires a coordinated effort to ensure that all young adults have the resources they need to develop the skills and support necessary to successfully engage and maintain engagement in adult health care systems, implement a healthy lifestyle, and, ultimately, maximize their lifelong functioning and potential.

Despite various guidelines that describe methods to address the health care transition needs of all youth, profound gaps persist in the delivery of health care transition services. Only 20.6% of parents of youth with special health care needs (YSHCN) report that their pediatric physician* has spoken to them about the need to eventually see an adult physician, thereby leaving an estimated 2.3 million youth potentially unaware of the need to identify an adult physician.[10] Among young adults more generally, only approximately 1 in 4 receives appropriate health care transition components.[11] Recent research indicates that many young adults struggle to receive primary and preventive care,[12,13] continue to receive care from a pediatrician,[14] rely on urgent care or emergency rooms for acute needs,[15] or disengage from health care completely.[12] YSHCN may experience additional gaps in preventive care services compared to their peers.[16] Furthermore, about one-half of internists and 3 of 5 pediatricians feel that adult primary care physicians and systems are unprepared to care for young adults with chronic conditions, making it difficult for young adults to find adult primary care physicians.[17] These data suggest that the current health care system is not prepared to provide the services or supports necessary to address the health care needs of this population, especially YSHCN.

IMPLEMENTATION OF HEALTH CARE TRANSITION RECOMMENDATIONS

The AAP/AAFP/ACP first addressed transition services for YSHCN in a 2002 consensus statement.[18] These recommendations were also endorsed by the Society for Adolescent Medicine.[19] Models for delivery of transition services often addressed condition-specific transition needs that applied predominantly to pediatric subspecialty clinics.[20-22] In 2011, the 2002 consensus statement was expanded to apply to *all* youth moving to adult health care.[1] The 2011 clinical report proposes an algorithm for implementing transition within a medical home. To support implementation of the report's recommendations into a variety of practice settings, Got Transition adapted the algorithm's action steps into the Six Core Elements of Healthcare Transition.[4] These elements include Transition Policy, Transition Tracking and Monitoring, Transition Readiness, Transition Planning, Transfer

* The use of physician was preferred by the journal. The authors wish to express that this process is relevant to and supported by a broader range of providers than just physicians. Subsequently, the word "physician" could often be substituted with the word "provider" to represent the broader applicability and relevance of the findings.

of Care, and Transfer Completion. Core elements are elaborated in the following sections. Current recommendations are based on expert opinion. When available, empirical evidence for any aspect of the recommendations is summarized in the appropriate section. Each physician is charged to adapt the general recommendations and algorithm in the report[1] to meet the needs of his or her specific system of care and patient population. As health care transition services are implemented by an increasing number of medical homes and subspecialty clinics, additional evidence will need to be gathered from these experiences to inform practice improvements that ultimately will lead to high-quality transition services and successful outcomes as youth transition to adult health care.

Transition Policy

As a first step in supporting health care transition, practices should develop and communicate a clearly defined written transition policy. This transition policy sets the expectation that all youth will transition to an adult model of health care, normalizes transition as a positive part of preparation for adult life, and provides a guide by which patients, families, and physicians can collaborate to plan and implement transition. A transition policy should apply to *all* youth within the practice and describe a consistent process by which patients shift to an adult model of care. Experts recommend the policy be developed with input from patients and families; policies should articulate the roles and responsibilities of the physician, the patient, and the family in the health care transition process. Additionally, policy statements should clarify expectations regarding privacy and consent for patients. At a minimum, the transition policy should include the components recommended in Table 1. Policies should be accessible through the various means in which practices disseminate materials (eg, Web, brochures). It is recommended that the written policy be provided to new patients, visibly posted for patients and families to read, and initially distributed to patients and their families when the patients are ages 12 to 14 years. Physicians should facilitate discussion of the policy's components, and the discussion should be documented.

Table 1
Recommended transition policy components

Expected age of patient at transfer to adult model of health care	Family responsibilities in preparing for transition
Expected point of transfer to new provider, if applicable.	
Medical physician's responsibilities in preparing for transition	Goal of health care transition
Patient's responsibilities in preparing for transition	Role of transition planning in movement from pediatric to adult health care model
Privacy and consent information	

Adapted from American Academy of Pediatrics, American Academy of Family Physicians, American College of Physicians, Transitions Clinical Report Authoring Group. Supporting the health care transition from adolescence to adulthood in the medical home. *Pediatrics*. 2011;128(1):182-200

Despite consensus that a transition policy is important,[1,4] limited data exist on the effect of a policy on experiences with the transition process or health outcomes. Studies have shown that physicians describe several transition approaches and policies and suggest that their patients experience an individualized approach to transition.[23,24] Lack of a transition policy may result in lack of transition planning, minimal preparation of youth and their families, confusion and anxiety surrounding the transition process, and, ultimately, patient, family, and physician dissatisfaction.[25]

Transition Tracking and Monitoring

The AAP recommends that practices use registries to track patients with special health care needs.[26] A patient registry is an organized system that collects uniform clinical data to evaluate identified outcomes for a defined population.[27] Got Transition expands the recommendations for a registry to include transition services for *all* youth.[4] However, the resources needed to build and maintain a registry may be prohibitive, in which case it is recommended that physicians create a flow sheet to track transition. Recommendations outline that pediatric physicians should establish criteria for identifying which patients should be in the process of transitioning to adult care and then incorporate that information into the registry or flow sheets, utilize a registry or flow sheet to track transition progress, and use the registry or flow sheet and electronic medical record to incorporate transition into clinical care.

In building a registry, a practice can create fields to indicate which components of transition have been completed. Within an existing registry, sorting by age can help to identify patients who should be receiving transition planning. Once patients are identified, the registry can assist physicians with implementing the clinical report's steps for transition planning by age.[1] A transition registry can also assist physicians in tracking which patients successfully transfer to adult physicians or are lost to follow-up. The flow sheet should track whether patients received specific elements of transition planning (described below) and can be kept on paper or in the electronic medical record. Registries or flow sheets can be expanded to track individual progress on recommended transition activities, such as discussing guardianship or identification of adult primary care and subspecialty physicians. Registries or flow sheets with accurate documentation can also notify physicians when a patient is due for follow-up transition counseling.

Evidence on the use of registries for improving patient care and evaluating outcomes in pediatrics comes from initiatives such as the Cystic Fibrosis Foundation Care Center Network,[28] Children's Oncology Group,[29] and ImproveCareNow,[30] which emphasize tracking patients and using registries at the point of care. Together, evidence across initiatives indicates improved care guidelines and outcomes when registries are used.[31] Whether a registry or flow sheet is used, carefully tracking and monitoring transitioning patients will help formalize the process of transition preparation, identify areas for improvement, and assist in preventing patients from "falling through the cracks."

Transition Readiness

The 2011 clinical report recommends that preparation begin no later than age 14 to 15 years with the development of a transition plan (discussed below).[1] An important component of the transition plan is assessment of transition readiness. The purpose of assessing readiness is to identify gaps in skills and knowledge, as well as to develop goals and action steps that prepare youth for transfer to the adult health care setting. Ideally, assessments help physicians identify when an adolescent is ready to transfer out of the pediatric setting. What constitutes true "transition readiness" and how to best assess readiness is an active area of research. In general, tools should measure self-efficacy and the acquisition of skill sets (eg, medication self-management, healthy behaviors),[32] identify a target population for whom the measure is intended before development (eg, adolescents with type 1 diabetes, adolescents with chronic conditions), and have meaningful results (ie, information derived from the measure should be valid and interpretable).[33] Information obtained from a tool can be used to counsel patients (eg, with motivational interviewing) and to develop systematic changes within the medical home. A transition readiness tool can track results longitudinally to determine youths' progress and evaluate whether systematic changes are successful. As discussed previously, maintaining a registry will make these data more accessible and applicable during transition planning.

Multiple transition readiness assessments are available, although few have been empirically validated in a scientific manner.[32] Online tools for parents and teens are available at www.gottransition.org. Most assessments with established validity based on content and internal consistency are disease specific and evaluate skill sets, self-management, and personal health and health care system knowledge.[32] In a review of 10 transition readiness assessment tools, the Transition Readiness Assessment Questionnaire (TRAQ) was considered the "best" overall assessment tool as evaluated by its content and construct delivery (Table 2). The TRAQ is suitable for all YSHCN[32,34] but is limited by its use of self-report. Other

Table 2
Example of TRAQ items

Domain 1: self-management	Domain 2: self-advocacy
Do you take medications correctly and on your own?	Do you answer questions that are asked by the doctor, nurse, or clinic staff?
Do you call the suppliers when there is a problem with the equipment?	Do you get financial help with school or work?

assessments developed for specific disease populations include a parent assessment[22,35]; all currently validated parent assessments are disease specific. Other readiness measures compare patient responses with the medical record to minimize reliance on self-report.[36] Another limitation of all readiness assessments is the lack of evidence that scores are associated with health outcomes. Furthermore, although the 2011 clinical report encourages physicians to implement transition services for youth without chronic illnesses, to date, no assessment of transition readiness has been developed for youth without chronic conditions.[1] Additionally, although Got Transition recommends the use of transition readiness assessments for identifying goals and action steps to include in the transition plan, few have clearly described how physicians can effectively incorporate findings from transition readiness assessments into transition plans.[4] Finally, readiness assessments may identify gaps in preparation but do not provide guidance on how physicians can address these gaps. Ongoing tool development and evaluation are necessary and should emphasize youth with and without chronic illnesses.

Transition Planning

As discussed earlier, transition planning should begin with discussion of the transition policy between the ages of 12 and 14 years, along with the initiation of a transition plan that is developed in collaboration with parents, patients, and physicians. The transition plan should promote uninterrupted comprehensive care as youth move to an adult health care model. Transition planning should generally address youths' developing independence, self-care, and decision-making skills in an effort to promote self-determination, autonomy, and positive health behaviors. Engagement of youth and their families in the process is essential to successful transition planning and requires focused efforts by physicians.

Although the optimal time for initiating transition planning discussions may be between the ages of 12 to 14 years, it is never too early for physicians to begin future-oriented planning discussions with parents and patients.[37] Development of a patient-specific plan should be initiated by age 14 years during a face-to-face office visit. The written transition plan includes assessments of transition readiness; written, actionable goals for transition; documented activities to ensure youth achieve established goals; and progress toward transition goals. The specifics of each component are listed in Table 3. During this process, differences between pediatric and adult health care models should be explained, and an adult physician who can be engaged in and support the process should be identified. Initial steps to identify an adult physician may begin with recommendations from current pediatric physicians or include adult physicians already known to the family. A plan for formally contacting the adult physician, scheduling initial appointments, and exchanging information should be developed during the transition planning process. A plan for determining the optimal time for transfer should also be documented. Subsequent follow-up for transition

Table 3
Four recommended transition plan components for all youth

Assess youth transition readiness
- Perform a person-centered assessment
- Articulate realistic goals
- Identify new skills that will be needed to meet goals
- Assess readiness in areas of education/vocation, independent living, and awareness of medical and preventive care needs

Plan dynamic, longitudinal process for achieving goals
- Establish jointly developed goals that promote a seamless transition
- Include specific actions needed to meet goals
- Develop a formal written plan that is documented in the chart
  At minimum, include:
  - Main goal
  - Identification of the professional in the medical home overseeing plan
  - Timeline for goals
  - Skills required for youth to achieve maximum self-management
  - Family/caregiver's role in process
  - Proposed financing of adult health care

Implement the plan
- Educate patient, parents, and other caregivers or medical professionals regarding transition
- Empower youth in self-care
- Initiate activities to facilitate the acquisition of needed skills (eg, schedule own appointments, dialogue with medical professional, familiar with own meds)
- Discuss transition plan at all adolescent health care visits
- See patient alone at visit
- Identify potential adult practices and suggest youth interview adult practice

Document progress
- Use transition checklist or tool and/or electronic health record to track progress
- Medical transition planning documents:
  - Transition plan
  - Documentation of transition readiness
  - Portable medical summary

Adapted from American Academy of Pediatrics, American Academy of Family Physicians, American College of Physicians, Transitions Clinical Report Authoring Group. Supporting the health care transition from adolescence to adulthood in the medical home. *Pediatrics.* 2011;128(1):182-200

planning should be accomplished through office visits, telephone calls, or other methods appropriate for a specific patient population. The written transition plan should be reviewed and updated as needed.

Transition planning for YSHCN typically requires additional effort and may involve supplementary components to those described earlier (Table 4). The plan should be tailored to youths' particular health care needs. The Chronic Care Management model (CCM) provides a useful framework for implementing transition planning.[38] Many YSHCN will already have an action-oriented care plan to address their health needs; by the age of 14 years, this care plan should include transition planning. To date, recommendations and consensus regard-

Table 4
Additional transition planning components for youth with special health care needs

Transfer documentation—data elements	Documentation of readiness
• Baseline functional status • Baseline neurologic status • Cognitive status (formal results) • Condition-specific emergency treatment plans and contacts • Patient's health education history and assessment of his or her understanding of condition • Advance directive planning • Identification of proxy decision maker • Patient's communication preferences • Anticipated needs for accommodations in communication and clinical care (eg, sign language)	*Insurance* • Discuss recent legislative changes for health care insurance • Changes in eligibility requirements • Evaluate future employment options based on health insurance coverage • Document plans for continued coverage *Self-advocacy* • Empowerment of youth • Plans for decision-making status • Initiate decision-making opportunities *Legal considerations* • Consent capacity • Support-service or program eligibility requirements • Selective service registration • Consent and confidentiality provisions • Potential need for guardianship • Health care proxy or power of attorney *Health education* • Periodic, updated health information about their condition • Knowledge of condition • Disease process and prognosis • Current treatment and treatment options • Medication knowledge • Self-assessment *Caregiver issues* • Family/caregiver adaptation and coping • Adapting to change in authority

Adapted from American Academy of Pediatrics, American Academy of Family Physicians, American College of Physicians, Transitions Clinical Report Authoring Group. Supporting the health care transition from adolescence to adulthood in the medical home. *Pediatrics*. 2011;128(1):182-200

ing transition planning for youth with and without chronic conditions have been established, but empirical support for the effect of individual elements of transition planning on health outcomes is lacking.

Transfer of Care

Transfer occurs when the adolescent or young adult fully participates in the adult health care model either in the current practice (family medicine or internal medicine/pediatrics) or with a new adult physician. By the time of transfer, the adolescent should feel empowered to participate in the adult health care model to their fullest potential, and all relevant medical information should be organized and accessible. Even if an adolescent does not need to change physicians, transfer of care is still relevant because physicians must shift their clinical approach when their patients become adults. Furthermore, adolescents may receive subspecialty care or need to meet new physicians for other reasons.

Transfer of care requires effective communication between physicians. This process can be expedited by pediatric physicians confirming the first appointment with the new adult physician, composing a transfer letter, and preparing a transition package.[4] The transition package (Table 5) is a potentially effective tool for easing passage to an adult physician; however, issues affecting some YSHCN may require an actual discussion between physicians before transfer.

Methods to support a successful transfer of care for YSHCN have been evaluated for differing patient populations.[39-41] Various approaches have been considered, including joint pediatric-adult clinics, young adult clinics, transition consult clinics,[42] and involvement of transition coordinators.[40] Joint pediatric-adult clinics introduce adolescents to adult physicians alongside their pediatric physicians, possibly improving continuity of care and decreasing anxiety for patients.[43] Young adult clinics may help young adults feel less awkward or out of place and allow for a more developmentally appropriate approach to health care delivery. Transition consult clinics work in tandem with pediatric physicians and patients to fashion a transition plan. Transition coordinators can perform tasks such as assessing transition readiness, managing a registry, and attending appointments with patients. They also may be effective in promoting a successful transfer to adult health care.[44] Ongoing research is needed to demonstrate the relative value of these approaches in improving health care transfer and health outcomes.

Transfer Completion

The final core element for improving the quality of transition services involves confirming completion of transfer. After a patient transfers to an adult practice, inadequate preparation and other barriers can lead to transfer failure with subsequent "bounce back" or complete loss to care.[1,45,46] To support successful completion of transfer, Got Transition recommends that, 3 to 6 months after transfer of care,

Table 5
Suggested components of a transition package

Summary letter	Plan of care (including pending actions)
Medical summary	Legal documents (eg, guardianship)
Emergency care plan	Condition fact sheet if needed

pediatric physicians communicate with adult physicians to confirm transfer of care responsibilities, ensure that patients are engaged, and obtain feedback from the adult physician on the transition process.[4] Pediatric physicians should offer consultation as needed and continue to build relationships with adult physicians. Ideally, the transition process should include an official comanagement period between pediatric and adult practices. During this time, the pediatric physician could support the adult physician in addressing any gaps in the patient's transition preparedness and offer guidance as needed regarding preventive care for young adults.[47] Ideally, each transfer of care should involve referral to a vetted adult physician whom the pediatric physician feels confident will continue to offer quality care.

Pediatric physicians also play a role in facilitating eventual success when transfer initially fails. The transition process must consider the patient's cognitive and social development and acknowledge that unsuccessful transfers may occur. The emotions and experiences surrounding transition should be normalized for the patient, family, and adult physicians. Discussing differences in the adult health care model with patients may encourage active participation and improve overall transition outcomes.

ADDRESSING BARRIERS AND THE FUTURE OF HEALTH CARE TRANSITION

Unfortunately, barriers arising from multiple sources may contribute to failure in implementing transition as part of clinical practice and thereby compromise the successful transfer of care. The current literature that addresses health care transition emphasizes the identification of barriers encountered; however, scant research informs the physician about how to successfully overcome those barriers. Our motivation for reviewing that literature is to help physicians anticipate issues that may arise during transition and to suggest methods to circumvent the negative effect of those barriers on transition for adolescent and young adult patients.

First, patients and families may express a desire to remain with their pediatric physicians, which may demotivate the young adult from transitioning to adult care. Both parents and patients have reported concerns about anticipated differences in health care support, adult physician knowledge of special health care needs, personal comprehension of specific medical conditions, and loss of meaningful relationships with pediatric physicians.[43,48-50] Anxiety about the transfer of care may stem from personal as well as others' negative experiences in adult care, from not knowing what to expect from adult care, from discomfort with an adult environment, and from having to restate health histories and transferring medical records.[43] Patients are often uncertain as to how to identify an adult physician.[25] Implementing a structured, well-planned transition process within the medical home, as outlined earlier, may alleviate many of these potential barriers.

Second, it may be challenging to discuss transition, assess readiness, prepare transition package, and communicate with receiving physicians within a busy clinic setting.[17,50-53] It can also can be challenging to identify adult physicians who are proficient in caring for young adults, particularly YSHCN. Young adults comprise a relatively small segment of most adult practices,[17,46,50,51] consequently adult physicians often lack experience with relatively rare pediatric conditions. Pediatric physicians have an opportunity to address these potential barriers by seeking educational opportunities that center on transition topics (eg, Got Transition provides training that awards continuing education credits[4]) and by networking with and subsequently educating adult physicians in their communities. Consideration should be given to the introduction of transition-related processes to all pediatrics, internal medicine, internal medicine/pediatrics, and family practice trainees.[54]

Finally, the lack of research dedicated to investigating clinical outcomes following transition to adult care presents a roadblock to establishing and fine-tuning best practices. Consensus is needed regarding the important outcomes on which to evaluate transition. Scant evidence is currently available that identifies effective processes for promoting optimal transition or the most efficacious methods for delivering services. It is our hope that physicians will implement the recommendations outlined in this article within their own practices and then contribute to the growing body of literature evaluating the effectiveness of health care transition, so as to optimize the safety and well-being of adolescents and young adults.

References

1. American Academy of Pediatrics, American Academy of Family Physicians, American College of Physicians, Transitions Clinical Report Authoring Group. Supporting the health care transition from adolescence to adulthood in the medical home. *Pediatrics*. 2011;128(1):182-200
2. Blum RW. Improving transition for adolescents with special health care needs from pediatric to adult-centered health care. *Pediatrics*. 2002;110(6):1301-1303
3. McDonagh JE, Kelly DA. Transitioning care of the pediatric recipient to adult caregivers. *Pediatr Clin North Am*. 2003;50(6):1561-1583
4. National Center for Health Care Transition Improvement. Six core elements of health care transition. January 2014. Available at: www.gottransition.org. Accessed January 23, 2014
5. Roisman GI, Masten AS, Coatsworth J, Tellegen A. Salient and emerging developmental tasks in the transition to adulthood. *Child Dev*. 2004;75(1):123-133
6. Burt KB, Masten AS. Development in the transition to adulthood: vulnerabilities and opportunities. In: Grant JE, Potenza MN, eds. *Young Adult Mental Health*. New York: Oxford University Press; 2010:5-18
7. Aud S, Kewal-Ramani A, Frohlich L; National Center for Education Statistics. *America's Youth: Transitions to Adulthood*. NCES 2012-026. Washington, DC: National Center for Education Statistics, US Department of Education; 2011
8. Mulye TP, Park MJ, Nelson CD, et al. Trends in adolescent and young adult health in the United States. *J Adolesc Health*. 2009;45(1):8-24
9. Stroud C, Mainero T, Olson S. *Improving the Health, Safety, and Well-Being of Young Adults*. Washington, DC: National Research Council of the National Academies; 2013

10. National Survey of Children with Special Health Care Needs. Youth's doctors discuss transition to providers who treat adults: child and Adolescent Health Measurement Initiative. Available at: childhealthdata.org/browse/survey/results?q=1729&r=1. Accessed January 6, 2014
11. Sawicki GS, Whitworth R, Gunn L, et al. Receipt of health care transition counseling in the National Survey of Adult Transition and Health. *Pediatrics*. 2011;128(3):e521-e529
12. Lau JS, Adams SH, Irwin CE Jr, Ozer EM. Receipt of preventive health services in young adults. *J Adolesc Health*. 2013;52(1):42-49
13. Okumura MJ, Hersh AO, Hilton JF, Lotstein DS. Change in health status and access to care in young adults with special health care needs: results from the 2007 National Survey of Adult Transition and Health. *J Adolesc Health*. 2013;52(4):413-418
14. Fortuna RJ, Halterman JS, Pulcino T, Robbins BW. Delayed transition of care: a national study of visits to pediatricians by young adults. *Acad Pediatr*. 2012;12(5):405-411
15. Fortuna R, Robbins B, Mani N, Halterman J. Dependence on emergency care among young adults in the United States. *J Gen Intern Med*. 2010;25(7):663-669
16. Bitsko RH, Visser SN, Schieve LA, et al. Unmet health care needs among CSHCN with neurologic conditions. *Pediatrics*. 2009;124:S343-S351
17. Okumura MJ, Kerr EA, Cabana MD, et al. Physician views on barriers to primary care for young adults with childhood-onset chronic disease. *Pediatrics*. 2010;125(4):e748-754
18. American Academy of Pediatrics, American Academy of Family Physicians, American College of Physicians–American Society of Internal Medicine. A consensus statement on health care transitions for young adults with special health care needs. *Pediatrics*. 2002;110(6 Suppl 3):1304-1306
19. Rosen DS, Blum RW, Britto M, Sawyer SM, Siegel DM. Transition to adult health care for adolescents and young adults with chronic conditions: position paper of the Society for Adolescent Medicine. *J Adolesc Health*. 2003;33(4):309-311
20. Smith GM, Lewis VR, Whitworth E, Gold DT, Thornburg CD. Growing up with sickle cell disease: a pilot study of a transition program for adolescents with sickle cell disease. *J Pediatr Hematol Oncol*. 2011;33(5):379-382
21. Nakhla M, Daneman D, To T, Paradis G, Guttmann A. Transition to adult care for youths with diabetes mellitus: findings from a Universal Health Care System. *Pediatrics*. 2009;124(6):e1134-e1141
22. Fredericks EM, Dore-Stites D, Well A, et al. Assessment of transition readiness skills and adherence in pediatric liver transplant recipients. *Pediatr Transplant*. 2010;14(8):944-953
23. Scal P. Transition for youth with chronic conditions: primary care physicians' approaches. *Pediatrics*. 2002;110(suppl 3):1315-1321
24. Shaw TM, DeLaet DE. Transition of adolescents to young adulthood for vulnerable populations. *Pediatr Rev*. 2010;31(12):497-505
25. Young NL, Barden WS, Mills WA, et al. Transition to adult-oriented health care: perspectives of youth and adults with complex physical disabilities. *Phys Occup Ther Pediatr*. 2009;29(4):345-361
26. American Academy of Pediatrics; for the Medical Home Initiatives for Children With Special Needs Project Advisory Committee. The medical home. *Pediatrics*. 2002;110(1 Pt 1):184-186
27. Registries for evaluating patient outcomes: a user's guide. In: Gliklich RE, Dreyer NA, eds. *AHRQ Methods for Effective Health Care*. 2nd ed. Rockville, MD: Agency for Healthcare Research and Quality, US Department of Health and Human Services; 2010
28. Cystic Fibrosis Foundation Care Center Network. 2014. Available at: www.cff.org/treatments/carecenternetwork/. Accessed January 25, 2014
29. Children's Oncology Group. Available at: www.childrensoncologygroup.org. Accessed January 25, 2014
30. ImproveCareNow. Available at: improvecarenow.org. Accessed January 25, 2014
31. Lannon CM, Peterson LE. Pediatric collaborative networks for quality improvement and research. *Acad Pediatr*. 2013;13(6 Suppl):S69-74
32. Zhang LF, Ho JS, Kennedy SE. A systematic review of the psychometric properties of transition readiness assessment tools in adolescents with chronic disease. *BMC Pediatr*. 2014;14(1):4
33. Terwee CB, Bot SD, de Boer MR, et al. Quality criteria were proposed for measurement properties of health status questionnaires. *J Clin Epidemiol*. 2007;60(1):34-42

34. Sawicki GS, Lukens-Bull K, Yin X, et al. Measuring the transition readiness of youth with special healthcare needs: validation of the TRAQ—Transition Readiness Assessment Questionnaire. *J Pediatr Psychol.* 2011;36(2):160-171
35. Gilleland J, Amaral S, Mee L, Blount R. Getting ready to leave: transition readiness in adolescent kidney transplant recipients. *J Pediatr Psychol.* 2012;37(1):85-96
36. Ferris ME, Harward DH, Bickford K, et al. A clinical tool to measure the components of health-care transition from pediatric care to adult care: the UNC TR(x)ANSITION scale. *Ren Fail.* 2012;34(6):744-753
37. Wolf-Branigin M, Schuyler V, White P. Improving quality of life and career attitudes of youth with disabilities experiences from the Adolescent Employment Readiness Center. *Res Soc Work Pract.* 2007;17(3):324-333
38. Coleman K, Austin BT, Brach C, Wagner EH. Evidence on the chronic care model in the new millennium. *Health Aff (Millwood).* 2009;28(1):75-85
39. Cadario F, Prodam F, Bellone S, et al. Transition process of patients with type 1 diabetes (T1 DM) from paediatric to the adult health care service: a hospital-based approach. *Clin Endocrinol.* 2009;71(3):346-350
40. Crowley R, Wolfe I, Lock K, McKee M. Improving the transition between paediatric and adult healthcare: a systematic review. *Arch Dis Child.* 2011;96(6):548-553
41. American Academy of Pediatrics Committee on Pediatric AIDS. Transitioning HIV-infected youth into adult health care. *Pediatrics.* 2013;132(1):192-197
42. Woodward JF, Swigonski NL, Ciccarelli MR. Assessing the health, functional characteristics, and health needs of youth attending a noncategorical transition support program. *J Adolesc Health.* 2012;51(3):272-278
43. Lugasi T, Achille M, Stevenson M. Patients' perspective on factors that facilitate transition from child-centered to adult-centered health care: a theory integrated metasummary of quantitative and qualitative studies. *J Adolesc Health.* 2011;48(5):429-440
44. Annunziato RA, Baisley MC, Arrato N, et al. Strangers headed to a strange land? A pilot study of using a transition coordinator to improve transfer from pediatric to adult services. *J Pediatr.* 2013;163(6):1628-1633
45. Huang JS, Gottschalk M, Pian M, et al. Transition to adult care: systematic assessment of adolescents with chronic illnesses and their medical teams. *J Pediatr.* 2011;159(6):994-998
46. Peter NG, Forke CM, Ginsburg KR, Schwarz DF. Transition from pediatric to adult care: internists' perspectives. *Pediatrics.* 2009;123(2):417-423
47. Ozer E, Urquhart JT, Brindis CD, Park M, Irwin CE. Young adult preventive health care guidelines: there but can't be found. *Arch Pediatr Adolesc Med.* 2012;166(3):240-247
48. Fredericks EM, Dore-Stites D, Lopez MJ, et al. Transition of pediatric liver transplant recipients to adult care: patient and parent perspectives. *Pediatr Transplant.* 2011;15(4):414-424
49. Henderson TO, Friedman DL, Meadows AT. Childhood cancer survivors: transition to adult-focused risk-based care. *Pediatrics.* 2010;126(1):129-136
50. Clarizia NA, Chahal N, Manlhiot C, et al. Transition to adult health care for adolescents and young adults with congenital heart disease: perspectives of the patient, parent and health care provider. *Can J Cardiol.* 2009;25(9):e317-e322
51. Sebastian S, Jenkins H, McCartney S, et al. The requirements and barriers to successful transition of adolescents with inflammatory bowel disease: differing perceptions from a survey of adult and paediatric gastroenterologists. *J Crohns Colitis.* 2012;6(8):830-844
52. Freyer DR. Transition of care for young adult survivors of childhood and adolescent cancer: rationale and approaches. *J Clin Oncol.* 2010;28(32):4810-4818
53. Eshelman-Kent D, Kinahan KE, Hobbie W, et al. Cancer survivorship practices, services, and delivery: a report from the Children's Oncology Group (COG) nursing discipline, adolescent/young adult, and late effects committees. *J Cancer Surviv.* 2011;5(4):345-357
54. Patel MS, O'Hare K. Residency training in transition of youth with childhood-onset chronic disease. *Pediatrics.* 2010;126(3):S190-S193

Adolesc Med 025 (2014) 438–454

Metabolic Syndrome in Adolescents

Manmohan K. Kamboj, MD[a*]; David R. Repaske, MD, PhD[b]

[a]Associate Professor, Wexner Medical Center at The Ohio State University, Section of Endocrinology, Metabolism and Diabetes, Department of Pediatrics, Nationwide Children's Hospital, Columbus, Ohio; [b]Professor, Wexner Medical Center at The Ohio State University, Section of Endocrinology, Metabolism and Diabetes, Department of Pediatrics, Nationwide Children's Hospital, Columbus, Ohio

BACKGROUND

There has been a rise in the overall prevalence of obesity over the last few decades. Along with the increase in obesity, particularly abdominal obesity, there has been recognition of a co-occurrence of multiple metabolic risk factors, including hyperglycemia/insulin resistance, hypertension, and dyslipidemia, all of which are seen to increase the risk of type 2 diabetes mellitus (T2DM) and cardiovascular disease (CVD).[1] The coexistence of these factors has been referred to as metabolic syndrome (MetS), syndrome X, or the insulin resistance syndrome.[2] It is reasonable to postulate that this constellation of conditions has common underlying pathophysiologic pathways. Concerns have been raised about the importance of predicting and recognizing an increased medical risk and predisposition for higher risk of morbidity and mortality in MetS and the consequent need for initiation of appropriate preventive and therapeutic measures.[3]

DEFINITION AND DIAGNOSTIC CRITERIA

The precise definition of MetS remains unclear. Multiple organizations have made efforts to develop a feasible definition for this syndrome in adults; however, there continue to be differences among the various defining criteria developed. The initial criteria were developed by World Health Organization (WHO) in 1998.[4] The most commonly used set of criteria are from the National Cholesterol Education Program Adult Treatment Panel III (NCEP:ATP III), which

*Corresponding author:
E-mail address: Manmohan.Kamboj@Nationwidechildrens.org

 ISSN 1934-4287

were developed in 2001 and updated in 2005. These criteria are believed to be more user-friendly at the physician level.[5] Other organizations, including the European Group for Study of Insulin Resistance (EGIR) in 1999, the International Diabetes Federation Criteria (IDF) in 2006, and the American Association of Clinical Endocrinologists (AACE) in 2003, have also developed their sets of criteria for the definition of MetS.[6-8] Table 1 summarizes the criteria included in these guidelines.[9] Recent efforts have been made to harmonize definitive criteria for MetS.[10] Furthermore, modifications of these definitions have been proposed for pediatrics and adolescents.[11-15] The common essential components of the MetS incorporated in all of these guidelines are obesity, glucose intolerance, hypertension, and dyslipidemia. However, the defining details of each of these criteria and the combinations/permutations required to make the diagnosis vary. It is evident that the existence of at least 5 different sets of diagnostic criteria creates lack of clarity, making the diagnosis of MetS a challenge. Additionally, it becomes difficult to decide when it is necessary to make therapeutic recommendations and management plans.

CHALLENGES IN MAKING THE DIAGNOSIS OF METABOLIC SYNDROME IN ADOLESCENTS

Based on the adult criteria noted earlier, 3 sets of modified diagnostic criteria for MetS have been proposed for children and adolescents and are summarized as follows:

1. The modified NCEP:ATP III criteria include the presence of ≥3 of the following features: triglycerides (>95th percentile); high-density lipoprotein (HDL; <5th percentile); hypertension (systolic blood pressure [SBP] or diastolic blood pressure [DBP] >95th percentile); impaired glucose tolerance.[12,13]
2. The National Health and Nutrition Examination Survey (NHANES) III criteria for adolescents require the presence of all of the following: waist circumference (≥90th percentile); triglycerides (>110 mg/dL); HDL (<40 mg/dL); hypertension (BP ≥90th percentile); glucose (fasting ≥110 mg/dL).[14]
3. The IDF criteria for pediatric patients have 3 different categories[15,16]

- Adolescents older than 16 years have the same diagnostic criteria for diagnosis of MetS as adults.
- For adolescents between 10 to 16 years of age, the criteria include waist circumference (90th percentile of ethnic-specific waist circumference) and ≥2 of the following: triglycerides (≥150 mg/dL); HDL (<40 mg/dL); hypertension (SBP ≥130 or DBP≥85 mmHg); glucose (fasting ≥110 mg/dL).
- For children younger than 10 years, there are no specific diagnostic criteria. Close follow-up is recommended for children whose waist circumference is ≥90th percentile.

Table 1
Various criteria for definition of metabolic syndrome in adults

Five definitions of the metabolic syndrome

	Required	Number of abnormalities	Glucose (fasting)	HDL cholesterol	Triglycerides	Obesity	Hypertension
NCEP STP3 2005*		≥3 of:	≥5.6 mmol/L (100 mg/dL) or drug treatment for elevated blood glucose	<1.0 mmol/L (40 mg/dL) (men); <1.3 mmol/L (50 mg/dL) (women) or drug treatment of low HDL-C¶	≥1.7 mmol/L (150 mg/dL) or drug treatment for elevated triglycerides¶	Waist ≥102 cm (men) or ≥88 cm (women)‖	≥130/85 mmHg or drug treatment for hypertension
IDF 2006	Waist ≥94 cm (men) or ≥80 cm (women)†	And ≥2 of:	≥5.6 mmol/L (100 mg/dL) or diagnosed diabetes	<1.0 mmol/L (40 mg/dL) (men); <1.3 mmol/L (50 mg/dL) (women) or drug treatment for low HDL-C	≥1.7 mmol/L (150 mg/dL) or drug treatment for high triglycerides		≥130/85 mmHg or drug treatment for hypertension
EGIR 1999	Insulin resistance or fasting hyperinsulinemia in top 25%	And ≥2 of:	6.1-6.9 mmol/ (110-125 mg/dL)	<1.0 mmol/L (40 mg/dL)	Or ≥2.0 mmol/L (180 mg/dL) or drug treatment for dyslipidemia	Waist ≥94 cm (men) or ≥80 cm (women)	≥140/90 mmHg or drug treatment for hypertension

WHO 1999	Insulin resistance in top 25%‡; glucose ≥6.1 mmol/L (110 mg/dL); 2-hour glucose ≥7.8 mmol/L (140 mg/dL)	And ≥2 of:		<0.9 mmol/L (35 mg/dL) (men); <1.0 mmol/L (40 mg/dL) (women)	Or ≥1.7 mmol/L (150 mg/dL)	Waist/hip ration >0.9 (men) or >0.85 (women) or BMI ≥30 kg/m²	≥140/90 mmHg
AACE 2003	High risk of insulin resistance§ or BMI ≥25 kg/m² or waist ≥102 cm (men) or ≥88 cm (women)	And ≥2 of:	≥6.1 mmol/L (110 mg/dL); ≥2-hour glucose 7.8 mmol/L (140 mg/dL)	<1.0 mmol/L (40 mg/dL) (men); <1.3 mmol/L (50 mg/dL) (women)	≥1.7 mmol/L (150 mg/dL)		≥130/85 mmHg

AACE, American Association of Clinical Endocrinologists; BMI, body mass index; EGIR, Group for the Study of Insulin Resistance; HDL, high-density lipoprotein; IDF, International Diabetes Federation; NCEP, National Cholesterol Education Program; WHO, World Health Organization.

*Most commonly agreed on criteria for metabolic syndrome (any 3 of 5 risk factors).

†For South Asia and Chinese patients, waist ≥90 cm (men) or ≥80 cm (women); for Japanese patients, waist ≥90 cm (men) or ≥80 cm (women).

‡Insulin resistance measured using insulin clamp.

§High risk of being insulin resistant is indicated by the presence of at least 1 of the following: diagnosis of cardiovascular disease (CVD), hypertension, polycystic ovary syndrome, nonalcoholic fatty liver disease or acanthosis nigricans; family history of type 2 diabetes, hypertension of CVD; history of gestational diabetes or glucose intolerance; nonwhite ethnicity; sedentary lifestyle; BMI 25 kg/m² or waist circumference 94 cm for men and 80 cm for women; and age 40 years.

¶Treatment with 1 or more of fibrates or niacin.

||In Asian patients, waist ≥90 cm (men) or ≥80 cm (women).

From Meigs JB. The metabolic syndrome (Insulin resistance syndrome or syndrome X). In: *UpToDate*. Nathan DM and Wolfsdorf JI (eds.), Waltham, MA. (Accessed January 20, 2014)

Therefore, as in adults, the lack of a unifying and common set of diagnostic criteria creates a challenge for addressing the diagnostic and therapeutic issues for MetS in the pediatric population (Table 2).

There is also ongoing disagreement on whether MetS is a clinical entity with a single underlying cause or whether the terminology simply represents a collection of independent risk factors for CVD.[17-19] Current therapy is directed exclusively at addressing the components of MetS and not at an underlying cause. There continues to be an ongoing controversy with regard to the additional benefits of the diagnosis of the cluster of components as a distinct syndrome. Although the presence of MetS does increase the risk of developing diabetes by 3 to 5 times, and of developing CVD by 1.5 to 2.2 times, this is not more than the sum of the risks of the component elements considered individually.[2,20,21]

EPIDEMIOLOGY

Varying prevalence rates for MetS are noted in the pediatric population based on the particular set of diagnostic criteria used. The lack of definitive diagnostic criteria prevents accurate estimations of prevalence and makes it difficult to compare outcomes of intervention strategies.[22] The development of MetS has been associated with several risk factors. A higher risk of adult MetS and adult CVD has been shown in individuals who had MetS during childhood and adolescence.[23,24] The prevalence of MetS is higher in obese individuals, and childhood obesity is noted to be predictive of adult MetS.[25] The NHANES data noted the overall prevalence of MetS to be 9% using the modified ATP III criteria in 12- to 19-year-olds.[13] However, the overweight and obese individuals in this study had a higher prevalence of 33%.[13] Weiss et al[26] demonstrated the absence of MetS in normal-weight children and adolescents, whereas 39% of moderately obese and 50% of severely obese individuals met the criteria for MetS. A direct

Table 2
Definitions of metabolic syndrome in adolescents

	Modified ATP	IDF (10-16 years)	NHANES III
Required: waist circumference		≥90th percentile, ethnic-specific	≥90th percentile
Plus: number of additional criteria	≥3	≥2	All
Triglycerides	>95th percentile	≥150 mg/dL	≥110 mg/dL
HDL	<5th percentile	<40 ng/dL	≤40 mg/dL
Blood Pressure	Either of:	Either of:	≥90th percentile
Systolic	>95th percentile	>130 mmHg	
Diastolic	>95th percentile	≥85 mmHg	
Glucose	IGT	≥100 mg/dL	≥110 mg/dL, fasting

HDL, high-density lipoprotein; IDF, International Diabetes Federation; ATP, Adult Treatment Panel; IGT, Impaired Glucose Tolerance; NHANES, National Health and Nutrition Examination Survey.

correlation between central adiposity and waist circumference has also been shown in 9- to 10-year-old girls, leading to a higher predisposition to develop MetS. An increase of 1 cm in waist circumference increased the risk of MetS by 7.4%, and the risk of MetS increased 1.3% for every 1 mg/dL increase in triglycerides.[27] Race and ethnicity also influence the predisposition to MetS. The prevalence of MetS was 8.4%, 9.4%, and 2.5% in US adolescent males and 4.4%, 6.4%, and 4.2% in females, among non-Hispanic whites, Mexican Americans, and non-Hispanic blacks, respectively, as analyzed in 3100 adolescents (aged 12-19 years) from the 1999 to 2006 NHANES.[28] Native Americans had the highest risk, with a reported prevalence of 18.6% in the 10- to 19-year-age group.[29]

Hormonal changes associated with puberty resulting in transient insulin resistance make the diagnosis of MetS in adolescence even more complex. A higher prevalence of MetS noted during puberty suggests that MetS resolves after completion of pubertal development in some adolescents, but in others, MetS may persist or develop after puberty.[30]

RISK FACTORS FOR METABOLIC SYNDROME

The presence of certain factors or behaviors may predispose some children and adolescents to developing MetS. Ethnic/racial/genetic factors, environmental circumstances, and certain lifestyle patterns are recognized to pose a higher risk than others (Table 3).[31-37] Early recognition of these factors may be instrumental in implementing healthy lifestyle changes, which may be helpful in somewhat mitigating the higher risk of morbidity in the long term. These may include an

Table 3
Genetic and lifestyle determinants for developing metabolic syndrome

- Positive family history of
  - ASCVD
  - Obesity
  - Diabetes mellitus
- Obesity
- Dyslipidemia
  - Low HDL
  - High triglycerides
- Hypertension
- Insulin resistance
  - Sedentary lifestyle–higher risk of obesity and MetS
- Nutrition/diet
  - Western dietary pattern: diet high in red meat, processed meat and foods, fried foods, high fat dairy, sugar beverages
    - Low dietary consumption of: whole grains, high fiber, nuts, fruits, vegetables, carotene, vitamin C, magnesium, long-chain fatty acids, fish, olive oil

HDL, high-density lipoprotein; MetS, metabolic syndrome; ASCVD, Atherosclerotic cardiovascular disease.

overall emphasis on healthy lifestyle behaviors, such as incorporation of regular physical activity in the daily routine in the home and school environment; an awareness of healthy and optimal nutritional intake; and the ease and affordability of making these options available to our children and families across all socioeconomic strata. In the future, it may be helpful to recognize these predisposing factors and establish a scoring/grading system for routine use by primary care physicians and pediatricians to allocate a higher risk.[38]

TREATMENT MODALITIES

Currently, there is no specific medication or treatment of MetS. Lack of clarity with regard to the underlying pathophysiology, diagnostic parameters, evolution of MetS over the life course, and implications of the presence and progression of the components of the condition leave us with insufficient evidence for making robust treatment recommendations for MetS at this time. However, gearing management strategies toward improving the individual component elements of obesity, hypertension, hyperlipidemia, and insulin resistance seem intuitive. It now is being recognized that the underlying pathophysiologic processes of the various components of the adult MetS are initiated during childhood and adolescence.

Obesity and central adiposity can be addressed with healthy lifestyle recommendations starting in infancy as a preventive strategy initially, but also as a therapeutic intervention when overweight and obesity are present. Close monitoring of weight and body mass index (BMI) at routine pediatric visits is the initial step toward this intervention. Healthy dietary practices, including limitation of caloric beverages and calorie-rich foods and attention to portion size, should be initiated as preventive strategies and should be implemented as therapeutic options when overweight or obesity is present as a component of MetS. Similarly, physical activity should be incorporated into the daily routine, starting in early childhood, in order to promote a healthy lifestyle. Incorporation of such healthy lifestyle modifications not only achieves weight control but more importantly results in improvement of glucose tolerance, insulin sensitivity, vascular endothelial function, hypertension, and hyperlipidemia.[37,39-42] Metformin use has also been shown to improve insulin sensitivity and decrease BMI in some studies, although it still is not recommended as standard of care therapy for MetS.[43,44] At this time it may be reasonable to extrapolate that implementation of these behaviors and therapies for weight control and treatment of MetS components early in the course of the disease process may result in improvement of cardiovascular risk profiles. The risk of developing diabetes may be decreased or delayed as well.[37,44-46] Table 4 summarizes recommendations to address obesity, hypertension, hyperlipidemia, and impaired glucose tolerance in a stepwise approach at the primary care level.[37] Referrals to cardiology, endocrinology, dietitians, behavioral medicine, and an exercise therapist may be undertaken as needed. Some institutions have incorporated this into a multidisciplinary clinic concept to address the complex needs of these patients.

OTHER CONDITIONS ASSOCIATED WITH METABOLIC SYNDROME

A few conditions are not a part of MetS but often occur in association with it

- Polycystic ovary syndrome (PCOS) and hyperandrogenism: Clinical and biochemical hyperandrogenism is an important diagnostic criterion for PCOS. Insulin resistance and hyperandrogenism often coexist, although the pathophysiology delineating the cause and effect between these 2 entities is still debated. The free testosterone levels (biologically active fraction) are elevated, predisposing adolescent females to PCOS with clinical presentation of amenorrhea/irregular menstrual periods, hirsutism, and acne. Metformin treatment may improve hyperinsulinemia and insulin resistance, and hormone therapy with oral contraceptive pills may be initiated for treatment of hyperandrogenemia and irregular menstrual periods.
- Nonalcoholic fatty liver disease (NAFLD): NAFLD seems to be the hepatic component of MetS. In a recent study, 25% of NAFLD patients (6-17 years old) met the diagnostic criteria for MetS.[47] The diagnosis of NAFLD remains a challenge; a liver biopsy is confirmatory but is not always undertaken. Liver enzyme levels are not always elevated and do not necessarily correlate with the severity of NAFLD.[48] The underlying pathophysiologic process is initiated by insulin resistance and imbalance of adipocytokines and results in increased hepatocellular lipids referred to as hepatic steatosis, which may evolve into liver cirrhosis.[49] Healthy lifestyle interventions to achieve weight loss remain the intervention of choice in these children. The focus of medical therapy in clinical trials includes use of metformin and antioxidants such as vitamin E.[37,50] Long-term therapeutic trials are necessary to study the response to treatment and disease progression.

LATEST DEVELOPMENTS IN METABOLIC SYNDROME AND FUTURE DIRECTIONS

MetS contributes significantly to morbidity and mortality and therefore has not only important health implications but also significant financial implications and burden on the health care system. A plethora of research is addressing the various aspects of MetS, ranging from the basic concept of establishing consistent and relevant diagnostic criteria, especially in the pediatric population, to investigating the underlying pathophysiologic mechanisms, and identifying and treating the various components of MetS.

Diagnostic Criteria in Metabolic Syndrome

Within the last decade, progress has been made in identifying modified diagnostic criteria specifically geared toward children and adolescents.[14,17] In 2009, a joint scientific statement addressing the progress and challenges of MetS in the

Table 4
Treatment recommendations for metabolic syndrome

Treatment recommendations		
General comments	Step 1	Step 2
Lifestyle		
Diet evaluation, diet education for all	Adequate calories for growth; total fat 25%-35% of calories, saturated fat <7% of calories, trans fat <1% of calories, cholesterol <300 mg/d	
BMI 85th-95th percentile	Maintain BMI with aging to reduce BMI to <85th percentile. If BMI >25 kg/m^2, weight maintenance 2- to 4-year-olds will achieve reductions in BMI by achieving a rate of weight gain <1 kg per 2 cm of linear growth. Children ≥4 years old will achieve reductions in BMI by BMI maintenance or more rapidly with weight maintenance during linear growth.	
BMI >95th percentile	Younger children: weight maintenance; adolescents: gradual weight loss of 1-2 kg/mo to reduce BMI	Dietitian referral
BMI ≥95th percentile plus comorbidity	Gradual weight loss (1-2 kg/mo) to achieve healthier BMI; assess need for additional therapy of associated conditions.	Dietitian referral ± pharmacologic therapy
Physical activity	Specific activity history for each child, focusing on time spent in active play and screen time (television + computer + video games). Goal is ≥1 h of active play each day; screen time limited to ≤2 h/d. Encourage activity at every encounter.	Referral to exercise specialist

Blood pressure		
SBP ± DBP = 90th-95th percentile or BP >120/80 mmHg (3 separate occasions within 1 mo) plus excess weight	Gradual weight loss (1-2 kg/mo) to achieve healthier BMI by decreased calorie intake, increased physical activity	Dietitian referral
Initial SBP ± DBP >95th percentile (confirmed within 1 wk) or 6-mo follow-up SBP or DBP >95th percentile		Pharmacologic therapy per Fourth Task Force recommendations
Lipids: TG		
TG = 150-400 mg/dL	Decrease simple sugars; low saturated and trans fats diet	
TG = 150-1000 mg/dL plus excess weight	Dietitian referral for weight loss management; energy balance training plus physical activity recommendations (see above)	TG 700-1000 mg/dL: consider fibrate or niacin if >10 y of age
TG ≥1000 mg/dL	Consider fibrate or niacin.	
Glucose		
FG = 100-126 mg/dL plus excess weight	Gradual weight loss (1-2 kg/mo) to achieve healthier BMI by decreased calorie intake, increased physical activity	
Repeat FG 100-126 mg/dL	Endocrine referral	Insulin-sensitizing medication per endocrinologist
Casual glucose >200 mg/dL or FG >126 mg/dL	Endocrine referral; treatment for diabetes	
Maintain HbA_{1C} <7%		

BP, blood pressure; DBP, diastolic blood pressure; FG, fasting glucose; HbA_{1c}, hemoglobin A_{1c}; SBP, systolic blood pressure; TG, triglycerides.

Body mass index (BMI) normal values for age/gender are available at www.cdc.gov/growthcharts.

Elevation of triglycerides to ≥1000 mg/dL is associated with significant risk for acute pancreatitis. A fasting triglyceride level of 700 mg/dL is likely to rise to >1000 mg/dL postprandially. Treatment recommendation is compatible with guidelines for management of dyslipidemia in diabetic children.

Reprinted with permission from Steinberger J, Daniels SR, Eckel RH, et al. Progress and challenges in metabolic syndrome in children and adolescents: a scientific statement from the American Heart Association Atherosclerosis, Hypertension, and Obesity in the Young Committee of the Council on Cardiovascular Disease in the Young; Council on Cardiovascular Nursing; and Council on Nutrition, Physical Activity, and Metabolism. *Circulation*. 2009;119(4):628-647 pediatric population was issued.[39] Consensus about diagnostic criteria did not result, but the difficulty in assigning the criteria was highlighted, including concerns about the availability of adequate data to evaluate if a cluster of characteristics, including abdominal obesity, insulin resistance, and hyperlipidemia, can predict the risk of future disease.[39] Many unanswered questions remain and serve as a direction for future research. Why do all obese adolescents not have a similar predisposition for MetS? What is the long-term outcome of adolescents with features of MetS as they mature into adulthood? What is the best way to predict risks of development of or resolution of MetS as an individual progresses through puberty? What is the status of insulin and glucose metabolism? MetS is a state of high risk for hyperinsulinemia and insulin resistance, but T2DM is not included in the diagnostic criteria per se. What happens to these individuals when there is disease progression from insulin resistance to development of T2DM? Does MetS remain a relevant diagnosis?

An additional area of investigation considers how best to stratify different phenotypic presentations of MetS to develop specific management strategies. Recent work by Gurka et al[51] formulated a confirmatory factor analysis of MetS in adolescents using the NHANES 1999 to 2000 data. The equation, developed from sex/ethnic-specific analysis, is useful for identifying children who are at high risk for developing adult MetS, and based on this identification they can be stratified toward appropriate intervention strategies.[51] Risk stratification based on more comprehensive criteria will be helpful in establishing a clinically relevant definition of MetS in the future.

Pathophysiologic Mechanisms (Inflammatory and Dietary Factors) of Metabolic Syndrome

Great strides have been made over the last few years in formulating a hypothesis for the underlying pathophysiologic mechanisms causing the clinical presentation associated with MetS. The net effect of complex interactive processes, including genetics and heredity, lifestyle, oxidative stress, cortisol, visceral adiposity, and inflammatory vascular markers of inflammation, ultimately determines individual predisposition and risk stratification for components of MetS. Altered adipose tissue metabolism is characterized by chronic inflammation with abnormal adipocytokine production, which has been shown to induce markers of chronic inflammation with macrophage and lymphocytic infiltration in the adipose tissue.[52] These in turn cause activation of the proinflammatory signaling pathways, resulting in activation of several transcription factors such as peroxisome proliferator-activated receptors (PPARs) and CCAAT-enhancer-binding proteins (C/EBPs). This results in control of expression of several genes of the intermediary pathways along with PPAR gamma coactivator-1-α (PGC-1) and the silent information regulator T1 (SIRT1). These regulate lipid metabolism, storage, and secretion by adipocytes. An understanding of these underlying pathophysiologic mechanisms ultimately may guide therapeutic targets.[52,53] Changes in circulating levels of adiponectin and leptin in obesity have been shown to be affected in a positive manner by treatment with omega-3, thus offering potential therapeutic implications for MetS patients.[54] Fibroblast growth factor 21 (FGF21) is an atypical member of the FGF family that has been shown to have the capability to normalize glucose, lipid, and energy metabolism. Novel biomedical engineering research may offer new, therapeutically feasible options for making FGF21 available in the form of more stable formulations or agonist antibodies for use in MetS.[55]

The extraskeletal role of vitamin D has been extensively studied over the last few years. Proponents have advocated its beneficial role in many human physiologic pathways, and MetS is no exception. However, no definite relationship between vitamin D and MetS has yet been established. Further targeted research and randomized controlled trials are needed to explore this relationship further.[56]

Dietary modulation of the proinflammatory state to lower oxidative stress and thereby lower cardiovascular risk has also been well studied. The benefits of the Mediterranean diet, which consists of high dietary intake of nuts, fruits, and vegetables; high intake of vitamins A and C; adequate intake of n-3 polyunsaturated fatty acids and monounsaturated fatty acids; avoiding high intake of saturated fatty acids and n-6/n-3 polyunsaturated fatty acids; preventing magnesium deficiency; and avoiding high fructose intake are all elements of dietary modulation that are being studied for their ability to lower cardiovascular risk and improve hyperglycemia, hyperlipidemia, and NAFLD. The benefits of high dietary fiber content were well elucidated in the recent RESMENA project in Spain, which compared the new dietary strategy for long-term treatment of MetS with guidelines from the American Heart Association.[57-62]

Brain Function in Metabolic Syndrome

Recent work from Yau et al[63] at the NYU School of Medicine highlighted rather startling findings in brain function in adolescents with MetS. Endocrine, magnetic resonance imaging, and neuropsychological evaluations were performed on 111 adolescents (49 with MetS, 62 without MetS). Findings from this study revealed lower cognitive performance (arithmetical score and verbal memory) and reduction in hippocampal volume in adolescents with MetS. Based on these data, a proposal was made for evaluation of brain function earlier in the course of obesity/MetS in the pediatric population.[63]

Relationship of Small-for-Gestational-Age Children and Metabolic Syndrome

Small-for-gestational age (SGA) children are at risk for both adolescent obesity and MetS. A study to determine whether it was obesity or SGA that predisposed to MetS indicated that overweight, former SGA children had an increased risk (40%) for MetS compared to overweight, former appropriate-for-gestational-age

(AGA) children (17%).[64] Unfortunately, a pathophysiologic mechanism was not uncovered, but these results suggest that careful screening for MetS in former SGA children and adolescents is warranted.

Role of Surgery in Metabolic Syndrome

Bariatric surgical procedures have been used to treat adult obesity for many years. Over the last few years, bariatric surgical procedures have been gaining popularity in the adolescent population with severe obesity and its associated morbidities. Roux-en-Y bypass and vertical sleeve gastrectomy have been shown to result in long-term weight loss and improvement in metabolic derangements, including insulin resistance, hyperglycemia, and hyperlipidemia.[65]

METABOLIC SYNDROME: IN THE FUTURE

It is very important for primary care physicians to identify early those children and adolescents with abdominal obesity and other features of MetS and to address their concerns aggressively to prevent complications. Furthermore, we as pediatric investigators need to develop a scoring system to facilitate risk stratification for MetS, starting as early as infancy. Factors such as genetics and family history of obesity, atherosclerotic cardiovascular disease (ASCVD), and diabetes place the patient at high risk for these conditions. The recent Prediction of Metabolic syndrome in Adolescence (PREMA) study concluded that the presence of all 3 predictors (birth weight <10th percentile, birth head circumference <10th percentile, and parental overweight/obesity in at least 1 parent) predicted MetS in adolescence with sensitivity of 91% and specificity of 98%.[66] The adverse pattern clustering of these features in some ethnic/racial groups versus others needs to be recognized, thus facilitating risk stratification. Ethnicity/race-specific reference data for the various anthropometric and biochemical markers for MetS may need to be developed for accurate assessment of risk. When high-risk children are identified early, preventive measures for a healthy lifestyle can be implemented early as well. The health care environment and public health policies should be directed toward encouraging a healthy lifestyle at all ages and levels, including the home environment and the school systems. Along with preventive strategies, once the components of MetS are identified in an individual child/adolescent, appropriate medication therapy may need to be instituted as well. Evidence-based, well-defined guidelines are needed to direct medication therapy for hypertension, hyperlipidemia, and insulin resistance, possibly based on risk stratification as well. Larger, long-term randomized, longitudinal trials are needed to follow the natural history and evolution of the cluster of features characteristic of MetS through childhood, adolescence, and adulthood. These studies may facilitate risk stratification and offer guidance on treatment strategies. Ongoing research needs to focus on the complex pathophysiologic molecular basis of the underlying disease process and offer explanations for the etiologic and pathophysiologic relationship between the various components of MetS.[37]

The unraveling of this mystery will provide clarification of MetS as an entity and help address various questions. Are these clusters of conditions simply coexisting, or are they basically related to each other? Does the cluster together present a higher risk of mortality and morbidity than the sum of the individual constituents? As more pathophysiologic questions are answered, further targeted therapeutic techniques may then be investigated.

References

1. Eckel RH, Grundy SM, Zimmet PZ. The metabolic syndrome. *Lancet.* 2005;365(9468):1415-1428
2. Grundy SM, Cleeman JI, Daniels SR, et al. Diagnosis and management of the metabolic syndrome: an American Heart Association/National Heart, Lung, and Blood Institute Scientific Statement. *Circulation.* 2005;112(17):2735-2752
3. Cameron AJ, Shaw JE, Zimmet PZ. The metabolic syndrome: prevalence in worldwide populations. *Endocrinol Metab Clin North Am.* 2004;33(2):351-375
4. Alberti KG, Zimmet PZ. Definition, diagnosis and classification of diabetes mellitus and its complications. Part 1: diagnosis and classification of diabetes mellitus provisional report of a WHO consultation. *Diab Med.* 1998;15(7):539-553
5. Expert Panel on Detection Evaluation, and Treatment of High Blood Cholesterol in Adults. Executive Summary of the Third Report of the National Cholesterol Education Program (NCEP) Expert Panel on Detection, Evaluation, and Treatment of High Blood Cholesterol in Adults (Adult Treatment Panel III). *JAMA.* 2001;285(19):2486-2497
6. Balkau B, Charles MA. Comment on the provisional report from the WHO consultation. European Group for the Study of Insulin Resistance (EGIR). *Diabet Med.* 1999;16(5):442-443
7. Alberti KG, Zimmet P, Shaw J. The metabolic syndrome: a new worldwide definition. *Lancet.* 2005;366(9491):1059-1062
8. Einhorn D, Reaven GM, Cobin RH, et al. American College of Endocrinology position statement on the insulin resistance syndrome. *Endocr Pract.* 2003;9(3):237-252
9. Meigs JB. The metabolic syndrome (Insulin resistance syndrome or syndrome X). In: *UpToDate.* Nathan DM and Wolfsdorf JI (eds.), Waltham, MA. (Accessed January 20, 2014)
10. Alberti KG, Eckel RH, Grundy SM, et al. Harmonizing the metabolic syndrome: a joint interim statement of the International Diabetes Federation Task Force on Epidemiology and Prevention; National Heart, Lung, and Blood Institute; American Heart Association; World Heart Federation; International Atherosclerosis Society; and International Association for the Study of Obesity. *Circulation.* 2009;120(16):1640-1645
11. Goodman E. Pediatric metabolic syndrome: smoke and mirrors or true magic? *J Pediatr.* 2006;148(2):149-151
12. Goodman E, Daniels SR, Morrison JA, Huang B, Dolan LM. Contrasting prevalence of and demographic disparities in the World Health Organization and National Cholesterol Education Program Adult Treatment Panel III definitions of metabolic syndrome among adolescents. *J Pediatr.* 2004;145(4):445-451
13. de Ferranti SD, Gauvreau K, Ludwig DS, et al. Prevalence of the metabolic syndrome in American adolescents: findings from the Third National Health and Nutrition Examination Survey. *Circulation.* 2004;110(16):2494-2497
14. Cook S, Weitzman M, Auinger P, Nguyen M, Dietz WH. Prevalence of a metabolic syndrome phenotype in adolescents: findings from the third National Health and Nutrition Examination Survey, 1988-1994. *Arch Pediatr Adolesc Med.* 2003;157(8):821-827
15. Zimmet P, Alberti G, Kaufman F, et al. The metabolic syndrome in children and adolescents. *Lancet.* 2007;369(9579):2059-2061
16. Fernandez JR, Redden DT, Pietrobelli A, Allison DB. Waist circumference percentiles in nationally representative samples of African-American, European-American, and Mexican-American children and adolescents. *J Pediatr.* 2004;145(4):439-444

17. Kahn R, Buse J, Ferrannini E, Stern M. The metabolic syndrome: time for a critical appraisal: joint statement from the American Diabetes Association and the European Association for the Study of Diabetes. *Diabet Care.* 2005;28(9):2289-2304
18. Grundy SM. Metabolic syndrome: a multiplex cardiovascular risk factor. *J Clin Endocrinol Metab.* 2007;92(2):399-404
19. Eckel RH, Kahn R, Robertson RM, Rizza RA. Preventing cardiovascular disease and diabetes: a call to action from the American Diabetes Association and the American Heart Association. *Circulation.* 2006;113(25):2943-2946
20. Sundstrom J, Vallhagen E, Riserus U, et al. Risk associated with the metabolic syndrome versus the sum of its individual components. *Diabet Care.* 2006;29(7):1673-1674
21. Bayturan O, Tuzcu EM, Lavoie A, et al. The metabolic syndrome, its component risk factors, and progression of coronary atherosclerosis. *Arch Intern Med.* 2010;170(5):478-484
22. Ford ES, Li C. Defining the metabolic syndrome in children and adolescents: will the real definition please stand up? *J Pediatr.* 2008;152(2):160-164
23. Morrison JA, Friedman LA, Gray-McGuire C. Metabolic syndrome in childhood predicts adult cardiovascular disease 25 years later: the Princeton Lipid Research Clinics Follow-up Study. *Pediatrics.* 2007;120(2):340-345
24. Morrison JA, Friedman LA, Wang P, Glueck CJ. Metabolic syndrome in childhood predicts adult metabolic syndrome and type 2 diabetes mellitus 25 to 30 years later. *J Pediatr.* 2008;152(2):201-206
25. Sun SS, Liang R, Huang TT, et al. Childhood obesity predicts adult metabolic syndrome: the Fels Longitudinal Study. *J Pediatr.* 2008;152(2):191-200
26. Weiss R, Dziura J, Burgert TS, et al. Obesity and the metabolic syndrome in children and adolescents. *N Engl J Med.* 2004;350(23):2362-2374
27. Morrison JA, Friedman LA, Harlan WR, et al. Development of the metabolic syndrome in black and white adolescent girls: a longitudinal assessment. *Pediatrics.* 2005;116(5):1178-1182
28. Walker SE, Gurka MJ, Oliver MN, Johns DW, DeBoer MD. Racial/ethnic discrepancies in the metabolic syndrome begin in childhood and persist after adjustment for environmental factors. *Nutr Metab Cardiovasc Dis.* 2012;22(2):141-148
29. Retnakaran R, Zinman B, Connelly PW, Harris SB, Hanley AJ. Nontraditional cardiovascular risk factors in pediatric metabolic syndrome. *J Pediatr.* 2006;148(2):176-182
30. Goodman E, Daniels SR, Meigs JB, Dolan LM. Instability in the diagnosis of metabolic syndrome in adolescents. *Circulation.* 2007;115(17):2316-2322
31. Hong Y, Pedersen NL, Brismar K, de Faire U. Genetic and environmental architecture of the features of the insulin-resistance syndrome. *Am J Hum Genet.* 1997;60(1):143-152
32. Pankow JS, Jacobs DR Jr, Steinberger J, Moran A, Sinaiko AR. Insulin resistance and cardiovascular disease risk factors in children of parents with the insulin resistance (metabolic) syndrome. *Diabet Care.* 2004;27(3):775-780
33. Chen W, Bao W, Begum S, et al. Age-related patterns of the clustering of cardiovascular risk variables of syndrome X from childhood to young adulthood in a population made up of black and white subjects: the Bogalusa Heart Study. *Diabetes.* 2000;49(6):1042-1048
34. Ekelund U, Brage S, Froberg K, et al. TV viewing and physical activity are independently associated with metabolic risk in children: the European Youth Heart Study. *PLoS Med.* 2006;3(12):e488
35. Steffen LM, Jacobs DR, Jr., Stevens J, et al. Associations of whole-grain, refined-grain, and fruit and vegetable consumption with risks of all-cause mortality and incident coronary artery disease and ischemic stroke: the Atherosclerosis Risk in Communities (ARIC) Study. *Am J Clin Nutr.* 2003;78(3): 383-390
36. Fung TT, Rimm EB, Spiegelman D, et al. Association between dietary patterns and plasma biomarkers of obesity and cardiovascular disease risk. *Am J Clin Nutr.* 2001;73(1):61-67
37. Steinberger J, Daniels SR, Eckel RH, et al. Progress and challenges in metabolic syndrome in children and adolescents: a scientific statement from the American Heart Association Atherosclerosis, Hypertension, and Obesity in the Young Committee of the Council on Cardiovascular Disease in the Young; Council on Cardiovascular Nursing; and Council on Nutrition, Physical Activity, and Metabolism. *Circulation.* 2009;119(4):628-647

38. Okosun IS, Lyn R, Davis-Smith M, Eriksen M, Seale P. Validity of a continuous metabolic risk score as an index for modeling metabolic syndrome in adolescents. *Ann Epidemiol.* 2010;20(11):843-851
39. Woo KS, Chook P, Yu CW, et al. Effects of diet and exercise on obesity-related vascular dysfunction in children. *Circulation.* 2004;109(16):1981-1986
40. Andersen CJ, Fernandez ML. Dietary strategies to reduce metabolic syndrome. *Rev Endocr Metab Disord.* 2013;14(3):241-254
41. Keane D, Kelly S, Healy NP, McArdle MA, Holohan K, Roche HM. Diet and metabolic syndrome: an overview. *Curr Vasc Pharmacol.* 2013;11(6):842-857
42. Reinehr T, Kleber M, Toschke AM. Lifestyle intervention in obese children is associated with a decrease of the metabolic syndrome prevalence. *Atherosclerosis.* 2009;207(1):174-180
43. Orchard TJ, Temprosa M, Goldberg R, et al. The effect of metformin and intensive lifestyle intervention on the metabolic syndrome: the Diabetes Prevention Program randomized trial. *Ann Intern Med.* 2005;142(8):611-619
44. Harden KA, Cowan PA, Velasquez-Mieyer P, Patton SB. Effects of lifestyle intervention and metformin on weight management and markers of metabolic syndrome in obese adolescents. *J Am Acad Nurse Pract.* 2007;19(7):368-377
45. Florez H, Temprosa MG, Orchard TJ, et al. Metabolic syndrome components and their response to lifestyle and metformin interventions are associated with differences in diabetes risk in persons with impaired glucose tolerance. *Diabetes Obes Metab.* 2014;16(4):326-333
46. Nemet D, Barkan S, Epstein Y, Friedland O, Kowen G, Eliakim A. Short- and long-term beneficial effects of a combined dietary-behavioral-physical activity intervention for the treatment of childhood obesity. *Pediatrics.* 2005;115(4):e443-e449
47. Patton HM, Yates K, Unalp-Arida A, et al. Association between metabolic syndrome and liver histology among children with nonalcoholic fatty liver disease. *Am J Gastroenterol.* 2010;105(9): 2093-2102
48. Alfire ME, Treem WR. Nonalcoholic fatty liver disease. *Pediatr Ann.* 2006;35(4):290-294, 297-299
49. Roden M. Mechanisms of Disease: hepatic steatosis in type 2 diabetes: pathogenesis and clinical relevance. *Nat Clin Pract Endocrinol Metab.* 2006;2(6):335-348
50. Pacifico L, Nobili V, Anania C, Verdecchia P, Chiesa C. Pediatric nonalcoholic fatty liver disease, metabolic syndrome and cardiovascular risk. *World J Gastroenterol.* 2011;17(26):3082-3091
51. Gurka MJ, Ice CL, Sun SS, Deboer MD. A confirmatory factor analysis of the metabolic syndrome in adolescents: an examination of sex and racial/ethnic differences. *Cardiovasc Diabetol.* 2012;11: 128
52. Fuentes E, Fuentes F, Vilahur G, Badimon L, Palomo I. Mechanisms of chronic state of inflammation as mediators that link obese adipose tissue and metabolic syndrome. *Mediators Inflamm.* 2013;2013:136584
53. Fuentes E, Guzman-Jofre L, Moore-Carrasco R, Palomo I. Role of PPARs in inflammatory processes associated with metabolic syndrome (review). *Mol Med Rep.* 2013;8(6):1611-1616
54. Gray B, Steyn F, Davies PS, Vitetta L. Omega-3 fatty acids: a review of the effects on adiponectin and leptin and potential implications for obesity management. *Eur J Clin Nutr.* 2013;67(12):1234-1242
55. Zhang J, Li Y. Fibroblast growth factor 21, the endocrine FGF pathway and novel treatments for metabolic syndrome. *Drug Discovery Today.* 2014;19(5):579-589
56. Gulseth HL, Gjelstad IM, Birkeland KI, Drevon CA. Vitamin D and the metabolic syndrome. *Curr Vasc Pharmacol.* 2013;11(6):968-984
57. de la Iglesia R, Lopez-Legarrea P, Abete I, et al. A new dietary strategy for long-term treatment of the metabolic syndrome is compared with the American Heart Association (AHA) guidelines: the MEtabolic Syndrome REduction in NAvarra (RESMENA) project. *Br J Nutr.* 2014;111(4):643-652
58. Esfahani A, Wong JM, Truan J, et al. Health effects of mixed fruit and vegetable concentrates: a systematic review of the clinical interventions. *J Am Coll Nutr.* 2011;30(5):285-294
59. Esposito K, Kastorini CM, Panagiotakos DB, Giugliano D. Mediterranean diet and metabolic syndrome: an updated systematic review. *Rev Endocr Metab Disord.* 2013;14(3):255-263

60. Fernandez-Garcia JC, Cardona F, Tinahones FJ. Inflammation, oxidative stress and metabolic syndrome: dietary modulation. *Curr Vasc Pharmacol.* 2013;11(6):906-919
61. Molendi-Coste O, Legry V, Leclercq IA. Dietary lipids and NAFLD: suggestions for improved nutrition. *Acta Gastroenterol Belg.* 2010;73(4):431-436
62. Rayssiguier Y, Gueux E, Nowacki W, Rock E, Mazur A. High fructose consumption combined with low dietary magnesium intake may increase the incidence of the metabolic syndrome by inducing inflammation. *Magnes Res.* 2006;19(4):237-243
63. Yau PL, Castro MG, Tagani A, Tsui WH, Convit A. Obesity and metabolic syndrome and functional and structural brain impairments in adolescence. *Pediatrics.* 2012;130(4):e856-864
64. Reinehr T, Kleber M, Toschke AM. Small for gestational age status is associated with metabolic syndrome in overweight children. *Eur J Endocrinol.* 2009;160(4):579-584
65. Stefater MA, Kohli R, Inge TH. Advances in the surgical treatment of morbid obesity. *Mol Aspects Med.* 2013;34(1):84-94
66. Efstathiou SP, Skeva, II, Zorbala E, Georgiou E, Mountokalakis TD. Metabolic syndrome in adolescence: can it be predicted from natal and parental profile? The Prediction of Metabolic Syndrome in Adolescence (PREMA) study. *Circulation.* 2012;125(7):902-910

Adolesc Med 025 (2014) 455–472

Mindfulness and Adolescence: A Clinical Review of Recent Mindfulness-Based Studies in Clinical and Nonclinical Adolescent Populations

Dzung X. Vo, MD[a]; Jacqueline Doyle, DClinPsych, PhD[b]; Deborah Christie, DipClinPsych, PhD[c*]

[a]*Assistant Clinical Professor, Division of Adolescent Health and Medicine, Department of Pediatrics, University of British Columbia and British Columbia Children's Hospital, Vancouver, British Columbia, Canada;* [b]*Clinical Psychologist, Department of Child and Adolescent Psychological Services, University College Hospital London NHS Foundation Trust, London, United Kingdom;* [c]*Consultant Clinical Psychologist & Reader in Paediatric and Adolescent Health, Department of Child and Adolescent Psychological Services, University College Hospital London NHS Foundation Trust, London, United Kingdom*

INTRODUCTION

Mindfulness practices are now being used extensively in large institutions, which range from technology companies such as Google and Twitter, to traditional companies in the automotive and energy sectors, state-owned enterprises in China, United Nations (UN) organizations, governments, the World Bank, prison populations, and active military units. Reported widely across the political spectrum by mainstream media such as *The Telegraph* and *The Guardian* in the United Kingdom to the *New York Times* and Fox News in the United States, mindfulness initiatives and apps are regularly posted on Twitter, Facebook and other social media sites. Sessions on Mindfulness and mindful leadership events were oversubscribed at the 2013 Davos World Economic Forum. Mindfulness has hit the tipping point, with claims of wide-reaching benefits for general health and well-being as well as specific effects on pain and stress-related physical and emotional symptoms. The concept has also been attractive to those interested in improving business skills or performance and job satisfaction in an increasingly

---

*Corresponding author:
E-mail address: Deborah.christie@uclh.nhs.uk

 ISSN 1934-4287

frantic, technology-driven world. This article summarizes studies of mindfulness and mindfulness-based interventions in children and adolescents published in the last 5 years (2008-2013). Studies were identified using a number of electronic databases, including ScienceDirect, PsyARTICLES, PsychINFO, and PubMed. The article draws on the extensive clinical and research experience of the 3 authors, but it is not a systematic review. Further extensive hand searching was not carried out, and it is possible that some studies may have been missed.

Mindfulness practices are connected to and derived from versions of meditation skills usually taught in Eastern spiritual and psychological practices. Buddhist psychology made reference to the concept of mindfulness more than 2500 years ago. However, before it hit the current crest of the wave, mindfulness and its associated meditation practices were seen as esoteric, bound to religious beliefs, and relevant to only a minority. The shift from contemplative practice to mainstream Western medicine and clinical practice began just over 40 years ago. The best recognized Western definition of mindfulness comes from Dr Jon Kabat-Zinn, who recognized the benefits of mindfulness for people with stress-related chronic health problems and pain, which were difficult to diagnose and treat. He defines mindfulness as, "paying attention in a particular way: on purpose, in the present moment, and nonjudgementally."[1] Marsha Linehan, who also was strongly influenced by Eastern meditation traditions, integrated mindfulness practice into Western psychotherapy in dialectical behavior therapy (DBT), which is now a well-established, evidence-based treatment for adult women with borderline personality disorder.[2] Conceptual definitions of mindfulness have been continuously revised and clarified; however, all reflect its linguistic roots of awareness circumspection, discernment, and retention.[3]

Mindfulness is a quality of consciousness that is alive to the present reality. It requires the individual to pay attention, observe, describe, participate, and focus in an effective way on the present. This attentional focus is intentional and single minded, with a complete awareness of being in the present moment—on a moment-to-moment basis—attending to what is occurring in one's immediate experience in an open, accepting way with care and discernment.[4,5] It requires the individual to remain present on purpose, without attachment to any particular point of view. We are to notice the clarity and vividness of our current experience, focusing on what is actually happening to us and in us at each successive moment.

A mindfulness stance is deliberately nonjudgmental and receptive to the whole field of awareness, remaining in an open state, directed to currently experienced sensations, thoughts, emotions, and memories.[6] It is argued that an ethical dimension is also inherent to the cultivation of mindfulness and, some argue, is necessary for its therapeutic and healing effect. Mindfulness practice cultivates not only a neutral, dispassionate, or amoral present-moment awareness but also an attitude or intention of compassion for oneself and for others.[7]

Mindfulness has slowly acquired the status of an "inherent quality of human consciousness," which is in direct contrast to mindlessness whereby attention and awareness capacities are scattered because of preoccupation with past memories or future plans.[8] It is the very antithesis to functioning on automatic pilot or responding in a habitual manner that may be a chronic way of being for many individuals.[9]

The degree to which we can develop this capacity of attention and awareness oriented to the present moment varies in degree within and between individuals. However, major strides have been made in the last decade to provide a valid operational definition of mindfulness and to show that the capacity for mindfulness can be assessed empirically and independent of religious, spiritual, or cultural beliefs.

A number of scales have been developed that claim to measure mindfulness as a dispositional characteristic, an outcome, or a practice.[10-14] Neuroscience has also started to provide evidence of changes in the brain's structure as a result of mindfulness practice.[15-20] The ability to examine both the associations and the influences of mindfulness on psychological, biologic, behavioral, and social variables has contributed to a greater ability to study mindfulness on a scientific level.

WHAT IS MINDFULNESS PRACTICE?

Mindfulness practices have been formally described in programs such as Mindfulness-Based Stress Reduction (MBSR) and Mindfulness-Based Cognitive Therapy (MBCT) as well as in a number of interventions described more generically as Mindfulness-Based Interventions (MBI), which use different aspects of MBSR and MBCT and incorporate meditation practices, yoga, and other therapeutic approaches.

The most well-known mindfulness based approaches are MBSR and MBCT. The MBSR program was developed by Jon Kabat-Zinn in 1979, at the University of Massachusetts Medical Center, for adults experiencing stress and pain related to chronic medical problems.[1] MBCT was developed as a modification of MBSR, with the goal of preventing depressive relapse in adults with chronic depression.[21] Both approaches follow a predefined 8-week course structure in which participants are taught key mindfulness practices. These include formal mindfulness practices that require dedicated time for meditation, such as the body scan, mindful movement, walking meditations, and sitting meditations, as well as informal mindfulness practices, in which participants are invited to bring the same nonjudgmental, present-moment awareness to daily activities such as walking, eating, chores, and work. In MBCT there are additional specific exercises, borrowed from cognitive therapy, designed to help participants identify habitual (and useless) thought patterns and ruminations that fuel anxiety and depression. There is an emphasis on developing a new relationship with the process of thinking, which involves mindfully observing thoughts as they come and go without necessarily believing, accepting, or getting carried away by them.

Sessions usually include

1. Didactic teaching related to mindfulness (eg, session 1 introduces the concept of automatic pilot).
2. A guided formal mindfulness meditation practice(s), often lasting up to 40 minutes each.
3. A facilitated inquiry process in which participants are invited to share their experiences of the meditation and make links between these experiences and their usual habitual patterns and behaviors.
4. Discussion of home-based practices, obstacles to practice, and what they reveal for every day life. MBSR and MBCT ask participants to commit to daily formal and informal mindfulness practices. Many programs also include a day-long retreat half way through the course, which is often conducted in silence for most of the day and offers an opportunity for participants to deepen their meditational practice.

Workbooks and audio CDs are included to support home practices. Despite its Buddhist roots and use of compassion-based and loving kindness meditations, neither MBSR nor MBCT is tied to a specific religious orientation. A recent meta-analysis of mindfulness-based interventions for youth in 20 studies reported that the interventions had a small-to-moderate effect. The greatest effect on psychological symptoms was in studies that used clinical samples.[22]

ADAPTING MINDFULNESS FOR ADOLESCENTS

Adaptations of traditional MBSR and MBCT interventions may offer an important addition to existing approaches for adolescents, although methodologically rigorous studies are lacking.[23-25] Reviews assessing the potential health benefits of mindfulness-based therapies report evidence supporting the merits of mindfulness-based interventions for adolescents to decrease anxiety, reduce stress, and improve general psychological well-being in both well and chronically ill adolescents.[26-28] Lagor et al[29] emphasize the need to address the frequency and number of sessions, the amount of between-session practice required, group size, and age rather than gender in creating groups, as well as the role of external rewards for participation when developing a mindfulness-based intervention for chronically ill youth. Most studies described here addressed these issues when adapting the adult-based programs. In some studies, home practice exercises were reduced to 10 to 35 minutes[30] and meditation sessions were made brief and frequent, using a range of methods to elucidate the concepts of mindfulness, such as mindful drawing, listening to music mindfully, and sculpting.[31] Most interventions did not include a daylong retreat or omitted certain practices. For example, Britton et al[30] did not make use of mindful movement/yoga sessions. In contrast, other studies placed a greater emphasis on the use of certain practices, for example, the use of the loving kindness meditation (an exercise of wishing well to self and others), to address low self-esteem in relation to attention-deficit/hyperactivity disorder (ADHD).[32]

Programs are also tailored to address issues relevant to specific clinic populations. For example, Biegel et al[31] included discussion of self-harm, image difficulties, and communication and interpersonal problems as an integral part of their program for adolescent psychiatric outpatients, whereas Britton et al[30] added sessions on sleep education and sleep hygiene in their mindfulness-based sleep intervention for adolescents attending substance abuse treatment centers. Several studies altered the overall number of sessions (5-20) as well as the duration of each session (1.5-2.5 hours).[31,33-36]

Mindfulness training has been used to specifically address issues of attention and impulsivity in adolescents. For example, in 1 task, adolescents were presented with half of their favorite bar of chocolate and told that they would receive the other half only if they waited until the trainers returned. Role play and exercises focusing on the sensation of breathing were encouraged to train attention and bring awareness to distracting thoughts feelings and sensations, which assisted participants in the process of waiting.[34] In another study of ADHD, adolescents were encouraged to practice focusing on their breath while being distracted by other participants, in order to become aware of distractibility in different situations.[37]

Thompson and Gauntlett-Gilbert[27] recommend developmentally appropriate clinical modifications for mindfulness with children and adolescents, including greater explanation and rationales, more emphasis on everyday informal mindfulness practices, developmentally appropriate metaphors and imagery, skillful use of variety and repetition, and shorter length of formal mindfulness practices. They emphasize the need to make written material accessible and appropriate for the developmental needs and reading age of the participants, such as simplifying the language used and making it more concrete.

Logistical adaptations to ensure participation (eg, sending reminders to participants to do home-based practices and to attend classes, and providing incentives for participation and cooperation) may help maximize adherence.[28] In 2 studies, mindfulness training was offered to parents in parallel with the sessions attended by the adolescents.[34,37] The standard MBCT course was adapted to encourage mindful and nonjudgmental observation and listening, with an emphasis on mindful parenting, communication, and cultivation of acceptance of the things about behavior that may remain unchanged. Parents were encouraged to practice daily, both as role models and for their own self-improvement. Increasingly it can be argued that mindfulness has a role with families and parents of adolescents.[38,39]

MINDFULNESS-BASED STRESS REDUCTION

Programs following the original MBSR structure have been used in nonclinical urban youth and college populations to lower stress and improve general psychological well-being. Participants report less anxiety, rumination, and negative coping mechanisms, as well as reductions in hostility and general and emotional discomfort.[40-42] For adolescents with a variety of mental health problems, a preliminary report suggested that a 5-week group mindfulness-based intervention led to significant decreases in psychological distress and increases in mindfulness and self-esteem.[32] MBSR modified for teens has also shown reduced anxiety and depression as well as improved global functioning in psychiatric outpatients[31] and has been described as an acceptable and feasible stress-reduction intervention for youth with human immunodeficiency virus (HIV).[35]

MINDFULNESS YOGA

Mindfulness yoga, which is based on MBSR, has been evaluated in 3 school-based study populations. It has been shown to enhance adaptive responses to stress and to increase self-esteem and self-regulation in these nonclinical populations.[43-45]

MINDFULNESS-BASED COGNITIVE THERAPY

A number of researchers have adapted MBCT for children and adolescents. Studies of mindfulness meditation training with adolescents having ADHD as well as a range of externalizing disorders such as oppositional defiant disorder, conduct disorder, and Asperger syndrome with externalizing behavioral problems found improvements in self-reported ADHD symptoms and performance in neurocognitive tasks (attention and set shifting), a reduction in attention and behavioral problems, and an increase in executive functioning.[33,34,37] MBCT has also been shown to improve emotional problems, depressive symptoms, anxiety, hopelessness, and perceived academic stress, and to increase academic performance in HIV-infected youth.[35,46] A randomized waitlist-controlled trial of MBCT for Children (MBCT-C) aged 9 to 13 years with reading problems, stress, and anxiety demonstrated improvements in anxiety symptoms, behavioral problems, and attention.[47] However, a randomized trial of young adults with social phobia did not show a benefit of MBCT relative to the group with cognitive behavior therapy (CBT).[48]

ACCEPTANCE AND COMMITMENT THERAPY

Acceptance and commitment therapy (ACT) has theoretical and philosophical roots similar to those for mindfulness and emphasizes increased psychological flexibility without active targeting of symptom reduction. ACT uses formal mindfulness practices and teaching; integrates acceptance training, values-based living, and behavioral change; and has been proposed as a therapeutic modality for children and adolescents.[49] ACT has been used with young adult woman attending college to help reduce sexual revictimization after childhood sexual abuse.[50] Pilot data and case reports suggest a potential role of ACT in the treatment of adolescent depression,[51,52] anorexia nervosa,[53] and chronic pain.[54] However, because many of these reports are single-case studies, there is little robust evidence for ACT in this age group.

DIALECTICAL BEHAVIOR THERAPY FOR ADOLESCENTS

Dialectical behavior therapy has been used for treatment of adolescents with borderline features[55] and suicidal adolescents.[56] It is an adaptation of CBT, which traditionally has focused on helping people change unhelpful ways of thinking and behaving. DBT helps people change, but it differs from CBT in that it focuses on accepting who you are at the same time. Therapists use mindfulness as part of the *acceptance techniques* that are balanced with *change techniques*. Developmentally appropriate modifications to DBT include emphasis on behavioral targets and emotional regulation rather than specific diagnoses (eg, borderline personality disorder), involvement of families and schools when appropriate, and use of age-appropriate language and skills training. Evidence supporting DBT in the adolescent population remains preliminary.

OTHER MINDFULNESS-BASED INTERVENTIONS FOR SPECIFIC CONDITIONS

Table 1 summarizes a number of studies on specific populations using adapted and modified mindfulness-based meditations.

MINDFULNESS IN SCHOOLS

A recent publication on mindfulness and schools clearly highlights the potential role of mindfulness within the school curriculum.[73] There is promising evidence that mindfulness training in educational settings can enhance a range of cognitive, social, and psychological outcomes across all grades and years, as well as improve teachers' well-being and classroom management.[74] One example is the Learning to Breathe mindfulness curriculum, which has shown improvements in emotion regulation and decreases in aches and pains and negative affect.[75,76] Other programs have found improved psychological well-being,[77] social and emotional competence,[78] and reductions in depression postintervention and at 6-month follow-up.[79,80] MindUP is a school-based mindfulness training program that has demonstrated improved social and emotional competence in 9- to 12-year olds.[78] Preliminary research has shown that Mindful Schools, another school-based program mostly in inner city schools in North America, shows promise for reducing depressive symptoms (www.mindfulschools.org/about-mindfulness/research/#research).[81] In the United Kingdom, the .b (dot b) program is a 9-lesson curriculum

Table 1
Studies on specific populations using adapted and modified mindfulness-based meditations

Population	Study type	Results	Reference
Individuals with mild to severe developmental disabilities (13-43 years)	Systematic review of 12 studies	Reduced behavioral and psychological problems	Hwang et al[57]
Adolescents with learning disabilities	Noncontrolled study	Reduction in anxiety, promotion of social skills, improved academic performance	Beauchemin et al[58]
Adolescent boys with learning disabilities and co-occurring attention-deficit/hyperactivity disorder and anxiety	20-week group program in clinical setting	No overall improvements in executive functioning or social skills; parent-rated improvements in externalizing behavior, oppositional defiant problems, and conduct problems; decreased anxiety in subgroups with elevated anxiety levels	Haydicky et al[36]
Aggression	Critical review of 11 studies	Group studies had weak design; single-subject studies showed encouraging results	Fix et al[59]
Asperger syndrome and autism	Clinical program "Soles of the Feet"	Decreased rates of aggression during training maintained at 4-year follow up	Singh et al[60,61]
Adolescent girls with sleep difficulties	Pilot of school based group intervention	Improved sleep onset latency, self-efficacy, total sleep time, earlier bedtime, smaller day-to-day bedtime variation	Bei et al[62]

Youth with substance use disorders	Outpatient multicomponent behavioral sleep intervention	Improvements in sleep and distress; increased sleep duration	Britton et al[30]
Adolescent with Prader-Willi syndrome	Single case study	Reduction in weight at 3-year follow-up	Singh et al[63]
Adolescents with cancer	Review of mindfulness studies and relationship to cancer	Concludes has capacity to help adolescents with cancer and improve psychosocial and quality-of-life outcomes	Jones et al[64]
Adolescents with cancer	Protocol for randomized controlled trial	Study design only	Malboef-Hurtboise et al[65]
Adolescent female with chronic pain	Single case study	Improved reporting of symptoms	Wicksell[54]
Pediatric chronic pain	Randomized controlled pilot study	Reduced reporting of pain	Jastrowski et al[66]
Incarcerated and homeless youth	Qualitative study	Youth reported positively on experience	Himelstein et al[67]
Incarcerated and homeless youth	Pilot of group program	Decrease in perceived stress and increased in healthy self regulation	Himelstein et al[68]
Incarcerated and homeless youth	Quasi-experimental pre-post study	Improved spirituality, mental wellness, psychological symptoms, resilience	Grabbe et al[69]
Incarcerated youth and substance abuse	Mixed methods pilot study	Decrease in impulsiveness, increase in risk of drug taking	Himelstein[70]
Young adult female marijuana users	Pilot study	Reduced marijuana use in intervention group	deDios et al[71]
College smokers	Randomized controlled trial	No difference in urge to smoke but intervention group showed reduction in smoking	Bowen et al[72]

developed by the Mindfulness in Schools project to promote mental health and well-being. A nonrandomized controlled trial demonstrated positive results, including less depression and stress and greater well-being reported in the intervention group (mindfulnessinschools.org/).[82]

YOUNG PEOPLE'S EXPERIENCE

Young people's qualitative experience of participating in mindfulness practice is extremely positive, with reports that mindfulness increases a sense of calm, balance, and control. They describe mindfulness as helping them develop a mindset that they associate with greater confidence and competence and less future distress.[83,84]

TEACHING MINDFULNESS

In-depth formal mindfulness training can be offered in systematic curricula such as MBSR, MBCT, DBT, or ACT, in an individual or family format as well as in a group format. In addition, it is possible to teach mindfulness in more informal ways in the medical or mental health clinic office setting. Pediatricians and primary care physicians can integrate brief mindfulness practices into clinic visits with youth suffering from chronic stress, anxiety, depression, or pain.[85] Physicians may consider modifying and adapting components of mindfulness-based interventions for more limited individual clinical applications; for example, focusing teaching for a youth with chronic pain on increasing awareness of all parts of their body, not just those where pain is located, and practicing mindfulness to cope with pain. There is little systematic evidence on brief individual mindfulness training in the medical or mental health office setting. However, there are several Web sites and mobile apps that physicians can use or refer to young people, which contain mindfulness practice instructions and guided mindfulness meditation recordings (Table 2).

Proponents of clinical mindfulness interventions argue that mindfulness instructors must have substantial personal experience with mindfulness practice and

Table 2
Website and mobile apps that contain guided mindfulness meditation recordings.

Stop Breathe & Think
stopbreathethink.org/
Smiling Mind
smilingmind.com.au/
Calm
www.calm.com
Mindshift
itunes.apple.com/ca/app/mindshift/id634684825?mt=8
play.google.com/store/apps/details?id=com.bstro.MindShift
Kelty Mental Health Resource Centre
keltymentalhealth.ca/healthy-living/mindfulness

should teach from their own direct experience of mindfulness.[7,86] The Center for Mindfulness in Medicine, Health Care, and Society at the University of Massachusetts, which includes many of the founders and leaders of MBSR, offers a structured MBSR teacher training pathway, which includes daily personal mindfulness practice, and practice in a residential retreat environment (www.umassmed.edu/cfm/oasis/indepth/index.aspx). The expectation that mindfulness teachers and instructors have their own regular mindfulness practice is grounded in the clinical experience that teaching mindfulness goes beyond sharing intellectual content or knowledge, exclusively relying on a written curriculum, or reading a script. Teaching mindfulness is a lived expression of mindfulness. It requires an element of role modeling and embodying a mindful presence, as well as having a lived experience of practicing mindfulness to cope with stress or pain. The Center for Mindfulness in Medicine, Health Care, and Society proposes that "Teaching MBSR is an expression of mindfulness as a way of being in wise relationship with your experience, and is never a matter of merely operationalizing techniques" (www.umassmed.edu/cfm/oasis/indepth/index.aspx).

Kabat-Zinn[86(p. xi)] has written that "...Our cardinal working principle is that the teaching has to come out of one's practice. Thus, to the bones of the curriculum need to be added the flesh and sinews of one's own experience with practice." Similarly, Segal et al[21(p. 419)] propose that for teachers of MBCT, "In order to do [teach MBCT], therapists should practice mindfulness themselves."

MINDFULNESS FOR PHYSICIANS

Mindfulness practice has received increasing attention as a tool for many, but particularly for health care professionals and their clients. In addition to being instrumental for teaching mindfulness in clinical settings as described earlier, mindfulness practice may improve patient care and help heath care professionals manage burnout. Mindfulness can be considered a core clinical skill for patient care professionals[87,88] and may help physicians increase patient-centered care and communication; improve physicians' critical self-reflection and clarity in decision-making; and help them clarify their own values to be able to act with more compassion. Mindfulness practice promotes qualities that patients value in their health care professionals, including attentiveness, nonjudgmental listening, compassion, presence, and creative and collaborative problem-solving. Conversely, lack of mindfulness (which we described earlier as *mindlessness*) may contribute to clinical errors, technical errors, lack of awareness of the physician's own bias, and poor communication.

Mindfulness practice may also be a powerful self-care and stress management tool for physicians to manage burnout and secondary trauma and to enhance work satisfaction. Physician burnout is associated with lower quality of care, patient dissatisfaction, increased medical errors, and decreased ability to communicate with empathy.[89] Physician burnout is also associated with significant personal and family morbidities.[89] A uncontrolled pilot study of physicians trained in mindful communication showed improvements in well-being with a more patient-centered orientation to clinical care. Thirty primary care physicians who underwent a short mindfulness training course showed improvements in job satisfaction and quality of life, as well as reduced levels of emotional exhaustion, depression, anxiety, and stress for up to 9 months after the course.[90] In a multicenter observational study of physicians caring for HIV-infected patients, the investigators measured physician mindfulness and patient satisfaction, as well as analyzing audio recordings of physician-patient interaction. Physicians who scored higher on the mindfulness scale had a more positive emotional tone, engaged in more patient-centered communication, and had more satisfied patients.[91] Despite the potential benefits of mindfulness for health care professionals, teaching and maintaining mindfulness practice in health training and clinical environments can be quite challenging.[87]

FUTURE DIRECTIONS

A number of research questions have been generated from these series of studies. Most critical is the lack of evidence from rigorous randomized controlled trials. There are a number of questions that more rigorous methodology may be able to answer.

Dosage

The relationship between outcome and the amount of meditation practice including overall length of interventions and number of sessions required is not clear). Furthermore, are there specific practices that might be more challenging for certain clinical groups? Bogels et al[34] talk of the dilemma of shorter versus longer practices. Children with a diagnosis of ADHD seemed to struggle with the longer practices, such as the body scan. Although shorter practices may have been more feasible and acceptable to the patients, learning to tolerate the potential boredom of longer exercises may have more relevance in real-life situations such as school.

What Specific Aspects of Mindfulness Practices Are Key?

Many interventions include multiple components, such as mindfulness meditation, CBT, and behavior modification. Interventions also may include social support, other psychological approaches, or training in communication techniques such as motivational interviewing. It is not clear which aspects of a given intervention are most likely to bring about change and the relative importance of the MBI elements used.

Translating Qualitative into Quantitative Outcomes

Process evaluations from adolescent participants are wholeheartedly positive, with some young people describing *transformational shifts*.[82] However, quantitative outcomes are less definitive, with small effect sizes often noted. In addition, the rhetoric used by some of the participants is about achieving enhanced self-control. The aim of MBSR/MBCT and other mindfulness practices such as ACT is not to fix or impose self-control (ie, in the form of suppression of thoughts and feelings) but to allow awareness and choice of ways to respond, rather than reacting habitually. These nuances are worthy of further attention.

Are There Populations In Whom Mindfulness Doesn't Work?

At the present time it is not clear whether there are groups of clinical populations for whom mindfulness may be contraindicated or for whom mindfulness-based group interventions may not be appropriate. For example, Bogels et al[34] described the training process as *hard work* because some of the adolescents with externalizing disorders in the study had difficulty concentrating and showed overt nonadherence. In the parent group, some of the parents came late, did not do the home-based tasks, or were themselves disruptive to the other parents. Although the authors talked about learning to trust the eventual effect of the group process, they also suggested that young people with a diagnosis of oppositional defiant disorder/conduct disorder might learn best by being taught mindfulness in an individual setting. There is evidence for mindfulness-based approaches for eating disorders in adult populations.[92] Although some suggestions have arisen from these adult studies on how mindfulness might be applied to children and adolescents, to date no methodologically sound studies have been reported for the younger age group. Finally, a possible area of investigation is the potential role of mindfulness in adolescents with acute depressive symptoms, anxiety, or pain. It is not clear whether mindfulness is only suited to adolescents with chronic or stable symptoms, or whether its use could be expanded into the acute setting.

CONCLUSION

Mindfulness with adolescents shows promise in a variety of settings and populations. Positive reports have been published describing improvements in mental health, executive functioning, and emotional regulation, in clinical as well as in school and community settings. Mindfulness practice also seems to be beneficial for adults who work and care for adolescents, including health care professionals, educators, and parents. Rigorous clinical research in the area is still in its early phases, and many questions remain. Professional and mainstream interest is exploding, and the potential for creative and original applications of mindfulness-based approaches is enormous. The time is now to rapidly develop practice and research in this area.

References

1. Kabat-Zinn J. *Full Catastrophe Living: Using the Wisdom of Your Body and Mind to Face Stress, Pain, and Illness.* New York, NY: Random House LLC; 2009

2. Linehan M. *Cognitive Behavioral Treatment of Borderline Personality Disorder.* New York, NY: Guilford Press; 1993
3. Shapiro SL. The integration of mindfulness and psychology. *J Clin Psychol.* 2009;65(6):555-560
4. Shapiro SL, Carlson LE. *The Art and Science of Mindfulness: Integrating Mindfulness Into Psychology and the Helping Professions.* Washington, DC: APA; 2009
5. Brown KW, Ryan RM. Perils and promise in defining and measuring mindfulness: observations from experience. *Clin Psychol Sci Pract.* 2004;11(3):242-248
6. Jha AP, Krompinger J, Baime MJ. Mindfulness training modifies subsystems of attention. *Cogn Affect Behav Neurosci.* 2007;7(2):109-119
7. Kabat-Zinn J. Some reflections on the origins of MBSR, skillful means, and the trouble with maps. *Contemp Buddhism.* 2011;12(1):281-306
8. Siegel DJ. Mindfulness training and neural integration: differentiation of distinct streams of awareness and the cultivation of well-being. *SCAN.* 2007;2(4):259-263
9. Brown KW, Ryan RM. The benefits of being present: mindfulness and its role in psychological well-being. *J Pers Soc Psychol.* 2003;84(4):822-848
10. Baer RA, Smith GT, Allen KB. Assessment of mindfulness by self-report: the Kentucky inventory of mindfulness skills. *Assessment.* 2004;11(3):191-206
11. Lau MA, Bishop SR, Segal ZV, et al. The Toronto Mindfulness Scale: development and validation. *J Clin Psychol.* 2006;62(12):1445-1467
12. Feldman G, Hayes A, Kumar S, et al. Mindfulness and emotion regulation: the development and initial validation of the Cognitive and Affective Mindfulness Scale—Revised (CAMS-R). *J Psychopathol Behav Assess.* 2007;29(3):177-190
13. Buchheld N, Grossman P, Walach H. Measuring mindfulness in insight meditation (vipassana) and meditation-based psychotherapy: the development of the Freiburg mindfulness inventory (FMI). *J Meditat Meditat Res.* 2001;1(1):11-34
14. Cardaciotto L, Herbert JD, Forman, EM, Moitra E, Farrow V. The assessment of present-moment awareness and acceptance: the Philadelphia mindfulness scale. *Assessment.* 2008;15(2):204-223
15. Hölzel BK, Carmody J, Evans KC, et al. Stress reduction correlates with structural changes in the amygdala. *Soc Cogn Affect Neurosci.* 2010;5(1):11-17
16. Hölzel BK, Carmody J, Vangel M, et al. Mindfulness practice leads to increases in regional brain gray matter density. *Psychiatry Res.* 2011;191(1):36-43
17. Luders E, Clark K, Narr KL, Toga AW. Enhanced brain connectivity in long-term meditation practitioners. *NeuroImage.* 2011;57(4):1308-1316
18. Lazar SW, Kerr CE, Wasserman RH, et al. Meditation experience is associated with increased cortical thickness. *Neuroreport.* 2005;16(17):1893-1897
19. Brefczynski-Lewis JA, Lutz A, Schaefer HS, Levinson DB, Davidson RJ. Neural correlates of attentional expertise in long-term meditation practitioners. *Proc Natl Acad Sci U S A.* 2007;104(27):11483-11488
20. Lutz A, Brefczynski-Lewis J, Johnstone T, Davidson RJ. Regulation of the neural circuitry of emotion by compassion meditation: effects of meditative expertise. *PloS One.* 2008;3(3):e1897. doi: 10.1371/journal.pone.0001897
21. Segal ZV, Williams JMG, Teasdale JD. *Mindfulness-Based Cognitive Therapy for Depression.* 2nd ed. New York, NY: Guilford Press; 2012
22. Zoogman S, Goldberg SB, Hoyt WT, Miller L. Mindfulness interventions with youth: a meta-analysis. *Mindfulness.* 2014;1-13
23. Burke CA. Mindfulness-based approaches with children and adolescents: a preliminary review of current research in an emergent field. *J Child Fam Stud.* 2010;19:133-144
24. Harnett PH, Dawe S. The contribution of mindfulness-based therapies for children and families and proposed conceptual integration. *Child Adolesc Mental Health.* 2012;17(4):195-308
25. Greenberg MT, Harris AR. Nurturing mindfulness in children and youth: current state of research. *Child Dev Perspect.* 2012;6(2):161-166
26. Shonin E, Van Gordon W, Griffiths MD. The health benefits of mindfulness-based interventions for children and adolescents. *Educ Health.* 2012;30:94-97

27. Thompson M, Gauntlett-Gilbert J. Mindfulness with children and adolescents: effective clinical application. *Clin Child Psychol Psychiatry.* 2008;13(3):395-407
28. Black DS, Milam J, Sussman S. Sitting-meditation interventions among youth: a review of treatment efficacy. *Pediatrics.* 2009;124(3):e532-e541
29. Lagor AF, Williams DJ, Lerner JB, McClure KS. Lessons learned from a mindfulness-based intervention with chronically ill youth. *Clin Pract Pediatr Psychol.* 2013;1(2):146
30. Britton WB, Bootzin RR, Cousins JC, et al. The contribution of mindfulness practice to a multicomponent behavioral sleep intervention following substance abuse treatment in adolescents: a treatment-development study. *Subst Abuse.* 2010;31(2):86-97
31. Biegel GM, Brown KW, Shapiro SL, Schubert CM. Mindfulness-based stress reduction for the treatment of adolescent psychiatric outpatients: a randomized clinical trial. *J Consult Clin Psychol.* 2009;77(5):855-866
32. Tan L, Martin G. Taming the adolescent mind: preliminary report of a mindfulness-based psychological intervention for adolescents with clinical heterogeneous mental health diagnoses. *Clin Child Psychol Psychiatry.* 2013;18(2):300-312
33. Zylowska L, Ackerman DL, Yang MH, et al. Mindfulness meditation training in adults and adolescents with ADHD: a feasibility study. *J Atten Disord.* 2008;11(6):737-746
34. Bögels S, Hoogstad B, van Dun L, de Schutter S, Restifo K. Mindfulness training for adolescents with externalizing disorders and their parents. *Behav Cogn Psychother.* 2008;36(2):193-209
35. Sibinga E, Stewart M, Magyari T, Welsh CK, Hutton N, Ellen JM. Mindfulness-based stress reduction for HIV-infected youth: a pilot study. *Explore J Sci Healing.* 2008;4(1):36-37
36. Haydicky J, Wiener J, Badali P, Milligan K, Ducharme JM. Evaluation of a mindfulness-based intervention for adolescents with learning disabilities and co-occurring ADHD and anxiety. *Mindfulness.* 2012;3(2):151-164
37. Van de Weijer-Bergsma E, Formsma AR, de Bruin EI, Bögels SM. The effectiveness of mindfulness training on behavioral problems and attentional functioning in adolescents with ADHD. *J Child Fam Stud.* 2012;21(5):775-787
38. Hastings RP, Singh NN. Mindfulness, children, and families. *J Child Fam Stud.* 2010;19(2):131-132
39. Sawyer Cohen JA, Semple RJ. Mindful parenting: a call for research. *J Child Fam Stud.* 2009;19(2):145-151
40. Anand U, Sharma MP. Impact of a mindfulness-based stress reduction program on stress and well-being in school going adolescents: a preliminary study. *Neuropsychiatr Enfance Adolesc.* 2012;60(5):S129
41. Oman D, Shapiro SL, Thoresen CE, Plante TG, Flinders T. Meditation lowers stress and supports forgiveness among college students: a randomized controlled trial. *J Am Coll Health.* 2008;56(5):569-578
42. Sibinga EM, Kerrigan D, Stewart M, Johnson K, Magyari T, Ellen JM. Mindfulness-based stress reduction for urban youth. *J Altern Complement Med.* 2011;17(3):213-218
43. Mendelson T, Greenberg MT, Dariotis JK, et al. Feasibility and preliminary outcomes of a school-based mindfulness intervention for urban youth. *J Abnorm Child Psychol.* 2010;38(7):985-994
44. White LS. Reducing stress in school-age girls through mindful yoga. *J Pediatr Health Care.* 2012;26(1):45-56
45. Gould LF, Dariotis JK, Mendelson T, Greenberg M. A school-based mindfulness intervention for urban youth: exploring moderators of intervention effects. *J Commun Psychol.* 2012;40(8): 968-982
46. Sinha UK, Kumar D. Mindfulness-based cognitive behaviour therapy with emotionally disturbed adolescents affected by HIV/AIDS. *J Indian Assoc Child Adolesc Mental Health.* 2010;6(1)19-30
47. Semple RJ, Lee J, Rosa D, Miller LF. A randomized trial of mindfulness-based cognitive therapy for children: Promoting mindful attention to enhance social-emotional resiliency in children. *J Child Family Stud.* 2010;19:218-229
48. Piet J, Hougaard E, Hecksher MS, Rosenberg NK. A randomized pilot study of mindfulness-based cognitive therapy and group cognitive-behavioral therapy for young adults with social phobia. *Scand J Psychol.* 2010;51(5):403-410

49. O'Brien KM, Larson CM, Murrell AR. Third-wave behavior therapies for children and adolescents: progress, challenges, and future directions. In: Greco LA, Hayes SC, eds. *Acceptance and Mindfulness Treatments for Children and Adolescents: A Practitioner's Guide*. Oakland, CA: New Harbinger Publications; 2008:15-35
50. Hill JM, Vernig PM, Lee JK, Brown C, Orsillo SM. The development of a brief acceptance and mindfulnessbased program aimed at reducing sexual revictimization among college women with a history of childhood sexual abuse. *J Clin Psychol.* 2011;67(9):969-980
51. Hayes L, Boyd CP, Sewell J. Acceptance and commitment therapy for the treatment of adolescent depression: a pilot study in a psychiatric outpatient setting. *Mindfulness.* 2011;2(2):86-94
52. Hayes L, Bach PA, Boyd CP. Psychological treatment for adolescent depression: perspectives on the past, present, and future. *Behav Change.* 2010;27(1):1-18
53. Heffner M, Sperry J, Eifert GH, Detweiler M. Acceptance and commitment therapy in the treatment of an adolescent female with anorexia nervosa: a case example. *Cogn Behav Pract.* 2002;9(3):232-236
54. Wicksell RK, Dahl J, Magnusson B, Olsson GL. Using acceptance and commitment therapy in the rehabilitation of an adolescent female with chronic pain: a case example. *Cogn Behav Pract.* 2005;12(4):415-423
55. Woodberry KA, Roy R, Indik J. Dialectical behaviour therapy for adolescents with borderline features. In: Greco LA, Hayes SC, eds. *Acceptance and Mindfulness Treatments for Children And Adolescents: A Practitioner's Guide*. Oakland, CA: New Harbinger Publications; 2008:115-138
56. Miller AL, Rathus JH, Linehan MM. *Dialectical Behavior Therapy with Suicidal Adolescents*. New York, NY: Guilford Press; 2006
57. Hwang YS, Kearney P. A systematic review of mindfulness intervention for individuals with developmental disabilities: long-term practice and long lasting effects. *Res Dev Disabil.* 2013;34(1): 314-326
58. Beauchemin J, Hutchins TL, Patterson F. Mindfulness meditation may lessen anxiety, promote social skills, and improve academic performance among adolescents with learning disabilities. *Complement Health Pract Rev.* 2008;13(1):34-45
59. Fix RL, Fix ST. The effects of mindfulness-based treatments for aggression: a critical review. *Aggress Violent Behav.* 2013;18(2):219-227
60. Singh NN, Lancioni GE, Singh AD, Winton AS, Singh AN, Singh J. Adolescents with Asperger syndrome can use a mindfulness-based strategy to control their aggressive behavior. *Res Autism Spectr Dis.* 2011;5(3):1103-1109
61. Singh NN, Lancioni GE, Manikam R, et al. A mindfulness-based strategy for self-management of aggressive behavior in adolescents with autism. *Res Autism Spectr Disord.* 2011;5(3):1153-1158
62. Bei B, Byrne ML, Ivens C, et al. Pilot study of a mindfulness-based, multi-component, in-school group sleep intervention in adolescent girls. *Early Interv Psychiatry.* 2013;7(2):213-220
63. Singh NN, Lancioni GE, Singh AN, Winton AS, Singh J, McAleavey KM, Adkins AD. A mindfulness-based health wellness program for an adolescent with Prader-Willi syndrome. *Behav Modif.* 2008;32(2):167-181
64. Jones P, Blunda M, Biegel G, et al. Can mindfulness-based interventions help adolescents with cancer? *Psychooncology.* 2013;22(9):2148-2151
65. Malboeuf-Hurtubise C, Achille M, Sultan S, Vadnais M. Mindfulness-based intervention for teenagers with cancer: study protocol for a randomized controlled trial. *Trials.* 2013;14(1):135
66. Jastrowski Mano KE, Salamon KS, Hainsworth KR, et al. A randomized, controlled pilot study of mindfulness-based stress reduction for pediatric chronic pain. *Altern Ther Health Med.* 2013; 19(6):8-14
67. Himelstein S, Hastings A, Shapiro S, Heery M. A qualitative investigation of the experience of a mindfulness-based intervention with incarcerated adolescents. *Child Adolesc Mental Health.* 2012;17(4):231-237
68. Himelstein S, Hastings A, Shapiro S, Heery M. Mindfulness training for self-regulation and stress with incarcerated youth: a pilot study. *Probat J.* 2012;59(2):151-165

69. Grabbe L, Nguy ST, Higgins MK. Spirituality development for homeless youth: a mindfulness meditation feasibility pilot. *J Child Fam Stud.* 2012;21(6):925-937
70. Himelstein S. Mindfulness-based substance abuse treatment for incarcerated youth: a mixed method pilot study. *Int J Transpers Stud.* 2011;30(1-2):1-10
71. de Dios MA, Herman DS, Britton WB, et al. Motivational and mindfulness intervention for young adult female marijuana users. *J Subst Abuse Treat.* 2012;42(1):56-64
72. Bowen S, Marlatt A. Surfing the urge: brief mindfulness-based intervention for college student smokers. *Psychol Addict Behav.* 2009;23(4):666-671
73. Frank JL, Jennings PA, Greenberg MT. Mindfulness-based interventions in school settings: An introduction to the special issue. *Res Hum Dev.* 2013;10(3). Available at: www.tandfonline.com/doi/abs/10.1080/15427609.2013.818480. Accessed July 7, 2014
74. Meiklejohn J, Phillips C, Freedman ML, et al. Integrating mindfulness training into K-12 education: fostering the resilience of teachers and students. *Mindfulness.* 2012;3(4):291-307
75. Broderick PC, Jennings PA. Mindfulness for adolescents: a promising approach to supporting emotion regulation and preventing risky behavior. *New Direct Youth Dev.* 2012;136:111-126
76. Broderick PC, Metz S. Learning to BREATHE: a pilot trial of a mindfulness curriculum for adolescents. *Adv School Mental Health Promot.* 2009;2(1):35-46
77. Huppert FA, Johnson DM. A controlled trial of mindfulness training in schools: the importance of practice for an impact on well-being. *J Posit Psychol.* 2010;5(4):264-274
78. Schonert-Reichl KA, Lawlor MS. The effects of a mindfulness-based education program on pre- and early adolescents' well-being and social and emotional competence. *Mindfulness.* 2010;1(3):137-151
79. Lau NS, Hue MT. Preliminary outcomes of a mindfulness-based programme for Hong Kong adolescents in schools: well-being, stress and depressive symptoms. *Int J Child Spirit.* 2011;16(4):315-330
80. Raes F, Griffith JW, Van der Gucht K, Williams JMG. School-based prevention and reduction of depression in adolescents: a cluster-randomized controlled trial of a mindfulness group program. *Mindfulness.* 2013;1-10
81. Liehr P, Diaz N. A pilot study examining the effect of mindfulness on depression and anxiety for minority children. *Arch Psychiatr Nurs.* 2010;24:69-71
82. Kuyken W, Weare K, Ukoumunne OC, et al. Effectiveness of the mindfulness in schools programme: non-randomised controlled feasibility study. *Br J Psychiatry.* 2013;203(2):126-131
83. Kerrigan D, Johnson K, Stewart M, et al. Perceptions, experiences, and shifts in perspective occurring among urban youth participating in a mindfulness-based stress reduction program. *Complement Ther Clin Prac.* 2011;17(2):96-101
84. Monshat K, Khong B, Hassed C, et al. A conscious control over life and my emotions: mindfulness practice and healthy young people. A qualitative study. *J Adolesc Health.* 2013;52(5):572-577
85. Vo DX. Mindfulness practice for resilience and managing stress and pain. In: Ginsburg KR, Kinsman SB, eds. *Reaching Teens: Strength-Based Communication Strategies to Build Resilience and Support Healthy Adolescent Development.* Elk Grove Village, IL: American Academy of Pediatrics; 2014:253-259
86. Kabat-Zinn J. Foreword. In: Segal ZV, Williams JMG, Teasdale JD, eds. *Mindfulness-Based Cognitive Therapy for Depression.* 2nd ed. New York, NY: Guilford Press; 2012
87. Epstein RM. Mindful practice. *JAMA.* 1999;282(9):833-839
88. Epstein RM. Mindful practice in action (I): technical competence, evidence-based medicine, and relationship-centered care. *Fam Syst Health.* 2003;21(1):1-9
89. Krasner MS, Epstein RM, Beckman H, et al. Association of an educational program in mindful communication with burnout, empathy, and attitudes among primary care physicians. *JAMA.* 2009;302(12):1284-1293
90. Fortney L, Luchterhand C, Zakletskaia L. Abbreviated mindfulness intervention for job satisfaction, quality of life, and compassion in primary care clinicians: a pilot study. *Ann Fam Med.* 2013;11(5):412-420

91. Beach MC, Sankar A. A multicenter study of physician mindfulness and health care quality. *Ann Fam Med.* 2013;11(5):421-428
92. DeSole L. Special issue: Eating disorders and mindfulness. Introduction. *Eat Disord.* 2011;19(1):1-5

Adolesc Med 025 (2014) 473–488

Twenty Questions About Media Violence and Its Effect on Adolescents

Victor C. Strasburger, MD*

Distinguished Professor of Pediatrics, Founding Chief, Division of Adolescent Medicine, Department of Pediatrics, University of New Mexico School of Medicine, Albuquerque, New Mexico

> *True, media violence is not likely to turn an otherwise fine child into a violent criminal. But, just as every cigarette one smokes increases a little bit the likelihood of a lung tumor someday, every violent show one watches increases just a little bit the likelihood of behaving more aggressively in some situation.*
>
> Psychologists Brad Bushman and Rowell Huesmann[1(p. 248)]

> *Media violence isn't going to disappear and most current efforts to stop it are unlikely to succeed. Like displays of material excess and gratuitous sex, violence exists within a commercial structure predicated on a powerful system of fantasies.*
>
> David Trend, *The Myth of Media Violence*[2(p. 10)]

Media violence has been around for a long time. Greek tragedy was steeped in it. Roman gladiators would have been right at home on reality TV, and some people feel that hockey and football players fulfill that role in modern society. Centuries later, penny novels and violent comic books alarmed the American public. Movies came next, followed by TV and now video games, the Internet, cell phones, and iPads—media 24/7.

Excuses have always been made to dismiss any possible harmful effects of media violence: Every new medium draws immediate criticism…it's harmless fantasy and entertainment…it's cathartic…the murder rate has gone down despite more graphic violence in the media…millions of kids play violent video games and don't turn into mass murderers…Hollywood is just imitating real life (Figure 1)—the list is nearly endless.

---

*Corresponding author:
E-mail address: VStrasburger@salud.unm.edu

 ISSN 1934-4287

"Contrary to the popular view our studies show that it is real life that contributes to violence on television."
PRODUCTIONS
S.Harris

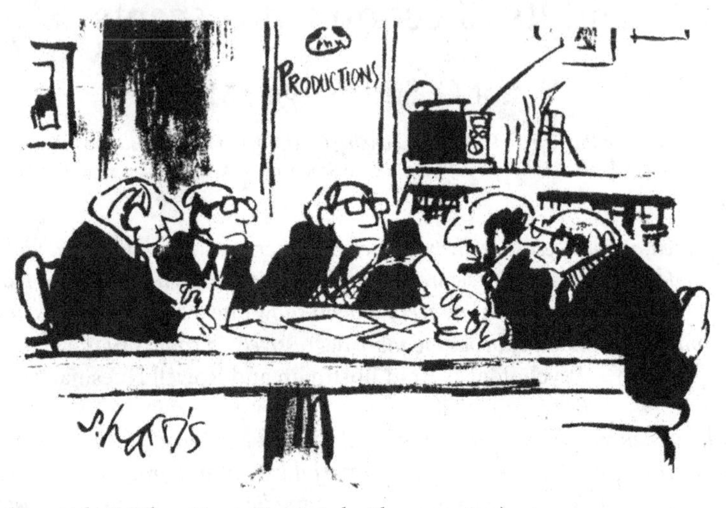

Fig 1. (Copyright © Sidney Harris. Reprinted with permission.)

The fact is, the media represent 1 of the most important—and underappreciated—known influences on child and adolescent development,[3] and the media *do* play a role in contributing to real-life violence. Is it the leading cause of violence in society? No. Other factors such as poverty, racism, and mental illness probably are far more important. Violence undoubtedly is multifactorial, and it is extremely doubtful that any single factor can explain horrific acts of violence. And yet the current amount of graphic violence available to children and adolescents is both concerning and potentially harmful, and warrants careful examination.

1. WHAT DOES THE RESEARCH SAY?

According to Harvard's Center on Media and Child Health, there are now more than 1000 studies in the research literature concerning media violence (www.cmch.tv). These range from early experiments such as Bandura's Bobo the Clown studies[4] to field studies, correlational studies, longitudinal studies, and meta-analyses (Table 1).[5] Although studies have sometimes been criticized for being too artificial (experiments) or having methodologic problems (correlational studies and meta-analyses), it is important to remember that researching media effects is like trying to study the air that people breathe.[5] Media are so ubiquitous that any significant findings are likely to be *highly* significant.[6] In addition, these

Table 1
A brief history of media violence research and responses

1933	Publication of the Payne Fund Studies, the first significant study on the effects of media on youth
1954	US Senate holds hearings on whether media violence contributes to juvenile delinquency
1960s	Classic experimental studies on media violence by Albert Bandura at Stanford using Bobo the Clown
1972	US Surgeon General issues a report on media violence Publication in *American Psychologist* of the first set of data from Eron and Huesmann's longitudinal study of 8-year-olds
1982	Publication of a 10-volume, comprehensive report on children and media by the National Institute of Mental Health
1984-1986	Huesmann, Eron, Lefkowitz, and Walder report on the results of their 22-year longitudinal study of 8-year-olds and media violence, which found a highly significant correlation between viewing TV violence in the 3rd grade and aggressive behavior 10 and 22 years later
1992	A review by the American Psychological Association estimates that the average American child or teenager sees 10,000 murders, rapes, and aggravated assaults per year on television alone
1993	After the release of "Death Race," an ultraviolent video game in which hit-and-run drivers obliterate wheelchair-bound octogenarians, the US Senate holds hearings on violent video games, leading to the development of a video game rating system
1994	Comstock and Paik publish a meta-analysis of more than 215 empirical studies, which found large effect sizes (r = 0.31, which means that media violence is responsible for 10% of real-life violence)
1998	The largest study ever undertaken of American television—the National Television Violence Study (NTVS)—examines nearly 10,000 hours of TV and finds that 60% of all programs contain violence and that children's programming is actually more violent than adults' programming
2000	The American Academy of Pediatrics (AAP) is joined by the American Medical Association, the American Academy of Child and Adolescent Psychiatry, and the American Psychological Association in issuing an unprecedented joint statement on the effect of entertainment violence on children in testimony before Congress
2003	A panel of media-violence experts convened by the National Institute of Mental Health, at the request of the US Surgeon General, publishes its comprehensive report on the effects of media violence on youth, which reveals media violence to be a significant causal factor in aggression and violence
2007	The Federal Communications Commission (FCC) releases its report on violent television programming and its effects on children and agrees with the Surgeon General that there is "strong evidence" that exposure to media violence can increase aggressive behavior in children

studies contain *epidemiologic* data, meaning that the media's effect on any given child or teen is impossible to predict.

To summarize this vast amount of research: Media violence can encourage aggressive thoughts, beliefs, and even actions in children and adolescents and may be responsible for perhaps 10% or more of real-life violence in society.[5-10] A correlation coefficient of 0.31 (found in several meta-analyses[11,12]) yields an effect size of

0.10 (0.31^2). However, some authors feel that a 0.31 correlation coefficient in social science research, which is difficult to achieve given the vagaries of human behavior, is equivalent to a 0.8 in medical research.[6] As it turns out, the relationship between media violence and real-life aggression is nearly as strong as the relationship between smoking and lung cancer and is stronger than many of the public health risks doctors and the general public take for granted (Figure 2).

2. WHY IS THIS STILL CONTROVERSIAL?

Why this remains controversial is a perplexing and complicated question, and the answer probably involves several factors.[13,14] Hollywood continues to deny any negative effects of any of its products yet will point to its finest TV shows and films as "ennobling" society. A 30-second Super Bowl ad now costs close to $4 million, and advertisers anticipate that it will boost sales; yet 7 hours of media a day for the average child is said to have no effects.

There are individual factors as well.[13,14] (1) The third-person effect: No one thinks that the media affect themselves (or their children). The media only affect *other* people.[15,16] (2) Faulty reasoning: Many people think that violent media have no effect on aggression and violence because they have never killed anyone after watching a violent TV show or film or playing a first-person shooter video game. (3) Refusal to believe or ignorance of the evidence: Many of the research studies are done in communications and psychology journals and are not immediately

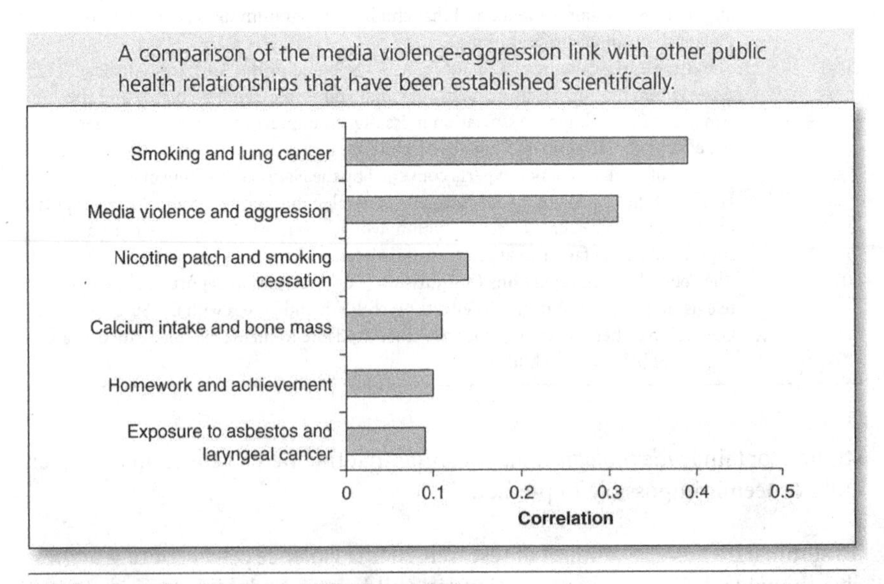

SOURCE: Adapted from Bushman and Huesmann (2001).

Fig 2. (From Strasburger VC, Wilson BJ, Jordan AB, eds. *Children, Adolescents, and the Media*. 3rd ed. Los Angeles, CA: Sage; 2014. Reprinted with permission.)

available to the general public or even to physicians. And many researchers have a difficult time effectively communicating their findings to the public, even when the media choose to publicize the results. (4) Cognitive dissonance: How could something so much fun and so entertaining, such like Oliver Stone's "Natural Born Killers," have led to a killing spree in France? (5) Finally, the Fairness Doctrine plays a crucial role in the public's misunderstanding of media effects.[13] Originally developed by the Federal Communications Commission (FCC) in 1949, it required broadcasters to present both sides of controversial issues and to do so in a manner that was honest, equitable, and balanced. However, the FCC eliminated the doctrine in 1987 and formally removed the language that implemented it in 2011. Despite this, broadcasters and journalists still believe that there are "2 sides to every story," including the issue of media violence. They give the nay-sayers (who can point to just a few nonsignificant studies) equal time with public health advocates and researchers who have thousands of studies to back up their assertions. Some issues simply do not have 2 equal sides. Broadcasters would never invite a Holocaust denier on a show about atrocities committed by Nazi Germany, yet they may choose to give airtime to Hollywood apologists asserting that media have no negative effects.

3. HOW "GOOD" IS THE RESEARCH?

No research is perfect, and social science research is particularly fraught with difficulty. Teasing out specific influences on human behavior is virtually a mission impossible. But the research is actually clear on this subject and has been for a long time.[5-10,17,18] Beginning with experimental studies in the 1960s, continuing with both field studies and longitudinal studies in the 1970s, and then with several meta-analyses later on, nearly every study has found a significant relationship between viewing media violence and the development of aggressive thoughts, beliefs, and even behavior. In fact, it is so clear that very little research is currently being done on the effect of media violence on TV or in films. Most of the research now is confined to video game effects and cyberbullying.

4. IS MEDIA VIOLENCE RESPONSIBLE FOR MURDERS AND MASS SHOOTINGS?

Here is where the general public, politicians, and even social scientists have difficulty: how to define aggression and measure it properly. Because murders and especially mass shootings are relatively rare, trying to pin them on the effects of media violence is a research mission doomed to failure. As a result, there are absolutely no studies on this subject.

But both murders and mass shootings are the wrong variables to be considering if one wants to determine the effect of media violence. First, medical advances in the past few years have saved thousands of lives of shooting victims—fewer people die from what would have been fatal wounds years ago. Second, very few people are murdered every year—fewer than 5 per 100,000 according to Federal Bureau of Investigation (FBI) crime statistics.[19] By contrast, interpersonal violence has increased dramatically in the latter half of the 20th century and far exceeds murder (Figure 3), just as media violence has increased and become more graphic. This is the type of violence that people are far more likely to experience or be exposed to and therefore should be used as the outcome variable whenever possible. Third, mass shootings are even rarer; and many factors contribute. It would require a longitudinal study of 10 to 20 years involving millions of subjects to even attempt to answer the question of whether media violence *causes* mass murders.

One of the newest and previously unconsidered aspects of media violence is relational aggression: acts that are intended to harm others emotionally rather than physically (eg, gossiping, rumor mongering, socially isolating others, insults). It is more common among girls than boys,[20] and several studies suggest that media violence may be contributing to real-life social aggression.[20-22]

5. ARE THERE GAPS IN THE RESEARCH?

As mentioned, media research is largely epidemiologic, so predicting the effect of any given media genre on any given individual is difficult. Not enough is

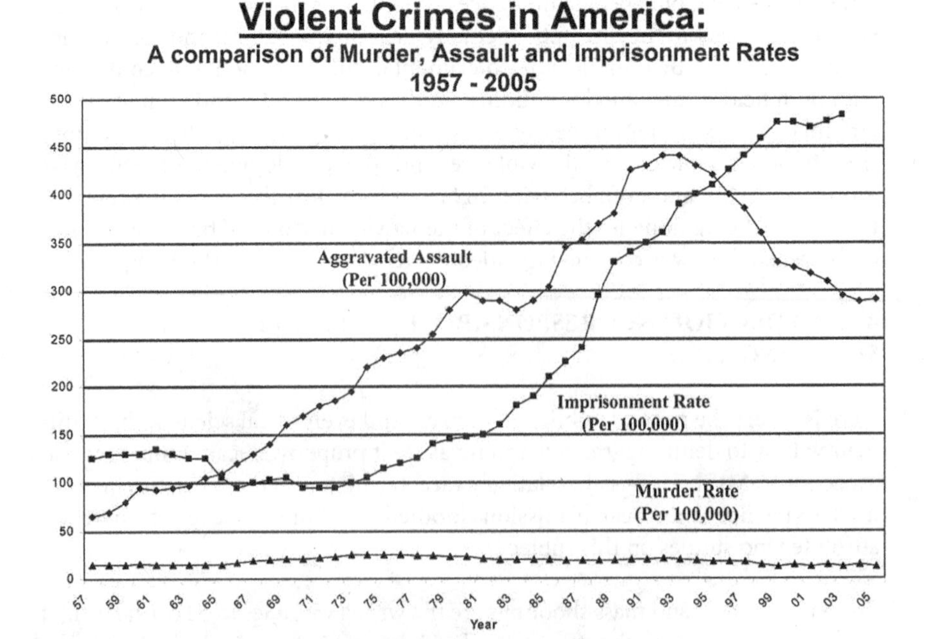

Fig 3. (From www.Killogy.com. Reprinted by permission.)

known about individual differences in processing media and being affected by it. Many variables can affect how a child or teen will or will not be affected by media: age, socioeconomic status, race, ethnicity, length and type of exposure to media, individual personality factors, parents' use of media, mother's educational level, etc. For example, black teens are relatively more resistant to tobacco advertising and to depictions of unhealthy body self-imagery,[23,24] but exactly why is unknown. Unfortunately, there is currently not much funding for media research, either from the federal government or from private foundations,[25] so many important questions like this go unanswered.

6. ISN'T WITNESSING REAL-LIFE VIOLENCE MORE HARMFUL?

Absolutely. Numerous studies document this.[26-28] But seeing murders, rapes, and assaults vicariously via the media has an effect as well. Children and adolescents can learn behavioral "scripts" about how to react in new situations.[29] Most damaging is the notion of "justifiable violence," which is the single most powerful reinforcement known in the research literature[5,17] and is very prevalent in American media.

A number of theories explain media effects. *Social learning theory* asserts that children learn new behaviors either by direct experience or by observing and imitating others in their social environment.[30] *Cognitive priming theory* asserts that violent stimuli activate aggressive thoughts in a viewer, which can then "prime" other thoughts, feelings, and actions when stored in a person's memory.[31] *Super-peer theory* hypothesizes that the media exert a form of peer pressure on children and teens by showing how other teens behave in "real-life" situations.[5] Equally important is how media violence is portrayed. Aggression is positively reinforced when "good guys" are the aggressors, when the violence is rewarded or goes unpunished, when there is no serious harm to the victim, and when the violence is made to look funny.[32]

7. HAS THE AMOUNT OF MEDIA VIOLENCE INCREASED?

Apparently so. Not only has the amount of violence increased, but it has become more graphic as well. For example, in a study of the 22 James Bond films between 1962 and 2008, portrayals of violence doubled over time, particularly portrayals of lethal violence, which tripled (Figure 4).[33] In a similar study of the top 30 films since 1950, the amount of violence has more than doubled, and gun violence in PG-13 films has more than tripled since 1985.[34] Another recent study of more than 800 top-grossing films from 1950 to 2006 found that 89% contained violence, and it has steadily increased over time.[35]

One other phenomenon has also occurred and is relevant: *ratings creep*. What used to be R-rated is now PG-13, and PG-13 has become PG.[36,37] A quantitative study of 45 PG-13 films from 1988 to 2006 found significant increases in violent

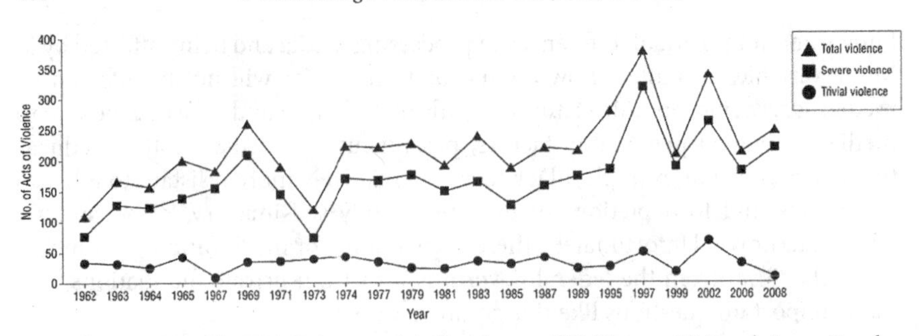

Fig 4. (From McAnally HM, Robertson LA, Strasburger VC, Hancox RJ. Bond, James Bond: a review of 46 years of violence in films. *Arch Pediatr Adolesc Med.* 2013;167:195-196. Copyright © JAMA Pediatrics. Reprinted with permission.)

content.[37] Unfortunately, the Motion Picture Association of America (MPAA) has always rated films more harshly for sexual content than for violent content, which is the opposite of what other western countries do. The communications research is clear that media violence is potentially far more harmful than sexual content is.[5]

8. ARE CARTOONS HARMFUL?

Potentially. The more realistic the violence being portrayed, the potentially more unhealthy it is. So, on the bright side, cartoons are obviously not very realistic. At the same time, the National Television Violence Study (NTVS) did find that children's programming actually is more violent than adult programming, with 70% of children's shows containing violence, and 1 incident occurring every 4 minutes (compared with 1 every 12 minutes for nonchildren's programming).[38] The study also found that children's programs were much more likely to depict unrealistically low levels of harm to victims compared with what would actually happen in real life. Given that children younger than 7 years have a difficult time distinguishing reality from fantasy, this may be especially problematic.[5]

9. WHEN DOES MEDIA VIOLENCE BEGIN AFFECTING KIDS?

One of the most powerful studies of media violence actually began as a study of parenting styles and aggressive behavior. In the 1960s, researchers Leonard Eron and Rowell Huesmann studied nearly 1000 3rd-graders in upstate New York. Initially, they thought they would collect data on TV use as a way of distracting parents from the real purpose of the study. But when they analyzed their data, TV violence proved to be a much stronger predictor of later aggressive behavior than parenting style. The researchers studied TV viewing habits and aggressive behavior at ages 8, 19, and 30 years. Among the boys, exposure to TV violence in early childhood was predictive of higher levels of aggression at ages 19 and 30, after controlling for IQ, socioeconomic status, and overall exposure to TV (Figure 5).[39-42] Exposure to violent TV also was predictive of serious criminal acts at

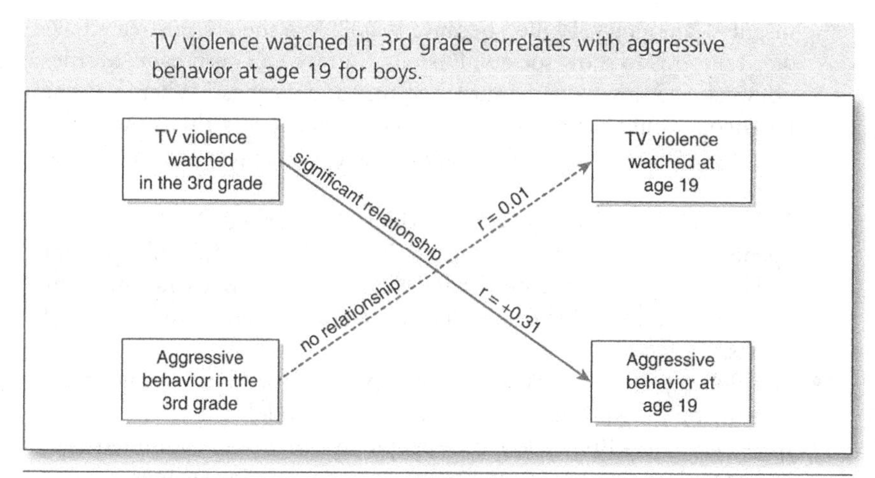

SOURCE: Reproduced from Liebert and Sprafkin (1988).

Fig 5. (From Strasburger VC, Wilson BJ, Jordan AB. *Children, Adolescents, and the Media*. 3rd ed. Los Angeles, CA: Sage; 2014. Reprinted with permission.)

age 30.[41] Subsequent studies found that this relationship holds for children in other countries[42,43] as well as for girls.[42] Researchers now think that there is a reciprocal relationship between viewing TV violence at a young age, aggressive behavior, and developing a taste for seeing even more media violence.[5] However, of most concern is the fact that the research indicates that people learn their attitudes about violence at a very early age—age 8 years or younger—and apparently, once learned, those attitudes are difficult to change.[5]

10. ARE VIDEO GAMES HARMFUL?

Just like the media in general, video games can be powerfully prosocial or seriously problematic. First-person shooter video games fall into the latter category. The research on video games is not nearly as voluminous as the research on media violence on TV or in movies, but it is equally clear: Violent video games can increase violent feelings, attitudes, and behavior, and reduce prosocial behavior.[44-46]

At the moment, no studies have linked violent video games with homicides or mass shootings. As discussed earlier, both are rare enough that to try to establish a link would be difficult if not impossible. However, a recent study has noted an association between violent video games and violent delinquency, even after controlling for the effects of screen time, years playing video games, age, sex, race, delinquency history, and personality traits.[47] In addition, there are several highly suggestive, media-related features of several of the mass shootings:

- After his arrest, 16-year-old Luke Woodham of Pearl, Mississippi (who killed 3 and wounded 7 classmates), was quoted as saying, “I am not insane. I am angry. I killed because people like me are mistreated every day. I did this to show society: Push us, and we will push back. Murder is not weak and slow-witted; murder is gutsy and daring."[48] Where else but in the media would he have learned such distorted ideas? This is the problem with the notion of justifiable violence that is so prevalent in American media.

- The Paducah, Kentucky, school killer, 14-year-old Michael Carneal, opened fire on a prayer group with 8 shots and had 8 hits—all upper torso and head—resulting in 3 deaths and 1 case of paralysis. He had never fired an actual gun in his life before that but had played point-and-shoot video games.[49]
- The Beltway Sniper, John Lee Malvo, prepared for his sniping spree by training on the Xbox game "Halo" in "sniper mode."[50]
- In 2011, Anders Breivik killed 69 people in Norway and admitted that he had specifically trained using first-person shooter video games.
- More recently, both the shooters involved in mass killings in Aurora, Colorado, and Newtown, Connecticut, were enamored of violent video games.

11. ARE VIOLENT VIDEO GAMES DIFFERENT FROM VIOLENT MOVIES OR TV SHOWS?

Most experts agree that violent video games differ significantly from movies and TV for a number of important reasons[44-46]: (1) the player identifies with the aggressor; (2) the games involve active participation and interaction; (3) the games involve repetitive sequences; (4) a hostile virtual reality is created; and (5) the games provide reinforcement for aggressive actions.

12. WHY DON'T ALL PARENTS AND THE GENERAL PUBLIC "GET" THIS?

Increasingly, people get their information from the media, especially TV. More people now get their news from TV and the Internet than from newspapers.[51] For obvious reasons, the broadcast media are loathe to report comprehensively about any negative effects their programming may have.

Desensitization also plays a role. People have become so accustomed to media violence that it doesn't register with them as being objectionable. It also takes more graphic violence to get people's attention, which may partially explain why media violence has become more explicit in the past several decades.[33-35]

13. IS CENSORSHIP THE ANSWER?

In a word, no (although European countries routinely edit out violent scenes in Hollywood movies and add in sexual content). The American Academy of Pediatrics strongly opposes censorship.[52] But self-censorship and good taste on the part of writers, directors, and producers are appropriate and could provide some benefit.

14. WHY DOESN'T HOLLYWOOD CLEAN UP ITS ACT?

The amount of money involved in creating entertainment programming is staggering. Films can cost $200 million or more to make (eg, "The Lone Ranger") and generate close to a $1 billion in revenues (eg, "Avatar"). TV series cost an average of $1.5 to 2 million per episode to make ("ER" cost $15 million per episode) but can generate huge revenues as well. For example, "Seinfeld" has generated $3.1 billion in rebroadcast fees since its final episode. When this amount of money is at stake, the entertainment industry tends to lose sight of any public health responsibility it may or may not have. Although Hollywood writers, directors, and producers tend to be more politically liberal than the American public, they also immediately rally behind their First Amendment rights when criticized and dismiss any notion that their products may be harmful to children or teens.

15. DO PEOPLE REALLY WANT TO SEE MORE VIOLENCE?

Absolutely not. Hollywood has had this misconception for decades, and there is no evidence to support it. What children, teenagers, and even adults like the most is *action*, but action doesn't have to be incredibly violent. For example, the car chases in Steve McQueen's classic movie "Bullit" or the Oscar-winning movie "The French Connection" were thrilling, but no one was injured, no gunfire erupted, and no bones were snapped.

Two recent sets of experiments demonstrate this. Researchers edited episodes from 5 different prime-time TV dramas (eg, *The Sopranos*, *Oz*, *24*) to create 1 version with graphic violence, 1 with sanitized violence, and 1 with no violence. Undergraduates enjoyed the nonviolent version significantly more than the violent ones.[53] In a related experiment, researchers created 4 different versions of an original slapstick cartoon: 1 low in both action and violence, 1 low in action but high in violence, 1 high in action but low in violence, and 1 high in both action and violence. A total of 128 grade-school students were randomly assigned to watch 1 of the 4 versions. The presence of violence had no effect on children's liking of the cartoons, and boys liked the high-action/low-violence version the best.[54]

16. CAN MEDIA VIOLENCE EVER BE CATHARTIC?

No, not in the traditional sense of the term. Aristotle originated the concept of catharsis, hypothesizing that people would be "purged" of their angry emotions by witnessing Greek tragedies. Media have obviously come a long way since then, but there is absolutely no evidence in the research literature that violent media makes people less aggressive; rather, the opposite is true. Despite this, Hollywood directors still seem to approve of the theory. For example, Alfred Hitchcock, director of the movie "Psycho," said, "One of television's greatest contributions is that it brought murder back into the home where it belongs. Seeing a murder on television can be good therapy. It can help work off one's antagonism." More recently, in 1992, Paul Verhoeven, director of the movie "Total Recall," said, "I think it's a kind of purifying experience to see violence."[55]

17. WHAT CAN PARENTS DO?

In a 2013 survey of 2300 parents of newborns to 8-year-old children nationwide, parents seemed almost lackadaisical about the effect of media on their children: 78% reported that their children's media use is not a source of family conflict, 55% say they are either not too concerned or not at all concerned about their children's media use (compared with 30% who are concerned), and their most consistent concern is about the effect on physical activity, not on aggressive attitudes or behavior. Only 38% were concerned about the effect of media on their children's behavior.[56] Again, this may reflect the third-person effect: "only those 'dumb kids' down the block are affected by media, not my beautiful, intelligent children."

Parents need to realize that their young children's attitudes and beliefs about social norms and aggressive behavior are being shaped in their childhood and preteen years and that the resulting behavior may not manifest itself until adolescence or young adulthood. In addition, the research clearly shows that media violence is potentially more harmful than sexual content,[5,17] which is the exact opposite of what most parents think.[57]

Consequently, parents need to think hard about observing the American Academy of Pediatrics' basic recommendations about media: (1) Avoid media use for infants younger than 2 years; (2) limit total entertainment screen time to less than 1 to 2 hours per day; (3) coview and discuss content with children; (4) keep screens and new technology out of children's bedrooms; and (5) avoid exposing children and teenagers to excessively graphic violence.[58]

18. WHAT CAN PHYSICIANS DO?

The American Academy of Pediatrics has strongly endorsed the need to ask 2 media-related questions at all well-child and well-adolescent health visits. (1) How many hours a day is spent with media? (2) Is there a TV or Internet-connected device in the child's bedroom?[58] These 2 questions take less than a minute to ask but could pay rich dividends. The research is clear that excessive screen viewing can contribute to obesity,[59-61] aggressive behavior,[17,18] and substance use.[61-63] In addition, the presence of a bedroom TV potentially increases the negative effect of media.[60,63]

19. WHAT CAN SCHOOLS DO?

Many schools are lagging in the technologic revolution.[64] Media can be used proactively and powerfully in ways that will engage young people and will mesh with the way they function outside of the classroom. For example, Ken Burns' "Civil War" series provides a far better way of teaching American history than any textbook. Thousands of middle-school students are forced to read *Romeo and Juliet* every year (despite it being about 2 teenagers who have sex and then kill themselves). Yet Shakespeare wrote his plays to be performed and seen, not to be read, and there now exist 10 video versions of *Romeo and Juliet* that would be far more appealing to 13-year-olds than wading through Elizabethan English on the printed page. Educators need to seriously consider a paradigm shift in their thinking about how new technology should be used and what it means to be an educated person in the 21st century.

Several studies have shown media literacy to be protective against harmful media effects.[65,66] Most western countries have incorporated media education into their normal curricula, yet it is rare in the United States. In 1914, to be literate meant that a person could read and write. In 2014, to be literate means that a person can read, write, text, download, and successfully navigate through the vast amount of information available on the Internet. One could easily argue that teaching media education is now at least as important as teaching the "3 R's."

20. WHAT CAN THE FEDERAL GOVERNMENT DO?

The federal government has neglected media influence for a long time. The last comprehensive report on media effects on children was issued in 1982, long before the Internet, cell phones, first-person shooter video games, and iPads.[67] A new comprehensive report is definitely needed and would stimulate new research ideas and new funding for research. In addition, very little research funding has been provided by either the federal government or even private foundations, despite the crucial role that media play in child and adolescent development and health-related behaviors. In 2005 when Hilary Clinton was in the Senate, she and Senator Joe Lieberman introduced the CAMRA (Children and Media Research Advancement) Act. It would have authorized funding for the establishment of a program on children and media with the National Institute of Child Health and Human Development (NICHD). Remarkably, no such program exists within the NICHD, elsewhere in the National Institutes of Health, or within the Centers for Disease Control and Prevention. Ongoing federal funding (and a home within the government's research agencies) is desperately needed for research on children, adolescents, and the media.

The bottom line is that the media represent 1 of the most important and under-recognized influences on children and adolescents today, insufficient research is being conducted and being funded, and the American public is being misled by inaccurate statements about how media affect young people.

References

1. Bushman BJ, Huesmann LR. Effects of televised violence on aggression. In Singer DG, Singer JL, eds. *Handbook of Children and the Media*. Thousand Oaks, CA: Sage; 2001;223-254
2. Trend D. *The Myth of Media Violence: A Critical Introduction*. Malden, MA: Blackwell; 2007
3. Strasburger VC, Jordan AB, Donnerstein E. Children, adolescents, and the media: health effects. *Pediatr Clin North Am*. 2012;59:533-587
4. Bandura A, Ross D, Ross SA. Imitation of film-mediated aggressive models. *J Abnorm Soc Psychol*. 1963;66:3-11
5. Strasburger VC, Wilson BJ, Jordan AB. *Children, Adolescents, and the Media*. 3rd ed. Los Angeles, CA: Sage; 2014
6. Comstock G, Strasburger V. Media violence: Q&A. *Adolesc Med State Art Rev*. 1993;4:495-509
7. Gentile DA, Bushman BJ. Reassessing media violence effects using a risk and resilience approach to understanding aggression. *Psychol Pop Media Cult*. 2012;1:138-151
8. Bushman BJ, Anderson CA. Media violence and the American public: scientific facts versus media misinformation. *Am Psychol*. 2001;56:477-489
9. Murray JP. Media violence: the effects are both real and strong. *Am Behav Sci*. 2008;51:1212-1230
10. Huesmann LR, Dubow EF, Yang G. Why it is hard to believe that media violence causes aggression. In: Dill K, ed. *The Oxford Handbook of Media Psychology*. New York: Oxford University Press; 2013;159-171
11. Hearold S. A synthesis of 1045 effects of television on social behavior. In: Comstock G, ed. *Public Communication and Behavior*, Vol. 1. New York, NY: Academic Press; 1986;65-133
12. Paik HJ, Comstock G. The effects of television violence on antisocial behavior: a meta-analysis. *Commun Res*. 1994;21:516-546
13. Bushman B. Why do people deny violent media effects? *Psychology Today*, February 18, 2013. Available at: www.psychologytoday.com/blog/get-psyched/201302/why-do-people-deny-violent-media-effects. Accessed July 7, 2014
14. Strasburger VC, Donnerstein E, Bushman BJ. Why is it so difficult to believe that media affect children and adolescents? *Pediatrics*. 2014;133:571-573
15. Eveland WP, Nathanson AI, Detenber AI, McLeod DM. Rethinking the social distance corollary: perceived likelihood of exposure and the third-person perception. *Commun Res*. 1999;26:275-302
16. Perloff RM. Mass media, social perception, and the third-person effect. In: Bryant J, Oliver MB, eds. *Media Effects: Advances in Theory and Research*. New York: Routledge; 2009:252-268
17. Strasburger VC; Council on Communications and Media. Media violence (policy statement). *Pediatrics*. 2009;124:1495-1503
18. Media Violence Commission, International Society for Research on Aggression. Report of the Media Violence Commission. *Aggress Behav*. 2012;38:335-341
19. US Federal Bureau of Investigation. Uniform Crime Reports. Washington, DC: US Government Printing Office; 2012
20. Spieker SJ, Campbell SB, Vandergrift N, et al. Relational aggression in middle childhood: predictors and adolescent outcomes. *Soc Dev*. 2012;21:354-375
21. Martins N, Wilson BJ. Mean on the screen: social aggression in programs popular with children. *J Commun*. 2012;62:991-1009
22. Martins, N, Wilson BJ. Social aggression on television and its relationship to children's aggression in the classroom. *Hum Commun Res*. 2012;38:48-71
23. West JH, Romero RA, Trinidad DR. Adolescent receptivity to tobacco marketing by racial/ethnic groups in California. *Am J Prev Med*. 2007;33:121-123
24. Padgett J, Biro FM. Different shapes in different cultures: body dissatisfaction, overweight, and obesity in African American and Caucasian females. *J Pediatr Adolesc Gynecol*. 2003;16(6):349-354

25. Strasburger VC. Why isn't there more media research? *Clin Pediatr.* 2013;52:583-584
26. Singer MI, Anglin TM, Song LY, Lunghofer L. Adolescents' exposure to violence and associated symptoms of psychological trauma. *JAMA.* 1995;273:477-482
27. Singer MI, Miller DB, Guo S, Flannery DJ, Frierson T, Slovak K. Contributors to violent behavior among elementary and middle school children. *Pediatrics.* 1999;104:878-884
28. Holmes M. The sleeper effect of intimate partner violence exposure: long-term consequences on young children's aggressive behavior. *J Child Psychol Psychiatry.* 2013;54:986-995
29. Huesmann LR. The role of social information processing and cognitive schemas in the acquisition and maintenance of habitual aggressive behavior. In: Geen RG, Donnerstein E, eds. *Human Aggression: Theories, Research, and Implications for Social Policy*. San Diego, CA: Academic Press; 1998:1120-1134
30. Bandura A. Social cognitive theory of mass communication. In: Bryant J, Oliver MB, eds. *Media Effects: Advances in Theory and Research.* New York: Routledge; 2009:94-124
31. Jo E, Berkowitz L. A priming effect analysis of media influences: an update. In: Bryant J, Zillmann D, eds. *Media Effects: Advances in Theory and Research.* Hillsdale, NJ: Lawrence Erlbaum; 1994:43-60
32. Wilson BJ, Smith SL, Potter W, et al. Violence in children's television programming: assessing the risks. *J Commun.* 2002;23: 446-460
33. McAnally HM, Robertson LA, Strasburger VC, Hancox RJ. Bond, James Bond: a review of 46 years of violence in films. *Arch Pediatr Adolesc Med.* 2013;167:195-196
34. Bushman BJ, Jamieson PE, Weitz I, Romer D. Gun violence trends in movies. *Pediatrics.* 2013;132:1-5
35. Bleakley A, Jamieson P, Romer D. Trends of sexual and violent content by gender in top-grossing U.S. films, 1950-2006. *J Adolesc Health.* 2012;51:73-79
36. Thompson KM, Yokota F. Violence, sex, and profanity in films: correlation of movie ratings with content. *MedGenMed.* 2004;6(3):3. Available at: www.medscape.com/viewarticle/480900. Accessed July 7, 2014
37. Leone R, Barowski L. MPAA ratings creep: a longitudinal analysis of the PG-13 rating category in US movies. *J Child Media.* 2011;5:53-68
38. Federman J, ed. *National Television Violence Study*, Vol. 3. Thousand Oaks, CA: Sage; 1998
39. Eron LD, Huesmann LR, Lefkowitz MM, Walder LO. Does television violence cause aggression? *Am Psychol.* 1972;27:253-263
40. Huesmann LR, Eron LD, Lefkowitz MM, Walder LO. Stability of aggression over time and generations. *Dev Psychol.* 1984;20:1120-1134
41. Huesmann LR, Miller LS. Long-term effects of repeated exposure to media violence in childhood. In: Huesmann LR, ed. *Aggressive Behavior: Current Perspectives.* New York: Plenum; 1994:153-186
42. Huesmann LR, Eron LD. The development of aggression in children of different cultures: psychological processes and exposure to violence. In: Huesmann LR, Eron LD, eds. *Television and the Aggressive Child: A Cross National Comparison.* Hillsdale, NJ: Lawrence Erlbaum; 1986;1-27
43. Krahe B, Moller I. Longitudinal effects of media violence on aggression and empathy among German adolescents. *J Appl Dev Psychol.* 2010;31:401-409
44. Anderson CA, Gentile DA, Buckley KE. *Violent Video Game Effects on Children and Adolescents.* New York: Oxford University Press; 2007
45. Anderson CA, Gentile DA, Dill KE. Prosocial, antisocial, and other effects of recreational video games. In: Singer DG, Singer JL, eds. *Handbook of Children and the Media.* 2nd ed. Thousand Oaks, CA: Sage; 2012:249-272
46. Krahe B. Video game violence. In: Dill KE, ed. *The Oxford Handbook of Media Psychology*. New York: Oxford University Press; 2013:352-372
47. DeLisi M, Vaughn MG, Gentile DA, Anderson CA, Shook JJ. Violent video games, delinquency, and youth violence: new evidence. *Youth Violence Juv Justice.* 2012;11:132-142
48. Teen accused in killings wrote note, officials say. *USA Today*, October 3, 1997. Available at: murderpedia.org/male.W/w/woodham-luke.htm. Accessed July 7, 2014

49. Strasburger VC, Grossman D. How many more Columbines? What can pediatricians do about school and media violence? *Pediatr Ann.* 2001;30:87-94
50. "Dateline." NBC Television, December 14, 2002. Available at: www.thefreeradical.ca/copycatCrimes/sniperTrainedOnVideoGame.html. Accessed July 7, 2014
51. Martins N, Weaver AJ, Yeshua-Katz D, et al. A content analysis of print news coverage of media violence and aggression research. *J Commun.* 2013;63:1070-1087
52. American Academy of Pediatrics Committee on Communications. Impact of music lyrics and music videos on children and youth (policy statement). *Pediatrics.* 1996;98:1219-1221
53. Weaver AJ, Wilson BJ. The role of graphic and sanitized violence in the enjoyment of television dramas. *Hum Commun Res.* 2009;35:442-463
54. Weaver AJ, Jensen JD, Martins N, Hurley R, Wilson BJ. Liking violence and action: an examination of gender differences in children's processing of animated content. *Media Psychol.* 2011;14:49-70
55. Net Industries. *Catharsis Theory and Media Effects.* Available at: encyclopedia.jrank.org/articles/pages/6455/Catharsis-Theory-and-Media-Effects.html. Accessed July 7, 2014
56. Wartella E, Rideout V, Lauricella AR, Connell AL. *Parenting in the Age of Digital Technology: A National Survey.* Evanston, IL: Northwestern University; 2013
57. Cheng TL, Brenner RA, Wright JL, Sachs HC, Moyer P, Rao MR. Children's violent television viewing: are parents monitoring? *Pediatrics.* 2004;114:94-99
58. American Academy of Pediatrics Council on Communications and Media. Children, adolescents, and media (policy statement). *Pediatrics.* 2013;132:958-961
59. Staiano AE, Harrington DM, Broyles ST, Gupta AK, Katzmarzyk PT. Television, adiposity, and cardiometabolic risk in children and adolescents. *Am J Prev Med.* 2013;44(1):40-47
60. Adachi-Mejia AM, Longacre MR, Gibson JJ, et al. Children with a TV in their bedroom at higher risk for being overweight. *Int J Obes (Lond).* 2007;31(4):644-651
61. Hanewinkel R, Sargent JD. Longitudinal study of exposure to entertainment media and alcohol use among German adolescents. *Pediatrics.* 2009;123(3):989-995
62. Gruber EL, Want PH, Christensen JS, Grube JW, Fisher DA. Private television viewing, parental supervision, and sexual and substance use risk behaviors in adolescents (abstract). *J Adolesc Health.* 2005;36(2):107
63. Jackson C, Brown JD, Pardun CJ. A TV in the bedroom: implications for viewing habits and risk behaviors during early adolescence. *J Broadcast Electron Media.* 2008;52(3):349-367
64. Strasburger VC. School daze: why are teachers and schools missing the boat on media? *Pediatr Clin North Am.* 2012;59:705-716
65. Potter WJ. *Media Literacy.* 7th ed. Los Angeles, CA: Sage; 2013
66. McCannon R. Media literacy/media education. In: Strasburger VC, Wilson BJ, Jordan AB, eds. *Children, Adolescents, and the Media.* 3rd ed. Los Angeles, CA: Sage; 2014:507-584
67. Pearl D, Bouthilet L, Lazar J. *Television and Behavior: Ten Years of Scientific Progress and Implications for the Eighties.* Rockville, MD: National Institute of Mental Health; 1982

Adolesc Med 025 (2014) 489–501

Human Papillomavirus and Oropharyngeal Squamous Cell Carcinoma of the Head and Neck: A Growing Epidemic

Jessica Bauman, MD[a*]; Lori Wirth, MD[b,c]

[a]*Fellow in Hematology-Oncology, Massachusetts General Hospital, Harvard Medical School, Boston, Massachusetts;* [b]*Medical Director of the Center for Head and Neck Cancers, Massachusetts General Hospital, Boston, Massachusetts;* [c]*Assistant Professor, Department of Medicine, Division of Medical Oncology, Massachusetts General Hospital, Boston, Massachusetts*

INTRODUCTION

Recently, human papillomavirus (HPV) has been identified as a major causative agent in oropharyngeal squamous cell carcinoma (OP-SCC) of the head and neck. HPV was already known to cause cervical, vulvar, anal, and penile cancers. Rates of HPV$^+$ OP-SCC are dramatically increasing in much of the world right now, and in the last 5 years the annual incidence of HPV$^+$ OP-SCC has overtaken the incidence of invasive cervical cancer in the United States.[1] Although HPV$^+$ OP-SCC is potentially curable at diagnosis and the prognosis is better than OP-SCC that is not associated with HPV, the morbidity related to treatment is high, with myriad of short- and long-term toxicities. Moreover, not every patient is cured. Hence, more can and needs to be done for HPV$^+$ OP-SCC. HPV vaccination is predicted to prevent HPV$^+$ OP-SCC, but current vaccination rates are too low to have a major effect on a population-wide level. In this review, we will summarize the current understanding of and latest developments in the clinical presentation, treatment, epidemiology, biology, and prevention of HPV$^+$ OP-SCC.

CLINICAL PRESENTATION OF HPV$^+$ OROPHARYNGEAL CANCER AND TREATMENT

There are approximately 55,070 cases of head and neck cancer annually in the United States.[2] Of these, more than 25% are cancers of the oropharynx (OP)

---

*Corresponding author:
E-mail address: jrbauman@partners.org

 ISSN 1934-4287

caused by HPV.[1] The OP includes cancers of the base of tongue, tonsils, soft palate, and walls of the pharynx, which is depicted in Figure 1.[3] People diagnosed with HPV$^+$ OP-SCC are 2 to 3 times more likely to be men (10511 vs. 3500 new cases annually in men and women, respectively), younger, white, have more education, and have a minimal history of smoking or drinking compared to those with HPV$^-$ OP-SCC.[1,4-6] HPV$^+$ OP-SCC begins as a primary tumor in the base of tongue, tonsil, soft palate, or pharyngeal wall, but it can spread regionally to the lymph nodes in the neck or distantly to organs such as the lungs, liver, and bone. HPV$^+$ OP-SCC most commonly presents as a locally advanced stage IV cancer with a painless mass discovered in the neck, which on biopsy shows a lymph node with metastatic squamous cell carcinoma that is nonkeratinizing, is poorly differentiated, and has basaloid morphology.[6] Follow-up examination of the OP then usually identifies the primary tumor, which often is small and asymptomatic despite the already involved lymph nodes.

Treatment for HPV$^+$ OP-SCC is intense and complex because of the advanced stage. It usually involves concurrent chemotherapy and daily radiotherapy for 6 to 8 weeks, as well as surgery in some cases. Throughout this period, patients become quite ill because a high symptom burden develops over the course of treatment. Treatment-related toxicities include severe mouth and throat pain requiring narcotic medication, difficulty swallowing with frequent need for a gastric feeding tube to maintain adequate nutrition, radiation dermatitis, nausea, dehydration, malnutrition, and weight loss.[7,8] Most of the time, patients are unable to work during treatment, and they experience a significant decline in overall quality of life. Additionally, patients commonly experience psychological

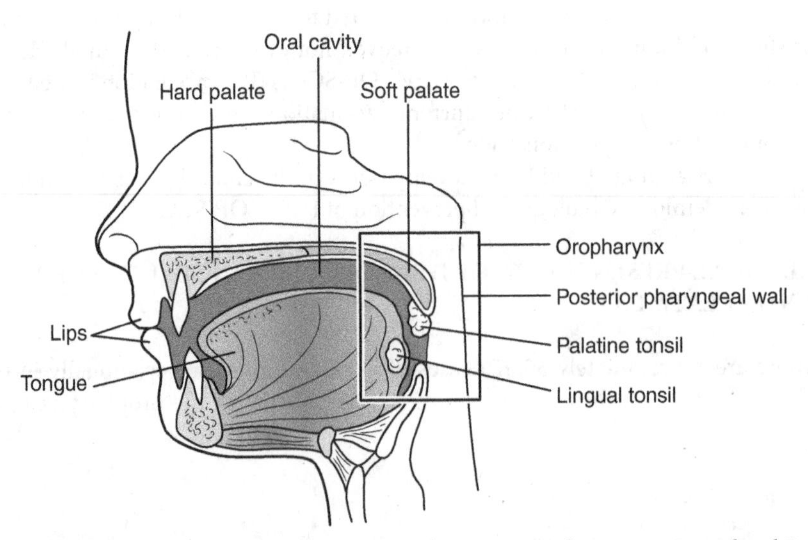

Figure 1 Anatomic depiction of the oropharynx. (From Centers for Disease Control and Prevention. The HPV-associated cancers page. Available at: www.cdc.gov/cancer/hpv/basic_info/cancers.htm. Accessed January 31, 2014.)

distress, with depression, anxiety, and posttraumatic stress syndrome (PTSD) both during and after treatment.[9,10] After this intense treatment finishes, recovery time for oropharyngeal cancer can last 6 months or longer, and common long-term side effects of treatment include dry mouth, dental complications, fibrosis in the radiated field, hypothyroidism, and psychological distress, as well as increased risk for more serious sequelae including osteoradionecrosis of the jaw, stroke, and second primary tumors induced by radiation.[7,8]

Although the treatment morbidity is high, HPV$^+$ OP-SCCs are potentially curable and have a better prognosis than non-HPV$^+$ OP-SCCs, even when they present at a locally advanced stage.[11-13] In 1 large study, patients with HPV$^+$ tumors had an 82.4% 3-year overall survival rate compared with patients with HPV$^-$ cancers, who had a 57.1% 3-year survival rate ($P < .001$).[11] This improvement in survival clearly indicates a different biology of HPV$^+$ OP-SCC compared to those driven by tobacco and alcohol.

Not all HPV$^+$ OP-SCCs have such an excellent prognosis, however. Both patient- and tumor-associated factors affect prognosis. One important patient factor is smoking status. Although smoking does not increase the risk of getting HPV$^+$ OP-SCC, it does affect prognosis.[11,14] A history of tobacco smoking of 10 pack-years or more significantly affects outcomes in patients with HPV$^+$ OP-SCC. For each pack-year, the rate of recurrence or death from HPV$^+$ OP-SCC increases by 1%.[11] Even patients with no additional risk factors, such as smoking status or large volume disease, can sometimes experience recurrence and die of their disease. Tumor-specific determinants of outcomes are not well understood at this point, but research is active in this area. To date, 2 findings have been linked to worse prognosis. One study showed that high expression of the antiapoptotic protein Bcl2 in HPV$^+$ OP-SCC tumors is associated with worse prognosis compared to specimens with low Bcl2 expression.[15] A different study showed that low levels of tumor-infiltrating lymphocytes (TILs) in HPV$^+$ OP-SCC were associated with worse prognosis, indicating that immune response may play a role in outcome.[16] Thus, although curability is high in HPV$^+$ OP-SCC, there is a subset of patients with a poor prognosis. Further elucidation of why some HPV$^+$ cancers have a worse prognosis than others will be critical to tailoring therapy to best suit the individual patient.

Although HPV$^+$ OP-SCC is generally highly curable, the cost of treatment in terms of morbidity and effect on quality of life is great. Thus, there is a desire to de-escalate the intensity of therapy. Because current treatment approaches were developed in an era of more classic and difficult-to-cure smoking- and alcohol-related head and neck cancers, treatment is likely more aggressive than necessary for some HPV$^+$ tumors. The field is now designing clinical trials for patients with HPV$^+$ OP-SCC to specifically compare less intense treatment strategies to the more aggressive standard of care.[17] The risk of de-escalation is, of course, loss of treatment efficacy. Therefore, the identification of patients with high-risk disease who would not be appropriate for de-escalation would be ideal in order to exclude them from de-escalation trials. Unfortunately, we do not yet know how to identify these patients. Thus, trials must be done carefully so as not to sacrifice cure just to make treatment better tolerated.

EPIDEMIOLOGY OF HPV INFECTION AND HPV$^+$ OROPHARYNGEAL CANCER

Although incidence and death rates for many cancers have decreased in recent years, OP-SCC incidence is on the rise, and HPV is the culprit.[1,2,4,18] HPV is associated with 3.3% of all cancers in women and 2.0% of cancers in men, for a total of approximately 34,788 new cases in the United States in 2009. Of these, 37.3% were OP-SCCs.[1] Although head and neck cancers in the past have been most commonly associated with tobacco and alcohol use, the epidemiology has been changing over the last 30 years because of HPV. In 1 study that determined the HPV status in OP-SCC from the Surveillance, Epidemiology, and End Results (SEER) tissue bank from 1984 to 2004, HPV prevalence in tumors grew dramatically, from 16.3% in 1984 to 1989 to 72.7% in 2000 to 2004.[18] HPV$^-$ OP-SCC decreased by half during this time, whereas HPV$^+$ OP-SCC increased by 225%.

There are more than 150 different human papillomaviruses, with 11 considered high-risk oncogenic viruses that cause HPV-driven cancers.[19] More than 90% of cases of OP-SCC are caused by HPV-16.[4,18] This is in contrast to cervical cancers, in which HPV-16 accounts for closer to 60% of cases, with the other 40% divided into other contributing high-risk types.[4] Comparisons between cervical cancer and OP-SCC epidemiology are given in Table 1.

With HPV at the center of this growing epidemic, several studies have sought to elucidate the relationship between OP-SCC and oral HPV infection. In a landmark case control study of 100 patients with OP-SCC compared with 200 controls, oral rinse and blood specimens were collected for markers of HPV infection.[20] The odds ratio for the association of oral HPV-16 infection with OP-SCC compared to controls was a striking 14.6 (95% confidence interval [CI], 6.3-36.6). Other markers of HPV infection were also highly associated with OP-SCC, such as HPV-16 L1 serologic positivity (odds ratio = 32.2; 95% CI, 14.6-71.3) and HPV-16 seropositivity for E6 or E7 (odds ratio = 58.4; 95% CI, 24.2-138.3). Overall, 55% of the OP-SCC cases were considered attributable to HPV-16.

With the link between OP-SCC and HPV identified, researchers have sought to determine the prevalence and risk factors of oral HPV. The largest of these studies collected oral rinse specimens from 5549 participants.[21] The overall prevalence of any oral HPV type was 6.9%, with high risk-HPV prevalence of 3.7%. Infection prevalence was higher in men than women at 10.1% and 3.6%, respectively. The prevalence of HPV 16 was 1% (which translates into approximately

Table 1
Comparison of the epidemiology of cervical cancer versus oropharyngeal cancer

Epidemiologic trait	Cervical cancer (CC)	Human papillomavirus-positive (HPV+) oropharyngeal squamous cell carcinoma (OP-SCC)
Annual incidence in the United States (in 2009)	11,388	12,989 10,511 (men) 3500 (women)
Gender	Only women	Men>women
Relative contribution to all HPV-related malignancies	32.7% (11,388/34,788)	37.3% (12,989/34,788)
Trends	Decreasing in most but not all developed and developing countries	Sharp increase, in contrast to other head and neck cancers
Relative contribution of HPV-16	61% (smaller than in OP-SCC)	90% (larger than in CC)
Relative contribution of HPV-18	10% (larger than in OP-SCC)	2% (smaller than in CC)
Relative contribution of HPV-16 and -18	71%	92%
Relative contribution of other HPV types	Between 2% and 6% each (31, 33, 35, 39, 45, 52, and 58 among many others)	<2% each (33, 35, 45, 59)
Screening	Papanicolaou smear and cervical HPV testing	None as of yet
Prevention	Bivalent or quadrivalent HPV vaccine can prevent vaccine-type premalignant cervical lesions and cancers	Likely will be able to prevent vaccine-type HPV+ OP-SCC

Adapted from Gillison ML, Castellsague X, Chaturvedi A, et al. Eurogin roadmap: comparative epidemiology of HPV infection and associated cancers of the head and neck and cervix. *Int J Cancer.* 2014;134:497-507, with permission from John Wiley & Sons Ltd; Jemal A, Simard EP, Dorell C, et al. Annual report to the nation on the status of cancer, 1975-2009, featuring the burden and trends in human papillomavirus(HPV)-associated cancers and HPV vaccination coverage levels. *J Natl Cancer Inst.* 2013;105:175-201.

2.1 million people infected in the United States). A bimodal age distribution for peak infection was observed, with a prevalence of 7.3% in those aged 30 to 34 years and 11.4% in those aged 60 to 64 years. Other studies have determined the prevalence of oral HPV infection to be similar,[22-24] although in a study of HIV-infected men, the oral HPV prevalence was higher at 16% for any HPV type and 4.9% for HPV-16 alone.[25] Overall, oral high-risk HPV prevalence is much lower than the prevalence of genital high-risk oncogenic HPV infections in 14- to 59-year-old US women at 29%.[26] However, given that more OP-SCCs than cervical cancers are diagnosed per year, even a relatively low prevalence of infection must be taken seriously.

Several studies have linked the risk of HPV$^+$ OP-SCC or oral HPV infection to sexual behavior. In 1 case control study, OP-SCC was associated with lifetime number of sexual partners and number of oral sex partners, with odds ratios of 3.1 (95% CI, 1.5-6.5) and 3.4 (95% CI, 1.3-8.8), respectively.[20] In another case control pooled population study, in addition to these risk factors, same sex contacts and younger age of sexual debut were also identified as risk factors for OP-SCC.[27] In studies of HPV infection, oral sex, number of lifetime sexual partners, open-mouth kissing, marijuana smoking, and tobacco smoking increased the risk of infection.[21,22,24,28] These associations provide strong evidence that oral HPV infection and HPV$^+$ OP-SCC must be considered a sexually transmitted infection. It is not yet known whether the increasing incidence of HPV$^+$ OP-SCC from the 1970s through the present day has to do with changing sexual practices in our population over time or with changes in the prevalence of and exposure to the virus across the population for other reasons.[18,27,29]

Although the prevalence of oral HPV is now better understood, most people who become infected with oral HPV will clear the infection within a year, just as with HPV infection of the cervix.[4,19,23] Several areas of HPV infection require further study. (1) Why do some people infected with oral HPV clear the infection but others do not? (2) Of the people who do not clear the infection, who is at highest risk for HPV$^+$ OP-SCC? (3) Why are men more likely than women to develop HPV$^+$ OP-SCC? (4) What is the role of the immune system and other factors in HPV infection and progression to cancer?

HPV AND CARCINOGENESIS

One might think that studying the natural history of HPV in the OP would be as easy as studying it in the cervix. However, anatomic differences have hindered natural history studies. The strong gag reflex in the OP prevents a test equivalent to the Papanicolaou smear, and visualization of the OP is limited compared to that of the cervix. Moreover, the OP mucosa consists of redundant folds of tissue with deep mucosal crypts that can easily conceal small abnormalities. We assume, however, that the natural history of HPV in the OP is similar to that of the cervix, in which the carcinogenesis of HPVs is well defined. Figure 2 shows the specialized epithelium of the OP and how HPV is thought to gain entry for infection.

HPV is a small, nonenveloped, circular, double-stranded DNA virus that encodes 3 oncoproteins (E5, E6, E7) and 2 capsid proteins (L1, L2) necessary for its oncogenic potential.[30,31] Capsid proteins facilitate HPV's entry into cells and can interfere with the cell cycle by binding to host proteoglycan moieties in the basement membrane and allowing for viral particle endocytosis. In the cervix, it

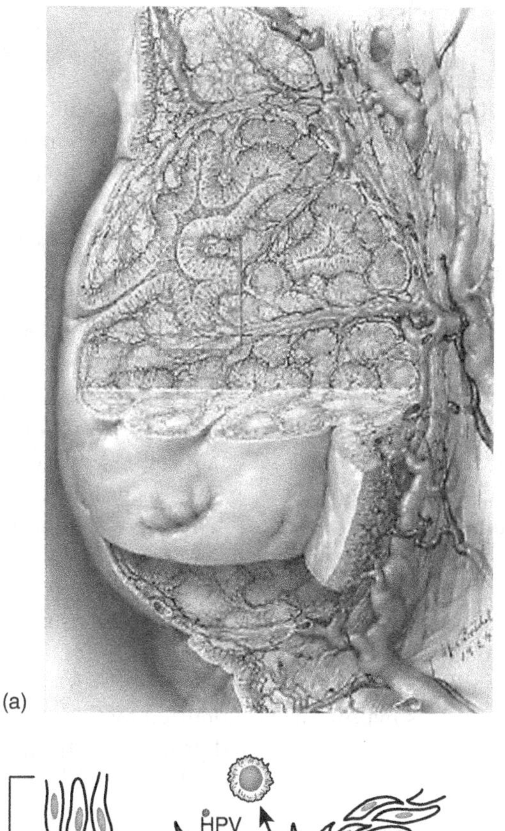

(a)

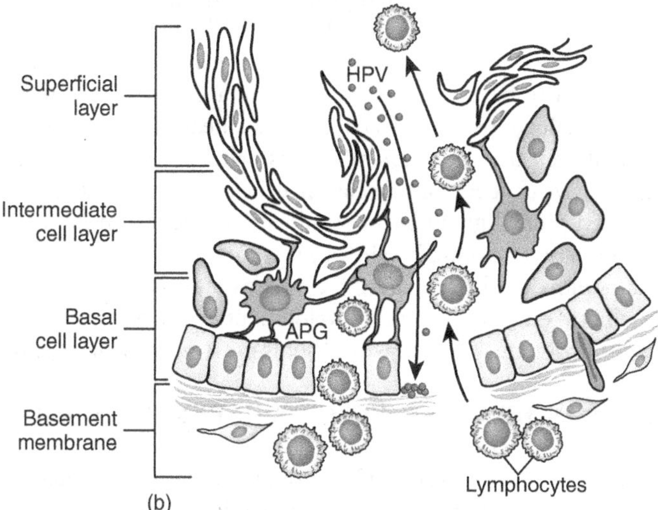

(b)

Figure 2 Schematic depiction of tonsillar epithelium. (a) Topography of the human palantine tonsil. The surface epithelium of the palatine tonsil deeply invaginates into a lymphoid stroma as blind-ending and ramifying crypts *(boxed area)* that increase the surface area of the tonsil by nearly 700%. (Drawing by Max Brödel.) (b) The specialized reticulated epithelium lining the tonsillar crypts. The zones of squamous epithelium—the basal, intermediate, and superficial layers—are interrupted by migrating nonepithelial cells, including lymphocytes and antigen-presenting cells. Loss of structural integrity leaves the basement membrane exposed to deposition of viral particles. (Drawing by T. Phelps.) APG = antigen-presenting group; HPV = human papillomavirus. (From Pai SI, Westra WH. Molecular pathology of head and neck cancer: implications for diagnosis, prognosis, and treatment. *Annu Rev Pathol.* 2009;4:49-70, with permission.)

is thought that trauma exposes the basement membrane to HPV, allowing for initial infection. Because the OP functions as a lymphoid organ, it is thought that the epithelium is more porous to allow for lymphocytes and other immune cells to traffic antigens more easily. As a result, HPV can gain access to the basal cell layer of the host mucosa and establish infection. This may explain in part HPV's tropism to the OP.

Once the virus enters the host basal cell, E6 and E7 are expressed. E6 and E7 target the classic tumor suppressor genes p53 and pRb, respectively, and thereby interfere with cell cycle regulation, DNA repair, cellular senescence, and apoptosis.[30-32] The result is uncontrolled cell growth, even in the face of DNA damage, which ultimately can lead to malignant cells. Cell line experiments support the critical roles played by E6 and E7 because cells that are made to express E6 and E7 constitutively are immortal.[33] Conversely, when these same cells are given an inhibitor of E6 or E7, they undergo apoptosis.[34]

As in cervical cancer, there is believed to be a lag time measured in decades from HPV infection to the development of OP-SCC.[22,32] Other molecular hits in addition to E6 and E7 expression likely are required to trigger transformation to malignancy.[30] This hypothesis is supported by the progression seen in cervical cancer, in which a well-documented progression from premalignant histologic changes occurs after HPV infection.[19] Normal cells develop atypia, which can progress to dysplasia. Dysplastic cells can then evolve into carcinoma in situ, which ultimately can become invasive carcinoma. In cervical cancer, not only can cancers be easily detected by Papanicolaou smears, but early detection then allows for treatment of premalignant lesions, which then prevents future progression to invasive cancer. For oropharyngeal carcinoma, the field of screening for HPV-related premalignant lesions and early cancers is in its infancy. Techniques to overcome anatomic barriers to screening and strategies to target the appropriate population for screening are under development.[4,11,30,31] Regardless, the lag time between infection and development of cancer provides an opportune space for early intervention, which holds great promise for the future.

PREVENTION OF HPV AND HPV$^+$ OROPHARYNGEAL CANCER

The rising number of HPV$^+$ OP-SCC coupled with the tremendous morbidity of cancer treatment provides strong rationale for making a concerted effort to prevent this cancer altogether. Prevention strategies can be either primary or secondary.

Secondary prevention of OP-SCC can be successful only if the following are achieved: (1) a test is developed that detects a cancer earlier than it typically is presenting now; (2) the test is used to screen an appropriate population of HPV-infected people at risk for cancer to detect premalignant lesions or an early cancer; (3) there is an effective treatment for the lesion; (4) the earlier cancer treatment carries less morbidity than treatment when the cancer is found later;

(5) there is reduced OP-SCC–specific mortality when the cancer is found earlier; and (6) there is more benefit to screening than there is harm.[35]

Several challenges lay ahead. No test yet detects cancers earlier, nor is there a detection strategy for identifying precursor lesions. Detection of HPV DNA in saliva may become 1 way of detecting HPV infection, but given that most people clear HPV infections within 1 year, this approach may not be specific enough to identify the high-risk subset of patients in need of further intervention. Another possibility is to test for HPV-specific antibodies. One case control study has shown that antibodies to HPV-E6 can be detected in 34.8% of patients with OP-SCC, whereas only 0.6% of controls were seropositive (adjusted odds ratio = 274; 95% CI, 110-681).[36] In cases with archival blood samples available, HPV-E6 antibodies could be detected in many of the earlier samples, some of which were obtained more than 10 years before the diagnosis of head and neck cancer. This may prove to be a useful screening test if used in the correct population to identify people at risk for HPV$^+$ OP-SCC.

Once a high-risk group is identified, studies to investigate the efficacy of early treatment can be conducted to establish more benefit than harm and a reduction in mortality with screening. Given the many unknowns, secondary prevention is not yet within our grasp.

Primary prevention, however, is much more promising at this point. Two highly effective vaccines are approved for HPV: Gardasil (HPV4), a quadrivalent vaccine for HPV-6, -11, -16, and -18; and Cervarix (HPV2), a bivalent vaccine for HPV 16- and -18.[32] Both vaccines are recombinant HPV virus–like particles that include the HPV capsid L1 protein as an antigen. The vaccines are approved for prevention of precancerous or cancerous lesions of the cervix (HPV2 and HPV4) and of the vulva, vagina, and anus (HPV4) caused by HPV-16 and -18. Neither vaccine is approved for prevention of HPV$^+$ OP-SCC because there is no evidence yet that vaccination can prevent it, but it is thought that it will. There is only 1 study to date that has investigated prevention of oral HPV infection.[37] The study did show a lower prevalence of oral HPV infection in women who received the HPV vaccine; however, there was no baseline comparison data for this population. Larger population studies are underway.

Vaccination is currently recommended for both boys and girls at ages 11 to 12 years, with catch-up vaccines in females aged 13 to 26 years who have not received the vaccine and in males aged 13 to 21 years with use permitted in males through age 26 years. The recommendation for girls was made in 2006 after the efficacy data from phase III clinical trials with HPV4 were presented and boys were included in the recommendation 5 years later. Only HPV4 is FDA-approved for both boys and girls, whereas HPV2 is approved only for girls.[38] The first trials with the HPV4 vaccines were FUTURE I and FUTURE II, both of which assessed the incidence of HPV-associated premalignant lesions or cancer in a randomized controlled trial of females who receive 3 doses of the quadrivalent vaccine against HPV-6, -11, -16, and -18 versus placebo.[39-41] Both studies showed seroconversion in participants receiving the vaccine with antibody titers that were much higher than seen in natural infection[32] and that remained high for up to 5.5 years of follow-up. Both FUTURE I and FUTURE II studies showed close to 100% efficacy of the vaccine in preventing precancerous vaginal, vulvar, perineal, and perianal epithelial lesions or warts caused by vaccine-type HPV in participants who appeared to be naïve to any HPV infection of the cervix at the time of vaccination. In both studies, intention-to-treat analysis showed efficacy was lower when analyzing the entire population studied, presumably because the participants who were infected with vaccine-type HPV at baseline were included. The primary study with the HPV2 vaccine paralleled these findings. HPV2 was also close to 100% effective in preventing vaccine-type HPV-associated cervical intraepithelial neoplasia 2+ or greater (CIN2); however, vaccine efficacy was similarly lower when participants who were positive for HPV-16 or -18 at baseline were included.[42] Since the HPV2 and HPV4 trials were published, a subsequent trial has also shown efficacy for the vaccine in preventing anal HPV infection and anal intraepithelial neoplasia, a precursor lesion to anal cancer.[43] All of the studies highlight the differences in vaccine efficacy across the population. The vaccine is not effective in people who have already been infected with vaccine-type HPV. Thus, it is important to vaccinate patients before HPV exposure, that is, before sexual debut.

Although the efficacy data for the HPV vaccines are excellent, successful prevention relies on vaccine delivery on a population level. The Advisory Committee on Immunization Practices (ACIP) recommends HPV vaccination for all children ages 11 to 12 years, and the federal government's Healthy People campaign calls for vaccination of at least 80% of all girls by 2020.[44,45] Yet, the current completion rates for the 3-vaccine series fall far short of these goals, with only 33.4% of girls and 6.8% of boys completing the vaccine series in 2012.[1,46] Despite the poor vaccine uptake, the prevalence of genital HPV infection already seems to be decreasing.[47] In the National Health and Nutrition Examination Surveys, the vaccine-type HPV prevalence in a cohort of 14- to 19-year-old females decreased by more than half, from 11.5% in 2003 to 2006 (prevaccination recommendations) to 5.1% in 2007 to 2010 (postvaccination recommendations).[46,47] This decrease was not seen in other age groups, which supports the notion that the decrease may result from HPV vaccination. Additionally, the vaccine-type prevalence was 3.1% in vaccinated females but was 12.6% in unvaccinated females. If the decreased HPV prevalence observed actually is the result of early effects of vaccination, increasing vaccine delivery to more people likely would result in an even more dramatic drop in prevalence.

Our current low vaccination rate likely is the result of a combination of factors, at the level of the parents and physicians.[1,48] In fact, physician recommendation is key to vaccine uptake. Still, physician recommendation is inconsistent.[1,48,49] When queried, vaccinated and unvaccinated women indicated that the strongest predictors of vaccination were physician discussion and the strength of the recommendation, with an odds ratio of 93.5 (95% CI, 39.1-223.6).[49] To further elucidate parental reasons for HPV vaccine refusal, the National Immunization Survey of Teens asked parents about vaccinating their teens.[48] The primary reasons given for choosing against vaccination fell into 2 categories: (1) lack of necessary information (including it was "not recommended," it was "not needed or not necessary," and "don't know"); and (2) concern over safety or appropriateness (including "not sexually active," "not age appropriate," and "safety concerns/side effects"). Answers varied by year, with parents who planned not to vaccinate increasing from 39.7% to 43.9%, and safety concerns as the reason for not vaccinating increasing from 4.5% to 16.4% from 2008 to 2010, despite the vaccine's outstanding safety profile. Thus, physicians need to offer all their young patients clear and consistent advice regarding HPV vaccination and effectively address safety and suitability concerns about the vaccine with parents and teens in order to succeed in this important mission to prevent HPV-associated cancers.

CONCLUSION

As a scientific community, we are developing a better understanding of the epidemiology and biology of the HPV$^+$ OP-SCC epidemic. Although many of these cancers are curable, the diagnosis and treatment cause a great deal of suffering, and there is a subset of people who die of this disease. Clinical trials are now focusing on de-escalating the intensity of treatment while still maintaining high cure rates, and development of screening strategies is underway. However, preventing HPV-positive cancers entirely is a loftier goal and one that is well within our reach for appropriate vaccination of our youth. HPV vaccines have already been shown to have the power to prevent most cervical and anal cancers, and evidence is mounting that the vaccines can prevent HPV$^+$ OP-SCC as well. Early epidemiologic results suggest that the prevalence of HPV may already be decreasing as a result of early vaccine uptake, but there still is significant room for improvement. Improving our efforts to vaccinate all girls and boys against HPV should, arguably, be one of the most important public health goals to prevent HPV-associated cancers at this time.

References

1. Jemal A, Simard EP, Dorell C, et al. Annual report to the nation on the status of cancer, 1975-2009, featuring the burden and trends in human papillomavirus (HPV)-associated cancers and HPV vaccination coverage levels. *J Natl Cancer Inst.* 2013;105:175-201
2. Siegel R, Ma J, Zou Z, et al. Cancer statistics, 2014. *CA Cancer J Clin.* 2014;64:9-29
3. Centers for Disease Control and Prevention. The HPV-associated cancers page. Available at: www.cdc.gov/cancer/hpv/basic_info/cancers.htm. Accessed January 31, 2014
4. Gillison ML, Castellsague X, Chaturvedi A, et al. Eurogin roadmap: comparative epidemiology of HPV infection and associated cancers of the head and neck and cervix. *Int J Cancer.* 2014;134:497-507
5. Gillison ML, D'Souza G, Westra W, et al. Distinct risk factor profiles for human papillomavirus type 16-positive and human papillomavirus type 16-negative head and neck cancers. *J Natl Cancer Inst.* 2008;100:407-420

6. Bonilla-Velez J, Mroz EA, Hammon RJ, et al. Impact of human papillomavirus on oropharyngeal cancer biology and response to therapy: implications for treatment. *Otolaryngol Clin North Am.* 2013;46:521-543
7. Murphy BA. Advances in quality of life and symptom management for head and neck cancer patients. *Curr Opin Oncol.* 2009;21:242-247
8. Murphy BA, Gilbert J, Cmelak A, et al. Symptom control issues and supportive care of patients with head and neck cancers. *Clin Adv Hematol Oncol.* 2007;5:807-822
9. Gil F, Costa G, Hilker I, et al. First anxiety, afterwards depression: psychological distress in cancer patients at diagnosis and after medical treatment. *Stress Health.* 2012;28:362-367
10. Kangas M, Milross C, Taylor A, et al. A pilot randomized controlled trial of a brief early intervention for reducing posttraumatic stress disorder, anxiety and depressive symptoms in newly diagnosed head and neck cancer patients. *Psychooncology.* 2013;22:1665-1673
11. Ang KK, Harris J, Wheeler R, et al. Human papillomavirus and survival of patients with oropharyngeal cancer. *N Engl J Med.* 2010;363:24-35
12. Posner MR, Lorch JH, Goloubeva O, et al. Survival and human papillomavirus in oropharynx cancer in TAX 324: a subset analysis from an international phase III trial. *Ann Oncol.* 2011;22:1071-1077
13. O'Rorke MA, Ellison MV, Murray LJ, et al. Human papillomavirus related head and neck cancer survival: a systematic review and meta-analysis. *Oral Oncol.* 2012;48:1191-1201
14. Maxwell JH, Kumar B, Feng FY, et al. Tobacco use in human papillomavirus-positive advanced oropharynx cancer patients related to increased risk of distant metastases and tumor recurrence. *Clin Cancer Res.* 2010;16:1226-1235
15. Nichols AC, Finkelstein DM, Faquin WC, et al. Bcl2 and human papilloma virus 16 as predictors of outcome following concurrent chemoradiation for advanced oropharyngeal cancer. *Clin Cancer Res.* 2010;16:2138-2146
16. Ward MJ, Thirdborough SM, Mellows T, et al. Tumour-infiltrating lymphocytes predict for outcome in HPV-positive oropharyngeal cancer. *Br J Cancer.* 2014;110:489-500
17. O'Sullivan B, Huang SH, Siu LL, et al. Deintensification candidate subgroups in human papillomavirus-related oropharyngeal cancer according to minimal risk of distant metastasis. *J Clin Oncol.* 2013;31:543-550
18. Chaturvedi AK, Engels EA, Pfeiffer RM, et al. Human papillomavirus and rising oropharyngeal cancer incidence in the United States. *J Clin Oncol.* 2011;29:4294-4301
19. Chung CH, Bagheri A, D'Souza G. Epidemiology of oral human papillomavirus infection. *Oral Oncol.* 2013;50(5):364-369
20. D'Souza G, Kreimer AR, Viscidi R, et al. Case-control study of human papillomavirus and oropharyngeal cancer. *N Engl J Med.* 2007;356:1944-1956
21. Gillison ML, Broutian T, Pickard RK, et al. Prevalence of oral HPV infection in the United States, 2009-2010. *JAMA.* 2012;307:693-703
22. Kreimer AR, Bhatia RK, Messeguer AL, et al. Oral human papillomavirus in healthy individuals: a systematic review of the literature. *Sex Transm Dis.* 2010;37:386-391
23. Kreimer AR, Pierce Campbell CM, Lin HY, et al. Incidence and clearance of oral human papillomavirus infection in men: the HIM cohort study. *Lancet.* 2013;382:877-887
24. Pickard RK, Xiao W, Broutian TR, et al. The prevalence and incidence of oral human papillomavirus infection among young men and women, aged 18-30 years. *Sex Transm Dis.* 2012;39:559-566
25. Darwich L, Canadas MP, Videla S, et al. Oral human papillomavirus type-specific infection in HIV-infected men: a prospective cohort study among men who have sex with men and heterosexual men. *Clin Microbiol Infect.* 2013 Dec 30. doi: 10.1111/1469-0691.12523. [Epub ahead of print]
26. Hariri S, Unger ER, Sternberg M, et al. Prevalence of genital human papillomavirus among females in the United States, the National Health And Nutrition Examination Survey, 2003-2006. *J Infect Dis.* 2011;204:566-573
27. Heck JE, Berthiller J, Vaccarella S, et al. Sexual behaviours and the risk of head and neck cancers: a pooled analysis in the International Head and Neck Cancer Epidemiology (INHANCE) consortium. *Int J Epidemiol.* 2010;39:166-181

28. D'Souza G, Agrawal Y, Halpern J, et al. Oral sexual behaviors associated with prevalent oral human papillomavirus infection. *J Infect Dis.* 2009;199:1263-1269
29. Caron SL, Moskey EG. Changes over time in teenage sexual relationships: comparing the high school class of 1950, 1975, and 2000. *Adolescence.* 2002;37:515-526
30. Howard JD, Chung CH. Biology of human papillomavirus-related oropharyngeal cancer. *Semin Radiat Oncol.* 2012;22:187-193
31. Pai SI, Westra WH. Molecular pathology of head and neck cancer: implications for diagnosis, prognosis, and treatment. *Annu Rev Pathol.* 2009;4:49-70
32. Moscicki AB. HPV vaccines: today and in the future. *J Adolesc Health.* 2008;43:S26-S40
33. Rampias T, Sasaki C, Weinberger P, et al. E6 and e7 gene silencing and transformed phenotype of human papillomavirus 16-positive oropharyngeal cancer cells. *J Natl Cancer Inst.* 2009;101:412-423
34. Smeets SJ, van der Plas M, Schaaij-Visser TB, et al. Immortalization of oral keratinocytes by functional inactivation of the p53 and pRb pathways. *Int J Cancer.* 2011;128:1596-1605
35. Kreimer AR. Prospects for prevention of HPV-driven oropharynx cancer. *Oral Oncol.* 2013;50(6):555-559
36. Kreimer AR, Johansson M, Waterboer T, et al. Evaluation of human papillomavirus antibodies and risk of subsequent head and neck cancer. *J Clin Oncol.* 2013;31:2708-2715
37. Herrero R, Quint W, Hildesheim A, et al. Reduced prevalence of oral human papillomavirus (HPV) 4 years after bivalent HPV vaccination in a randomized clinical trial in Costa Rica. *PLoS One.* 2013;8:e68329
38. Centers for Disease Control and Prevention (CDC). Recommendations on the use of quadrivalent human papillomavirus vaccine in males—Advisory Committee on Immunization Practices (ACIP), 2011. *MMWR Morb Mortal Wkly Rep.* 2011;60(50):1705-1708
39. Garland SM, Hernandez-Avila M, Wheeler CM, et al. Quadrivalent vaccine against human papillomavirus to prevent anogenital diseases. *N Engl J Med.* 2007;356:1928-1943
40. Future I/II Study Group, Dillner J, Kjaer SK, et al. Four year efficacy of prophylactic human papillomavirus quadrivalent vaccine against low grade cervical, vulvar, and vaginal intraepithelial neoplasia and anogenital warts: randomised controlled trial. *BMJ.* 2010;341:c3493
41. Future II Study Group. Quadrivalent vaccine against human papillomavirus to prevent high-grade cervical lesions. *N Engl J Med.* 2007;356:1915-1927
42. Paavonen J, Naud P, Salmeron J, et al. Efficacy of human papillomavirus (HPV)-16/18 AS04-adjuvanted vaccine against cervical infection and precancer caused by oncogenic HPV types (PATRICIA): final analysis of a double-blind, randomised study in young women. *Lancet.* 2009;374: 301-314
43. Palefsky JM, Giuliano AR, Goldstone S, et al. HPV vaccine against anal HPV infection and anal intraepithelial neoplasia. *N Engl J Med.* 2011;365:1576-1585
44. Centers for Disease Control and Prevention. The vaccine recommendations of the Advisory Committee for Immunization Practices (ACIP) page. Available at: www.cdc.gov/vaccines/hcp/acip-recs/vacc-specific/hpv.html. Accessed January 31, 2014
45. Healthy People 2020. The immunization and infectious disease page. Available at: healthypeople.gov/2020/topicsobjectives2020/objectiveslist.aspx?topicid=23. Accessed January 31, 2014
46. Centers for Disease Control and Prevention (CDC). National and state vaccination coverage among adolescents aged 13-17 years—United States, 2012. *MMWR Morb Mortal Wkly Rep.* 2013;62(34):685-693
47. Markowitz LE, Hariri S, Lin C, et al. Reduction in human papillomavirus (HPV) prevalence among young women following HPV vaccine introduction in the United States, National Health and Nutrition Examination Surveys, 2003-2010. *J Infect Dis.* 2013;208:385-393
48. Darden PM, Thompson DM, Roberts JR, et al. Reasons for not vaccinating adolescents: National Immunization Survey of Teens, 2008-2010. *Pediatrics.* 2013;131:645-651
49. Rosenthal SL, Weiss TW, Zimet GD, et al. Predictors of HPV vaccine uptake among women aged 19-26: importance of a physician's recommendation. *Vaccine.* 2011;29:890-895

Adolesc Med 025 (2014) 502–519

Update on Attention-Deficit/ Hyperactivity Disorder

Earl J. Soileau, Jr., MD

Assistant Professor of Family Medicine, Louisiana State University Health Sciences Center, New Orleans at Lake Charles, Louisiana

INTRODUCTION

Attention deficit/hyperactivity disorder (ADHD) is a condition that has many facets. The bottom line is that it affects every area of life. Referrals to adolescent physicians are often made by a school counselor, therapist, or teacher who says "I don't think ADHD has any bearing on these behaviors—these are just his or her choices." However, ADHD does affect multiple life domains. For adolescents it represents an enigma of past disappointments, hurts, and failures that have resulted in lack of confidence and difficulty sustaining motivation, as well as easy frustration and expectancy of failure. Many feel that everything attempted is more difficult, more complicated, and more likely to end with disappointing results. However, some are looking on the brighter side and using ADHD to an advantage. The boundless energy and thought processes some experience may be harnessed for great creativity and productivity.

A battle is still going on in American culture as to whether seeking treatment for ADHD is taking the easy way out or is a responsible thing to do. Much of this controversy is fueled by those who have not taken the time to understand our current knowledge of ADHD and the extent to which it causes morbidity and mortality, as well as how available therapies can improve ADHD symptoms such as educational and relationship success. Positive outcomes are dependent on improving brain function to a level as close to normal as possible, as quickly as possible. Preventing negative outcomes, such as substance abuse, accidents, depression, anxiety disorders, and suicide, is also an important goal.

*Corresponding author: Earl J. Soileau, Jr, MD
E-mail address: jsoileau@lcmh.com

 ISSN 1934-4287

It is becoming clear through molecular neurophysiology and neuro-imaging studies that the brain continues to mature through early adulthood. Age-related cognitive gains are mediated by the effects of white matter development on brain network integration.[1-3] Adolescents and young adults with ADHD may have more difficulty than those without ADHD in avoiding the pitfalls of transitioning into mature adulthood. Negative outcomes, which are much more probable in adolescents and young adults with inadequately treated ADHD, include a significantly increased risk of accidental death and injury, development of addiction, sexual sequelae such as unplanned pregnancy and sexually transmitted infections, lower levels of educational and occupational achievement, and decreased marital success.[4] This article addresses some of the latest developments in the area of ADHD in adolescent patients.

EVALUATION AND DIAGNOSIS

Neurophysiology

In the last several years, neuroimaging has advanced our understanding of ADHD. Testing capabilities that provide an objective diagnosis of ADHD has been 1 goal. The first potentially diagnostic test for ADHD is the EEG standard. On July 15, 2013, the Neuropsychiatric EEG-Based Assessment Aid (NEBA) System was approved by the Food and Drug Administration (FDA) and licensed to NEBA Health of Atlanta, Georgia. The test takes 15 to 20 minutes and calculates the theta to beta power ratio of brain waves given off each second. This ratio is significantly higher in individuals with ADHD.[5] Prerelease studies reported 275 children and adolescents ranging from 6 to 17 years old with attention or behavioral concerns. Physicians evaluated all 275 patients using standard diagnostic protocols, including the *Diagnostic and Statistical Manual of Mental Disorders* (Fourth Edition, Text Revision) (*DSM-IV-TR*) criteria, the NEBA System, behavioral questionnaires, and behavioral and IQ testing, to confirm a diagnosis of ADHD. An independent group of ADHD experts reviewed the data and came to a consensus diagnosis regarding whether the research subject indeed met clinical criteria for ADHD or a different condition. Use of NEBA and the clinical evaluation together was superior to the clinical evaluation alone. Reliability of the diagnosis was reported as increasing from 61% for clinical diagnosis to 88% with clinical diagnosis plus NEBA testing.[6] Because this is new technology, widespread clinical experience with this diagnostic tool is not yet available. However, this objective NEBA test is the first of its kind for ADHD. Among 12- to 18-year-olds, the specificity and sensitivity of NEBA are 87% and 89%, respectively.[6] The FDA approval specifies that it is not to be used as a standalone diagnostic tool but as part of a clinical evaluation. Loo and Makeig[7] reviewed the literature and discussed the utility of this tool for most patients whose clinical evaluation would be sufficient to make a sound diagnosis. One source reported a cost of up to $425 per test.[8] A laboratory, hospital, or physician must lease or purchase the EEG unit, the supplies, and the software analyses, and produce a printable report. However, this could be helpful in patients who cannot be definitively diagnosed with ADHD using current clinical evaluation tools. There still remains a concern for those who may have ADHD and are found falsely negative on the NEBA and thus are denied necessary treatment.[9] More study is needed to determine the utility of NEBA in actual clinical practice.

What Has Changed in the *Diagnostic and Statistical Manual of Mental Disorders* (Fifth Edition)

Changes in the new *Diagnostic and Statistical Manual of Mental Disorders*, Fifth Edition (*DSM-5*) include the addition of wording that allows for more accurate diagnosis of ADHD in adolescents and adults.[10] *DSM-5* retains the 2 major categories of inattentive and hyperactive/impulsive symptoms.

For children, adolescents, and adults, several of the criteria for inattention are the same in that it must be present for 6 months, must be impairing, and must not be accounted for by other conditions. For children and adolescents younger than 17 years, inattention requires 6 symptoms, whereas for older adolescents and adults (age 17 and older), at least 5 symptoms are required. *DSM-5* provides new examples for each criterion that pertain more to adolescent and adult ADHD.

Other changes from *DSM-IV* include a change in the latest age of onset of symptoms from age 7 years to 12 years. Many adolescents and young adults do not recall the presence or absence of symptoms before age 7 years, or they did not manifest symptoms before that age. This does not mean that they must have a diagnosis before 12 years of age but that youth should have exhibited symptoms that became evident by then. The presence of symptoms in 2 or more life domains, such as school, home, social events, or work, still is necessary, but the newer category "other specified ADHD" may be used for those who have symptoms in only 1 area but the symptoms are severe enough to warrant a diagnosis even though they do not meet the full criteria for ADHD.

Evaluation Tools

Evaluation instruments or checklists for children have been available for many years, based on the DSM criteria in use at the time. Because the DSM originally targeted patients up to 12 years of age, the symptoms criteria were not entirely applicable to adolescents or young adults, and well-accepted checklists for these groups are lacking. Behavior rating scales and symptoms checklists have always been considered a tool to aid in the diagnosis of ADHD, but they do not make the diagnosis. The accepted standard for diagnosis is still the clinical interview, which delineates a persistent pattern of ADHD symptoms over a long period of time and preferably from 2 or more informants in 2 or more life domains.[11,12]

Unlike younger patients, older adolescents and young adults may present by themselves and may not have someone, such as a teacher or parent, to fill out questionnaires or behavior checklists. Objective observers such as teachers, parents, or employers may not see the adolescent except in limited situations, such as in the classroom or in the food production line. Parents may not see them as much because they may attend school and then go to a job afterward. The teens themselves may be the only ones who see themselves in multiple domains of life. The Brown ADD Scales for Adolescents or the Conners-Wells Adolescent Self-Report Scale are 2 scales that have been validated for adolescents and can be purchased online.[13,14] Even though research has indicated that adolescents and young adults tend to significantly underreport ADHD symptoms, these scales may be helpful in supporting the diagnosis.[15,16]

The World Health Organization ADHD Self-Report Scale (ASRS) has been validated in populations 18 to 44 years of age.[17] It is available in many languages at www.hcp.med.harvard.edu/ncs/asrs.php. It can be used free of charge as long as the source credit is maintained and the scale is not modified. It is based on *DSM-IV-TR* criteria but has been altered for adult symptoms sets. Although there are many other scales for adults, they are not necessarily aimed at the young adult spectrum. The Brown Scale and the Wender Utah Scale[18] are other proprietary scales that are available online and, although targeted at adults, seem to have more relevance to young adults than the childhood scales.[18]

MANAGEMENT

Nonmedical Interventions

Many forms of psychotherapy and behavioral therapies have been helpful for those with ADHD. The Multimodal Treatment Study of ADHD (MTA) trials and follow-up evaluations showed benefit from behavioral therapy, although expert medication management was very similar to medication plus behavioral therapy, and both were significantly better than behavioral therapy alone.[19,20] The initial age of the study group was 7 to 9.9 years. The age range of the follow-up group 8 years later in 2009 was 15 to 18 years. Continued overall improvement was reported above baseline, but not remission. In most areas of function, there were deficits that fell below those of the control group at completion of the follow-up study. However, behavioral therapy was not continued after the initial intervention, and medication management was followed as an open-label naturalistic study rather than a controlled study.

There are many emotional and behavioral symptoms associated with ADHD, and in many individuals behavioral therapies can improve quality of life and performance in several domains of life. It is important to note that although behavioral therapies seem to have some long-term benefits, they do not normalize these individuals. In addition, although behavior modification is much more challenging in adolescents because they have more autonomy, less contact with parents, and increased peer influence, there is increasing evidence that cognitive behavioral therapies (CBTs) are useful in improving function in those with ADHD.[21] CBT focuses on the role cognition plays in both behavior and emotional control. It is targeted at particular thought patterns (eg, distractibility, procrastination), the emotions associated with them, and the need for individuals to take charge of their thoughts in order to become competent in dealing with them.

Most of the research on CBT has been conducted in adults but is applicable to older adolescents and young adults.[22] There are various approaches, but 1 that has yielded significant improvement as an adjunct to medication incorporates 3 core modules: psychoeducation and organizing/planning; coping with distractibility; and adaptive thinking. Optional modules that can be very helpful address procrastination and involvement of a partner or spouse (or, for adolescents, a parent or coach).[23] Some medical professionals have learned brief CBT techniques to help their patients, and many useful videos demonstrating CBT are available on YouTube. However, for most medical professionals this may be impractical for relatively short patient encounters. As training has become more prevalent, CBT-trained therapists often are available to provide these services.

Nutritional Supplementation

Although evidence has been meager, there have been suggestions that some nutritional treatments might be helpful in patients with ADHD. There has been a thread of research related to iron deficiency and ADHD symptoms. In 2004, it was reported that children with ADHD had lower serum ferritin levels than controls.[24] Other studies reported less robust or no difference in ferritin levels in ADHD-affected individuals versus normal controls. But at the same time, there was evidence of increased sensitivity to amphetamine treatment such that a lower dose of amphetamine was needed to successfully treat ADHD after treatment with iron.[25-27] Iron supplementation has some risks, including iron accumulation with subsequent neuro-degeneration. Therefore, it is very important to evaluate iron levels before recommending therapeutic doses for more than several months, and levels should be monitored over time.

Several studies have implicated omega-3 fatty acids, including eicosapentaenoic acid (EPA) and docosahexaenoic acid (DHA), in ADHD. Children and adolescents with learning problems, including ADHD, have been noted to have lower levels of essential fatty acids compared to normal controls.[28,29] Furthermore, supplementation with essential fatty acids such as EPA (in most studies) and DHA (in some studies) has been shown to relieve ADHD symptoms.[30] A small but significant benefit of omega-3 fatty acid supplementation was reported in a systematic review and meta-analysis in 2011.[31] Doses of EPA ranging from 500 to 1000 mg daily have been shown to be helpful.[32]

Pharmacogenomics

New avenues are opening up for guiding ADHD treatments. Pharmacogenomics is the study of genetic variability as it relates to medication response in an individual. By studying individual candidate genes, the probability of side effects or the failure to respond can be linked to gene variants that specifically affect drug-metabolizing enzymes, receptors, or transporters.[33] We know that gene systems significantly contribute to the development of ADHD symptoms,[34] and this information may assist in identifying treatments that are more likely to work (or not to work) in particular individuals, as well as suggest the most likely effective dose range for a given medication. Although this information has been building for more than 10 years, clinical application is still evolving for ADHD and other psychotropic medications.

Several genes modulate attention, and some modulate responsiveness to medication.[35] For example, SLC6 A3 encodes a presynaptic protein that causes reuptake of dopamine from the synapse, which is where the major actions of both methylphenidate and amphetamine occur. Stein et al[36] found that the presence of 2 of the 10 repeat alleles correlated with higher rates of symptom reduction and reduced impairment when treated with Osmotic Release Oral (Delivery) System (OROS) MPH. Individuals with 2 of the less common 9-repeat alleles had a nonlinear dose-response curve and more side effects to stimulants as well as more residual impairment during treatment than did those without this gene variation. In another double-blind placebo controlled study, those with ADHD with 9/9 genotype had more negative parent symptoms but not teacher-rated symptoms than did those with ADHD but without the 9/9 genotype.[37] Although there has not been agreement in all studies, what has emerged is a trend toward evaluation of these gene systems and their effects more systematically and with more reproducibility over time. Pharmacogenomic tests are performed by taking swabs of the buccal mucosa on each side of the mouth and sending them to the reference laboratory, which characterizes the genetic material. The laboratory then provides the physician with a report on metabolizer status (slow, normal, or very rapid) as well as the presence of variants of specific gene systems such as ADRA2 A, which codes for binding affinity polymorphism and, if homozygous, causes decreased binding, rendering the patient less responsive to some ADHD medications.

At this time, pharmacogenomic testing is not indicated in all patients, although it may be recommended in the future if reliability and utility continue to improve. The FDA has already suggested testing in patients with other psychiatric conditions to prevent dangerously high blood levels of medications in those who may have unknown slow metabolizer status.[38] This testing may be particularly useful in patients for whom stimulant medications do not work adequately in order to guide decisions about which adjunctive therapy might be most likely to succeed. For now, further test development and clinical experience are needed to assess the usefulness of pharmacogenomics testing for treating ADHD.

Change Points

Although not specifically studied, it has become clear to many physicians who prescribe medicines to adolescent and young adults that there are transitional times in the lives of ADHD-affected individuals during which treatment is more likely to be neglected, recently referred to as "change points.[39] The most common change points are the transitions from elementary school to middle school, middle school to high school, high school to college/post-high school training or career, and college to employment. At each of these change points the potential is very high for individuals who are not highly invested in their own treatment to drop out. All of these time frames seem to be critical. Beginning in middle school, peer influences may play a large role in risk-taking behaviors. Impulsive individuals who are not doing well in school tend to find things they enjoy doing and may try chemical use, sexual exploration, and possibly antisocial behaviors. This behavior intensifies at the beginning of high school when many seem to drop out of treatment and alternatively may self-medicate with substances such as alcohol or marijuana. There is a very striking derailment of treatment upon graduating from high school and going on to college or technical school or going into the work force. At a time when a higher level of mental concentration is needed, young adults feel a desire to be free of constraints such as therapy sessions, environmental modifications, and medications. Even when going directly from high school to full-time employment, many have difficulty with punctuality, consistency, reliability, and accuracy in their work, which negatively affects their ability to achieve advancement and maintain employment.

Although not well studied, it is the experience of experts caring for these youth that counseling patients and parents before these change points may help. Youth may be better able to handle change points when they are connected with treatment providers so that they feel more invested in treatment and realize that both the present and the future will be better if they engage in treatment. Parents need to support the whole treatment paradigm, including medication, therapy, and life/educational modifications. This is particularly true for younger adolescents who tend to depend on parents to make treatment decisions. If parents are ambivalent about treatment, their son or daughter likely will be ambivalent as well. The youth also may be more easily influenced by pressure from others or by their internal desire to be free of ADHD, and ultimately they may sabotage their treatment. Many physicians in college health have recognized the need to keep students with ADHD engaged in treatment, especially at the outset of college. ADHD coaching has been studied more in the past several years.[40,41] Many universities have instituted programs to provide coaches for incoming freshmen, which seems to help the students make a successful transition to college life.

MEDICATION

We know that brain chemistry is affected in those with ADHD and that neurologic function correlates with these effects, which can be seen behaviorally in life settings and can be evaluated by the physician. It seems that brain function is improved by medication. This improvement has been shown in many studies from the American Academy of Pediatrics (AAP), the Academy of Child and Adolescent Psychiatry (ACAAP), and the Texas Childrens Medical Project suggesting that medication is the most helpful option.[11,12,42] The ACAAP in its practice parameter states, "It seems established that a pharmacological intervention for ADHD is more effective than a behavioral treatment alone." There have been many outcome studies related to ADHD medications, but the difficulty in studying individuals over time has yielded different results. The 8-year follow-up of the MTA study indicated that all patients who had medication treatment were doing better than they were at baseline. However, the MTA study also found that many individuals in the middle to late teen years did not follow through consistently with medication treatment, with 62% of the original group having stopped taking their medication. Follow-up study patients had poorer performance for 91% of the variables followed compared to the non-ADHD control group.[20]

When the decision is made to use medication therapy, the most robust response has been seen with stimulant medication. In ADHD without comorbidity, the use of stimulants is preferred. The longer-acting stimulants have been shown to be more effective than shorter-acting stimulants for adolescents. Adherence is better, and the effect on driving performance is substantial.[43,44] The guidelines and other major publications underscore the need for treatment to cover most of the waking hours throughout the year.[45] It is important to consider whether a medication will have its effect at a particular time of day and to match the time the medication will work to the tasks that need to be accomplished. For teens who participate in evening activities and who drive, it is important that the medication have its effect late in the day. For patients who are making decisions regarding sexual activity, drug use, or other possible risk behaviors, it would be most helpful for the medication to cover these at-risk times of day. Stimulant effects will not continue at high levels of efficacy for academic study into the late evening hours, even with the long-acting preparations. However, the driving studies mentioned earlier (eg, OROS MPH) showed significant driving improvement long past the 12-hour expected duration. This indicates that although the effect of these longer-acting medications may wane in the evening hours, there still may be enough of an effect to allow better performance in some domains.[46]

There are many exhaustive sources of information on how to initiate and manage ADHD medications. This section will only discuss the updates to medication therapy from the last several years. There are 3 categories of stimulant medications: short-acting, which last only 3 to 5 hours; intermediate-acting, which last 8 to 9 hours; and long-acting, which are targeted to last 12 hours. Generally it is best to start with longer-acting preparations, which are more likely to ensure effective medication during most of the waking hours. These medications also have better adherence and fewer side effects. In any population there are individuals who metabolize ADHD medications at a slow rate, an intermediate (average) rate, or a very fast rate. There are also those who are highly sensitive or are relatively insensitive to medications at a receptor level, resulting in some individuals who are very sensitive to low doses of medication and others who require much larger doses to have the desired positive effects. Therefore, a low starting dose is recommended to avoid intense startup side effects in slow metabolizers. Common titration times in practice range from every 3 days to every week. ADHD-affected adolescents and young adults are, by nature, not very patient. They have low frustration tolerance, including waiting for a positive effect from medication. That being the case, it is prudent to titrate at shorter intervals such as every 3 days. Many use an auto-titration plan based on a maximum allowable increase in dose before the next visit. Because the contents of the capsule for lisdexamfetamine do not have to be in the capsule to have sustained action, it can be mixed with a drink of choice. For younger and smaller patients, mix half of the contents of the 20-mg capsule with a juice of their choice (except for grapefruit juice) each morning. Every 3 to 4 days, increase by half of a capsule (10 mg) until the desired dose is reached. Once the dose that works best is determined, a single capsule can be given. In this way, titration can be achieved without multiple prescriptions for drugs of different strengths, which patients often find difficult to fill because of insurance restrictions. With OROS methylphenidate, the extended-release mechanism is an osmotic pump that is destroyed if the capsule is cut in half, so the pill can only be titrated in whole-pill increments. For smaller patients 18 mg is an appropriate starting dose, increasing every 3 to 4 days until optimal benefit or 54 mg is reached. Further titration may be accomplished then if needed.

Methylphenidate long-acting liquid is the newest preparation of longer-acting methylphenidate. It is composed of 20% immediate-release MPH and 80% bound in cationic polymer matrix particles. Like most other extended-release preparations, it allows rapid progression to a therapeutic level with maintenance of that level over an extended period of time. With the limited experience so far, it seems to work well. It has been studied in adolescents 13 to 15 years old as well as younger children in the laboratory classroom, and the pharmacodynamics seemed to be the same for both groups.[47] Symptom reduction was maintained over a 12-hour period. Although it is approved for 12 hours, the Swanson, Kotkin, Agler, M-Flynn, and Pelham Scale (SKAMP) data demonstrate significance only up through 8 hours. This preparation is a powder that is mixed with water to make a solution that is 25 mg/5 mL. It is available in 300-mg, 600-mg, 750-mg, and 900-mg bottles, which yield 60 mL, 120 mL, 150 mL, and 180 mL of final product when diluted. Prescriptions must be written for 1 of these specified amounts. Some patients have found this to be a smoother alternative when some of the other extended-release preparations do not provide optimal symptom control or cause side effects. In addition to being useful in patients who are not able to swallow pills, this preparation is useful for the rare patient who has a very narrow therapeutic window and requires a dose between the available strengths of other timed-release medications. Another potential use is for oppositional patients who cheek medications as a method of assuring adherence to the regimen because it is more difficult to feign swallowing a liquid and hold it in the mouth to be spit out later.

Dexmethylphenidate is one of the later additions to the armamentarium. In the 1990s, the FDA began an initiative to produce medications that contain only the pharmacologically active stereoisomers/enantiomers. Studies have indicated that the D-isomer of methylphenidate is the pharmacologically active form. Improvement in ADHD symptoms is similar with the single isomer or the racemic mixture, and there is some evidence that the L-form may interfere with the positive action of D-methylphenidate.[48-50] In clinical practice, many patients have failed D,L-methylphenidates and have done much better on the single isomer D-methylphenidate. With the emergence of pharmacogenomics we may discover why some patients respond better to one preparation than another of the same basic compound.

Atomoxetine is one of 3 nonstimulants approved for treatment of ADHD. It has been shown to be effective for both impulsiveness/hyperactivity and attention symptoms. Review of several studies indicated the response to mixed amphetamine salts (Adderall XR) and osmotically released methylphenidate was significantly greater improvement in ADHD symptom scores in head-to-head trials compared to atomoxetine.[51-53] It takes 6 to 8 weeks of titration to see the full benefit with atomoxetine, and a cross-taper strategy should be used when switching from a stimulant to atomoxetine. Side effects of the change will be minimized if the switch is done over several weeks. Long-acting α_2-agonists are nonstimulant medications for ADHD that have recently been brought to market. These medications have a very low peak concentration in the blood, which makes them very different from immediate-release preparations. Clonidine and guanfacine in their immediate-release forms are known for making individuals very sleepy and are not helpful for ADHD because of the drowsiness. This is often used to advantage in those who have difficulty initiating sleep. However, extended-release guanfacine (Intuniv) and clonidine (Kapvay) are primarily targeted for use as ADHD treatment because of their ability to treat impulsive and overactive symptoms of ADHD. They are most often used in combination with other ADHD medications because they do not significantly improve cognitive symptoms and therefore are rarely effective enough on their own.

A troubling development in the last few months is the marketing of what seem to be nonequivalent generics of ADHD medications. There is now a generic drug that is approved as an equivalent to OROS MPH, which has an osmotic pump release system, and at least 1 generic indeed is equivalent; it has been as effective as the original branded medication because it has the same release system. Another generic drug that is considered equivalent by the FDA has 2 sets of beads compressed into a tablet. Anecdotally, patients who had been stable on the original preparation have not had similar efficacy with this different release type preparation at the same milligram dose.

Doses of stimulants for adolescents and young adults may be larger than they are for children. Preclinical trials were performed for most ADHD stimulants using dosages that might be expected to work on 6- to 12-year-olds because that was the age group generally targeted in the past. When trials were done with adolescents, the same dosages were used. The accepted recommendation is to titrate up to the dose of medication that gives optimal relief of symptoms with no intolerable side effects. If the patient has not reached optimal benefit and has not had intolerable side effects, then it is necessary to continue titrating upward until either of these points is reached.[11] ACAAP guidelines include a table of FDA-approved doses and dosages that are not uncommonly needed to achieve resolution of symptoms (Table 1, p. 514). The ACAAP practice parameter also restates the ideal that the dose of medication must be individualized to meet each patient's need and takes into account the risk-to-benefit ratio. In the last few years, insurers have tried to limit the dosages of medications to only what is FDA approved, imposing limits that unduly discriminate against those who have a fast metabolism or receptor-relative insensitivity. The prescribing physician may need to advocate for the patient with the insurer to ensure coverage of an appropriate dose. When prescribing more than an FDA-approved dosage, it is prudent to note it in the patient chart and to discuss it with the patient as well. The notation should include the fact that there are no intolerable side effects and that optimal effect was not reached at a lower dose. If the common maximum noted in the table is reached, then it may be best to try a different medication. This attempt, if still not effective, should be documented; the prescriber then may return to the prior medication and increase the dose. Adhering to the guideline of advancing to the optimal dose that does not cause intolerable side effects is most likely to result in better control.

SPECIAL SITUATIONS

There are patients who have ADHD symptoms and met criteria in earlier years who later become very motivated, are more mature in high school, and are able to keep up grades very well without medication. However, when they take college entrance exams, which are very long and arduous, fatigue may set in after an hour or 2, and efficiency decreases. In these individuals who score quite low despite being prepared, it may be necessary to treat again for testing purposes. They also may need treatment again for university courses in general. The same may be true of those who have a family history of ADHD but have not been diagnosed previously. The increased cognitive function level required for entrance exams and college courses may require treatment if environmental modifications do not help enough.

Diversion and Misuse

Current research about diversion and abuse shows that lifetime nonmedical use of prescription ADHD stimulants was reported by 3.4% of those aged 12 years and older.[54] Of that group, 95.3% reported also use of drugs such as marijuana, cocaine/crack, heroin, hallucinogens, or inhalants, or nonmedical use of medications such as tranquilizers, pain relievers, or sedatives. The illicit drug use came before any stimulant use in 77.6% of cases. Those who used stimulants illicitly but had prescriptions for them were more likely to have been diagnosed in college, whereas those who were treated early were more likely to have no involvement in illicit use of ADHD stimulants. From other studies it has become clear that most of those taking ADHD stimulants do so for academic performance needs, such as studying and improving memory organization.[55] Some patients who have ADHD but are not diagnosed obtain their own treatment either from friends or peers, or "on the street." Most of those who persistently use prescription stimulants nonmedically were found to have ADHD symptoms that predated their illicit or nonmedical drug use.[56] This is not surprising because there seems to be an increased incidence of substance abuse among those who were undiagnosed and/or untreated as children and younger adolescents, and treatment reduces the likelihood of later substance abuse by 50%.[57]

What are we to do then to help those with ADHD while not playing into the hands of those wanting to abuse and/or divert the stimulant medications? Recommendations have included denying stimulants to college students or having them come back every month so that they can be monitored more closely. However, both of these recommendations represent significant obstacles to treatment for those who really need help. How much are these misused stimulants hurting the general population? It is hard to tell. It is important to take steps toward due diligence in preventing abuse and diversion of these medications without impeding legitimate use.

Heart Issues

In the 2011 practice guidelines for ADHD treatment, the AAP noted that the risk of sudden cardiac death in patients, including adolescents, taking stimulant medications is extremely rare, and it is not clear that there is any increased risk with stimulant use in the general population.[58] This finding was in line with the 2009 AAP position statement that there is minimal cardiovascular risk from stimulants in healthy patients but recommended screening only in the presence of strong family history or symptoms of heart disease.[12] The ACAAP also recommended against routine screening in their 2007 practice parameter.[11] No increase in cardiac death was found in several other large population studies.[58-60] The recommendations are to evaluate cardiac risk, as any physician would for youth without ADHD.[61-63]

Table 1
Medications approved by the FDA for ADHD (alphabetical by class)

Generic class/ Brand name	Dose form	Typical Starting Dose	FDA max/day	Off-label max/ day	Comments
Amphetamine preparations					
Short-acting					Short-acting stimulants often used as initial treatment in small children (<16 kg) but have disadvantage of bid–tid dosing to control symptoms throughout day
Adderall[a]	5-, 7.5-, 10-, 12.5-, 15-, 20-, 30-mg tab	3–5 y: 2.5 mg qd ≥6 y: 5 mg qd–bid	40 mg	>50 kg: 60 mg	
Dexedrine*	5-mg cap	3–5 y: 2.5 mg qd			
DextroStat*	5-, 10-mg cap	≥6 y: 5 mg qd–bid			
Long-acting					
Dexedrine	5-, 10-, 15-mg cap	≥6 y: 5–10 mg qd–bid	40 mg	>50 kg: 60 mg	Longer-acting stimulants offer greater convenience, confidentiality, and adherence with single daily dosing but may have greater problematic effects on evening appetite and sleep
Spansule				>50 kg: 60 mg	
Adderall XR	5-, 10-, 15-, 20-, 25-, 30-mg cap	≥6 y: 10 mg qd	30 mg		
Lisdexamfetamine	30-, 50-, 70-mg cap	30 mg qd	70 mg	Not yet known	
Methylphenidate preparations					
Short-acting					Short-acting stimulants often used as initial treatment in small children (<16 kg) but have disadvantage of bid–tid dosing to control symptoms throughout day
Focalin	2.5-, 5-, 10-mg cap	2.5 mg bid	20 mg	50 mg	
Methylin*	5-, 10-, 20-mg tab	5 mg bid	60 mg	>50 kg: 100 mg	
Ritalin*	5-, 10-, 20-mg tab	5 mg bid	60 mg	>50 kg: 100 mg	

Intermediate-acting					
Metadate ER	10-, 20-mg cap	10 mg qam	60 mg	>50 kg: 100 mg	Longer-acting stimulants offer greater convenience, confidentiality, and adherence with single daily dosing but may have greater problematic effects on evening appetite and sleep
Methylin ER	10-, 20-mg cap	10 mg qam	60 mg	>50 kg: 100 mg	
Ritalin SR*	20-mg cap	10 mg qam	60 mg	>50 kg: 100 mg	
Metadate CD	10-, 20-, 30-, 40-, 50-, 60-mg cap	20 mg qam	60 mg	>50 kg: 100 mg	Metadate CD and Ritalin LA caps may be opened and sprinkled on soft food
Ritalin LA	10-, 20-, 30-, 40-mg cap	20 mg qam	60 mg	>50 kg: 100 mg	
Long-acting					
Concerta	18-, 27-, 36-, 54-mg tab	18 mg qam	72 mg	108 mg	Swallow whole with liquids Nonabsorbable tablet shell may be seen in stool
Daytrana patch	10-, 15-, 20-, 30-mg patches	Begin with 10-mg patch qd, then titrate up by patch strength	30 mg	Not yet known	
Focalin XR	5-, 10-, 15-, 20-mg cap	5 mg qam	30 mg	50 mg	
Selective norepinephrine reuptake inhibitor					
Atomoxetine					Not a schedule II medication
Strattera	10-, 18-, 25-, 40-, 60-, 80-, 100-mg cap	Children and adolescents <70 kg: 0.5 mg/kg/day for 4 days; then 1 mg/kg/day for 4 days; then 1.2 mg/kg/day	Lesser of 1.4 mg/kg or 100 mg	Lesser of 1.8 mg/kg or 100 mg	Consider if active substance abuse or severe side effects of stimulants (mood lability, tics); give qam or divided doses bid (effects on late evening behavior); do not open capsule; monitor closely for suicidal thinking and behavior, clinical worsening, or unusual changes in behavior

*Generic formulation available.

ADHD = attention-deficit/hyperactivity disorder; FDA = US Food and Drug Administration.

Priapism

On December 17, 2013, the FDA posted a Drug Safety Communication about risk of long-lasting erections in males taking methylphenidate medications and proposed label changes to medications containing methylphenidate.[64] Adverse event reporting noted 15 cases that met the definition of priapism reported from 1997 to 2012 associated with patients having taken a methylphenidate product. Only 2 required surgical intervention. In 1 patient, a shunt was required; in the other patient, corpus cavernosum aspiration was necessary. No other information was presented. The mean age of patients with priapism was 12.5 years. Prolonged erections are common in this age group with emerging pubertal changes. The significance of the 14 reported cases of priapism can be questioned when one considers the number of patient-years of stimulant treatment encompassed during that 15-year timeframe. In a study by Eland et al,[65] 1.5 cases of ischemic priapism per 100,000 person-years was reported in the general population of The Netherlands during the years from 1995 to 1999. It would be helpful to see a ratio of cases to patient-years for the general population versus the treated population, much the same as the heart-related deaths were evaluated. This would allow physicians and patients to determine whether there is a significantly increased risk of priapism in those treated with ADHD stimulants. It is recommended that physicians speak to their patients about priapism before initiating stimulant therapy with MPH.

References

1. Stevens MC, Skudlarski P, Godfrey D, et al. Age-related cognitive gains are mediated by the effects of white matter development on brain network integration. *Neuroimage.* 2009;48(4):738-746
2. Chambers RA, Taylor JR, Potenza MN. Developmental neurocircuitry of motivation in adolescence: a critical period of addiction vulnerability. *Am J Psychiatry.* 2003;160(6):1041-1052
3. Geier C, Luna B. The maturation of incentive processing and cognitive control. *Pharmacol Biochem Behav.* 2009;93(3):212-221
4. Soileau EJ Jr. Medications for adolescents with attention-deficit/hyperactivity disorder. *Adolesc Med State Art Rev.* 2008;19(2):254-267
5. Snyder SM, Hall JR. A meta-analysis of quantitative EEG power associated with attention-deficit hyperactivity disorder. *J Clin Neurophysiol.* 2006;23:440-455
6. De novo application with FDA. Available at: www.accessdata.fda.gov/cdrh_docs/reviews/K112711.pdf. Accessed July 8, 2014
7. Loo SK, Makeig S. Clinical utility of EEG in attention-deficit/hyperactivity disorder: a research update. *Neurotherapeutics.* 2012;9(3):569-587
8. NEBA Health. FAQ. Available at: nebahealth.com/faq.html. Accessed July 8, 2014
9. Brauser D. Mixed reaction to FDA approval of ADHD brain-wave test. *Medscape Medical News.* Available at: www.medscape.com/viewarticle/809079. Accessed July 10, 2014
10. *Diagnostic and Statistical Manual of Mental Disorders.* 5th ed. Washington, DC: American Psychiatric Association; 2013
11. Pliszka S, AACAP Work Group on Quality Issues. Practice parameter for the assessment and treatment of children and adolescents with attention-deficit/hyperactivity disorder. *J Am Acad Child Adolesc Psychiatry.* 2007;46(7):894-921
12. American Academy of Pediatrics Subcommittee on Attention-Deficit/Hyperactivity Disorder, Steering Committee on Quality Improvement and Management, Wolraich M, et al. ADHD: clinical

practice guideline for the diagnosis, evaluation, and treatment of attention-deficit/hyperactivity disorder in children and adolescents. *Pediatrics.* 2011;128(5):1007-1022

13. Rucklidge JJ, Tannock R. Validity of the Brown ADD scales: an investigation in a predominantly inattentive ADHD adolescent sample with and without reading disabilities. *J Atten Disord.* 2002;5(3):155-164
14. Conners CK, Wells KC, Parker JD, et al. A new self-report scale for assessment of adolescent psychopathology: factor structure, reliability, validity, and diagnostic sensitivity. *J Abnorm Child Psychol.* 1997;25(6):487-497
15. Romano E, Tremblay RE, Vitaro F, et al. Prevalence of psychiatric diagnoses and the role of perceived impairment: findings from an adolescent community sample. *J Child Psychol Psychiatry.* 2001;42:451-462
16. Smith B, Pelham WE Jr, Gnagy E, et al. The reliability, validity, and unique contributions of self-report by adolescents receiving treatment for attention-deficit/hyperactivity disorder. *J Consult Clin Psychol.* 2000;68:489-499
17. Kessler RC, Adler L, Gruber MJ, et al. Validity of the World Health Organization Adult ADHD Self-Report Scale (ASRS) Screener in a representative sample of health plan members. *Int J Methods Psychiatr Res.* 2007;16(2):52-65
18. McCann BS, Scheele L, Ward N, et al. Discriminant validity of the Wender Utah Rating Scale for attention-deficit/hyperactivity disorder in adults. *J Neuropsychiatry Clin Neurosci.* 2000;12:240-245
19. The MTA Cooperative Group. A 14-month randomized clinical trial of treatment strategies for attention-deficit/hyperactivity disorder. *Arch Gen Psychiatry.* 1999;56(12):1073-1086
20. Molina BS, Hinshaw SP, Swanson JM, et al. The MTA at 8 years: prospective follow-up of children treated for combined type ADHD in a multisite study. *J Am Acad Child Adolesc Psychiatry.* 2009;48(5):484-500
21. Antshel KM, Faraone SV, Gordon M. Cognitive behavioral treatment outcomes in adolescent ADHD. *FOCUS.* 2012;10:334-345
22. Emilsson B, Gudjonsson, Sigurdsson J, et al. Cognitive behaviour therapy in medication-treated adults with ADHD and persistent symptoms: a randomized controlled trial. *BMC Psychiatry.* 2011;11:116
23. Sprich S, Knouse L, Cooper-Vince C, et al. Description and demonstration of CBT for ADHD in adults. *Cogn Behav Pract.* 2010;17(1):9-15
24. Konofal E, Lecendreux M, Arnulf I, et al. Iron deficiency in children with attention-deficit/hyperactivity disorder. *Arch Pediatr Adolesc Med.* 2004;158:113-115
25. Calarge C, Farmer C, DiSilvestro RL, et al. Serum ferritin and amphetamine response in youth with attention-deficit/hyperactivity disorder. *J Child Adolesc Psychopharmacol.* 2010;20(6):495-502
26. Donfrancesco R, Parisi P, Vanacore N. Iron and ADHD: time to move beyond serum ferritin levels. *J Atten Disord.* 2013;17(4):347-357
27. Cortese S, Angriman M, Lecendreux M, et al. Iron and attention deficit/hyperactivity disorder: what is the empirical evidence so far? A systematic review of the literature. *Expert Rev Neurother.* 2012;12(10):1227-1240
28. Mitchell EA, Aman MG, Turbott SH, et al. Clinical characteristics and serum essential fatty acid levels in hyperactive children. *Clin Pediatr (Phila).* 1987;26:406-411
29. Colter A, Cutler C, Meckling K. Fatty acid status and behavioural symptoms of attention deficit hyperactivity disorder in adolescents: a case-control study. *Nutr J.* 2008;7:8
30. Grassmann V, Santos-Galduróz R, José Galduróz C. Effects of low doses of polyunsaturated fatty acids on the attention deficit/hyperactivity disorder of children: a systematic review. *Curr Neuropharmacol.* 2013;11:186-196
31. Bloch MH, Qawasmi A. Omega-3 fatty acid supplementation for the treatment of children with attention-deficit/hyperactivity disorder symptomatology: systematic review and meta-analysis. *J Am Acad Child Adolesc Psychiatry.* 2011;50(10):991-1000
32. Ageranioti Bélanger S, Vanasse M, Spahis S, et al. Omega-3 fatty acid treatment of children with attention-deficit hyperactivity disorder: a randomized, double-blind, placebo-controlled study. *Paediatr Child Health.* 2009;14(2):89-98

33. Froehlich T, McGough J, Stein M, et al. Progress and promise of attention-deficit hyperactivity disorder pharmacogenetics. *CNS Drugs.* 2010;24(2):99-117
34. Farroan S, Mick E. Molecular genetics of attention deficit hyperactivity disorder. *Psychiatr Clin North Am.* 2010;33(1):159-180
35. Arcos-Burgos M, Castellanos FX, Pineda D, et al. Attention-deficit/hyperactivity disorder in a population isolate: linkage to loci at 4q13.2, 5q33.3, 11q22, and 17p11. *Am J Hum Genet.* 2004;75(6):998–1014
36. Stein MA, Waldman ID, Sarampote CS, et al. Dopamine transporter genotype and methylphenidate dose response in children with ADHD. *Neuropsychopharmacology.* 2005;30(7):1374-1382
37. Joober R, Grizenko N, Sengupta S, et al. Dopamine transporter 30-UTR VNTR genotype and ADHD: a pharmaco-behavioural genetic study with methylphenidate. *Neuropsychopharmacology.* 2007;32(6):1370-1376
38. Rogers HL, Bhattaram A, Zineh I, et al. CYP2 D6 genotype information to guide pimozide treatment in adult and pediatric patients: basis for the U.S. Food and Drug Administration's new dosing recommendations. *J Clin Psychiatry.* 2012;73(9):1187-1190
39. Robin A, Soileau EJ, Thomas MH. Navigating changepoints: improving ADHD care in our nation's adolescents. Presentation to Society for Adolescent Medicine and Health; October 20, 2011
40. Parker D, Hoffman S, Sawilowsky S. An examination of the effects of ADHD coaching on university students' executive functioning. *J Postsecond Educ Disabil.* 2011;24(2):115-132
41. Murphy K, Ratey, N, Maynard S, et al. Coaching for ADHD. *J Atten Disord.* 2010;13(5):546-552
42. Pliszka SR, Crismon ML, Hughes CW, et al. The Texas Children's Medication Algorithm Project: revision of the algorithm for pharmacotherapy of attention-deficit/hyperactivity disorder. *J Am Acad Child Adolesc Psychiatry.* 2006;45(6):642-657
43. Wilens TE, McBurnett K, Bukstein O, et al. Multisite controlled study of OROS methylphenidate in the treatment of adolescents with attention-deficit/hyperactivity disorder. *Arch Pediatr Adolesc Med.* 2006;160:82-90
44. Biederman J, Fried R, Hammerness P, et al. The effects of lisdexamfetamine dimesylate on driving behaviors in young adults with ADHD assessed with the Manchester driving behavior questionnaire. *J Adolesc Health.* 2012;51(6):601-607
45. Cox DJ, Merkel RL, Penberthy JK, et al. Impact of methylphenidate delivery profiles on driving performance of adolescents with attention-deficit/hyperactivity disorder: a pilot study. *J Am Acad Child Adolesc Psychiatry.* 2004;43(3):269-275
46. Cox DJ, Merkel RL, Moore M, et al. Relative benefits of stimulant therapy with OROS methylphenidate versus mixed amphetamine salts extended release in improving the driving performance of adolescent drivers with attention-deficit/hyperactivity disorder. *Pediatrics.* 2006;118(3):e704-e710
47. Wigal SB, Childress AC, Belden, H, et al. NWP06, an extended-release oral suspension 0 f methylphenidate, improved attention-deficit/hyperactivity disorder symptoms compared with placebo in a laboratory classroom study. *J Child Adolesc Psychopharmacol.* 2013;23(1):3-10
48. Quinn D. Does chirality matter? Pharmacodynamics of enantiomers of methylphenidate in patients with attention-deficit/hyperactivity disorder. *J Clin Psychopharmacol.* 2008;28(3 Suppl 2):S62-S66
49. Heal DJ, Pierce DM. Methylphenidate and its isomers: their role in the treatment of attention-deficit hyperactivity disorder using a transdermal delivery system. *CNS Drugs.* 2006;20(9):713-738
50. Markowitz JS, Patrick KS. Differential pharmacokinetics and pharmacodynamics of methylphenidate enantiomers: does chirality matter? *J Clin Psychopharmacol.* 2008;28(3 Suppl 2):S54-S61
51. Garnock-Jones KP, Keating GM. Atomoxetine: a review of its use in attention-deficit hyperactivity disorder in children and adolescents. *Paediatr Drugs.* 2009;11(3):203-226
52. Prasad S, Steer C. Switching from neurostimulant therapy to atomoxetine in children and adolescents with attention-deficit hyperactivity disorder: clinical approaches and review of current available evidence. *Paediatr Drugs.* 2008;10(1):39-47
53. Niederkirchner K, Slawik L, Wermelskirchen D, et al. Transitioning to OROS® methylphenidate from atomoxetine is effective in children and adolescents with ADHD. *Exp Rev Neurother.* 2011;11(4):499-508

54. Sweeney C, Sembower M, Ertischek M. Nonmedical use of prescription ADHD stimulants and preexisting patterns of drug abuse. *J Addict Dis.* 2013;32:1-10
55. Bogle KE, Smith BH. Illicit methylphenidate use: a review of prevalence, availability, pharmacology, and consequences. *Curr Drug Abuse Rev.* 2009;2(2):157-176
56. Arria A, Garnier-Dykstra L, Caldeira K, et al. Persistent nonmedical use of prescription stimulants among college students: possible association with ADHD symptoms. *J Atten Disord.* 2011;15(5): 347-356
57. Faraone SV, Wilens T. Does stimulant treatment lead to substance use disorders? *J Clin Psychiatry.* 2003;11(Suppl 64):9-13
58. Perrin JM, Friedman RA, Knilans TK, Black Box Working Group; Section on Cardiology and Cardiac Surgery. Cardiovascular monitoring and stimulant drugs for attention-deficit/hyperactivity disorder. *Pediatrics.* 2008;122(2):451-453
59. Warren AE, Hamilton RM, Bélanger SA, et al. Cardiac risk assessment before the use of stimulant medications in children and youth: a joint position statement by the Canadian Paediatric Society, the Canadian Cardiovascular Society, and the Canadian Academy of Child and Adolescent Psychiatry. *Can J Cardiol.* 2009;25(11):625-630
60. Winterstein AG, Gerhard T, Kubilis P, et al. Cardiovascular safety of central nervous system stimulants in children and adolescents: population based cohort study. *BMJ.* 2012;345:e4627
61. Habel LA, Cooper WO, Sox CM, et al. ADHD medications and risk of serious cardiovascular events in young and middle-aged adults. *JAMA.* 2011;306(24):2673-2683
62. Schelleman H, Bilker WB, Strom BL, et al. Cardiovascular events and death in children exposed and unexposed to ADHD agents. *Pediatrics.* 2011;127(6):1102-1110
63. Huang C, Gerhard T, Olfson M, et al. Stimulants and cardiovascular events in youth with attention-deficit/hyperactivity disorder. *J Am Acad Child Adolesc Psychiatry.* 2012;51(2):147-156
64. FDA Drug Safety Communication. FDA warns of rare risk of long-lasting erections in males taking methylphenidate ADHD medications and has approved label changes. Safety Announcement. December 17, 2013. Available at: www.fda.gov/downloads/Drugs/DrugSafety/UCM378835.pdf. Accessed July 8, 2014
65. Eland IA, van der Lei J, Stricker BH, et al. Incidence of priapism in the general population. *Urology.* 2001;57:970-972

Adolesc Med 025 (2014) 520–531

Note: Page numbers of articles are in **boldface** type. Page references followed by "*f*" and "*t*" denote figures and tables, respectively.

A

 ISSN 1934-4287

B

C

D

E

N

R

S

T